PHYSIOLOGY

CASES AND PROBLEMS

3RD EDITION

BOARD
REVIEW
SERIES

PHYSIOLOGY

CASES AND PROBLEMS

3RD EDITION

Linda S. Costanzo, Ph.D.
Professor of Physiology and Biophysics
Medical College of Virginia
Virginia Commonwealth University
Richmond, Virginia

Wolters Kluwer | Lippincott Williams & Wilkins
Health
Philadelphia • Baltimore • New York • London
Buenos Aires • Hong Kong • Sydney • Tokyo

Executive Editor: Betty Sun
Managing Editor: Stacey Sebring
Marketing Manager: Emilie Moyer
Designer: Holly McLaughlin
Compositor: International Typesetting and Composition
Printer: Data Reproductions Corporation

Third Edition

Library of Congress Cataloging-in-Publication Data

Costanzo, Linda S., 1947-
    Physiology : cases and problems / Linda S. Costanzo. — 3rd ed.
        p. ; cm. — (Board review series)
    Includes bibliographical references and index.
    ISBN-13: 978-0-7817-8871-7
    ISBN-10: 0-7817-8871-4
  1. Physiology, Pathological—Problems, exercises, etc.   2. Physiology, Pathological—Case studies.   3. Human physiology—Problems, exercises, etc.   4. Human physiology—Case studies.
I. Title.   II. Series.
    [DNLM: 1. Physiology–Examination Questions.   2. Physiology–Outlines.
    QT 18.2 C838b 2009]
    RB113.C787 2009
    616.07—dc22

                                                                                    2008010588

The publishers have made every effort to trace the copyright holders for borrowed material. If they have inadvertently overlooked any, they will be pleased to make the necessary arrangements at the first opportunity.

To purchase additional copies of this book, call our customer service department at **(800) 638-3030** or fax orders to **(301) 824-7390.** International customers should call **(301) 714-2324.**

Visit Lippincott Williams & Wilkins on the Internet: http://www.LWW.com. Lippincott Williams & Wilkins customer service representatives are available from 8:30 am to 6:00 pm, EST.

For my students

Contents

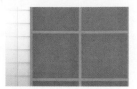

Preface

This book was written for first- and second-year medical students who are studying physiology and pathophysiology. In the framework of cases, the book covers clinically relevant topics in physiology by asking students to answer open-ended questions and solve problems. This book is intended to complement lectures, course syllabi, and traditional textbooks of physiology.

The chapters are arranged according to organ system, including cellular and autonomic, cardiovascular, respiratory, renal and acid–base, gastrointestinal, and endocrine and reproductive physiology. Each chapter presents a series of cases followed by questions and problems that emphasize the most important physiologic principles. The questions require students to perform complex, multistep reasoning and to think integratively across the organ systems. The problems emphasize clinically relevant calculations. Each case and its accompanying questions and problems are immediately followed by complete, stepwise explanations or solutions, many of which include diagrams, classic graphs, and flowcharts.

This book includes a number of features to help students master the principles of physiology.

- Cases are shaded for easy identification.
- Within each case, questions are arranged sequentially so that they intentionally build upon each other.
- The difficulty of the questions varies from basic to challenging, recognizing the progression that most students make.
- When a case includes pharmacologic or pathophysiologic content, brief background is provided to allow first-year medical students to answer the questions.
- Major equations are presented in boldface type, followed by explanations of all terms.
- Key topics are listed at the end of each case so that students may cross-reference these topics with indices of physiology texts.
- Common abbreviations are presented on the inside front cover, and normal values and constants are presented on the inside back cover.

Students may use this book alone or in small groups. Either way, it is intended to be a dynamic, working book that challenges its users to think more critically and deeply about physiologic principles. Throughout, I have attempted to maintain a supportive and friendly tone that reflects my own love of the subject matter.

I welcome your feedback, and look forward to hearing about your experiences with the book. Best wishes for an enjoyable journey!

Linda S. Costanzo, Ph.D.

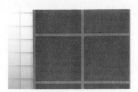

Acknowledgments

I could not have written this book without the enthusiastic support of my colleagues at Lippincott Williams & Wilkins. Nancy Duffy and Stacey Sebring provided expert editorial assistance, and Matthew Chansky served as illustrator.

My colleagues at Virginia Commonwealth University have graciously answered my questions and supported my endeavors. In particular, I would like to thank Drs. Clive Baumgarten, Roland Pittman, and Raphael Witorsch.

Special thanks to my students at Virginia Commonwealth University School of Medicine for their helpful suggestions and to the students at other medical schools who have written to me about their experiences with the book.

Finally, heartfelt thanks go to my husband, Richard, and our children, Dan and Rebecca, for their love and support.

Linda S. Costanzo, Ph.D.

Cellular and Autonomic Physiology

Case 1

Permeability and Simple Diffusion

Four solutes were studied with respect to their permeability and rate of diffusion in a lipid bilayer. Table 1–1 shows the molecular radius and oil–water partition coefficient of each of the four solutes. Use the information in the table to answer the following questions about diffusion coefficient, permeability, and rate of diffusion.

TABLE 1–1	Molecular Radii and Oil–Water Partition Coefficients of Four Solutes	
Solute	Molecular Radius, Å	Oil–Water Partition Coefficient
A	20	1.0
B	20	2.0
C	40	1.0
D	40	0.5

 QUESTIONS

1. What equation describes the diffusion coefficient for a solute? What is the relationship between molecular radius and diffusion coefficient?

2. What equation relates permeability to diffusion coefficient? What is the relationship between molecular radius and permeability?

3. What is the relationship between oil–water partition coefficient and permeability? What are the units of the partition coefficient? How is the partition coefficient measured?

4. Of the four solutes shown in Table 1–1, which has the highest permeability in the lipid bilayer?

5. Of the four solutes shown in Table 1–1, which has the lowest permeability in the lipid bilayer?

6. Two solutions with different concentrations of Solute A are separated by a lipid bilayer that has a surface area of 1 cm². The concentration of Solute A in one solution is 20 mmol/mL, the concentration of Solute A in the other solution is 10 mmol/mL, and the permeability of the lipid bilayer to Solute A is 5×10^{-5} cm/sec. What is the direction and net rate of diffusion of Solute A across the lipid bilayer?

7. If the surface area of the lipid bilayer in Question 6 is doubled, what is the net rate of diffusion of Solute A?

8. If all conditions are identical to those described for Question 6, except that Solute A is replaced by Solute B, what is the net rate of diffusion of Solute B?

9. If all conditions are identical to those described for Question 8, except that the concentration of Solute B in the 20 mmol/mL solution is doubled to 40 mmol/mL, what is the net rate of diffusion of Solute B?

ANSWERS ON NEXT PAGE

ANSWERS AND EXPLANATIONS

1. The **Stokes–Einstein equation** describes the **diffusion coefficient** as follows:

$$D = \frac{K\,T}{6\,\pi\,r\,\eta}$$

where

D = diffusion coefficient
K = Boltzmann's constant
T = absolute temperature (K)
r = molecular radius
η = viscosity of the medium

The equation states that there is an inverse relationship between molecular radius and diffusion coefficient. Thus, small solutes have high diffusion coefficients, and large solutes have low diffusion coefficients.

2. **Permeability** is related to the diffusion coefficient as follows:

$$P = \frac{K\,D}{\Delta x}$$

where

P = permeability
K = partition coefficient
D = diffusion coefficient
Δx = membrane thickness

The equation states that permeability (P) is directly correlated with the diffusion coefficient (D). Furthermore, because the diffusion coefficient is inversely correlated with molecular radius, permeability is also inversely correlated with molecular radius. As the molecular radius increases, both the diffusion coefficient and permeability decrease.

3. The oil–water **partition coefficient** ("K" in the permeability equation) describes the solubility of a solute in oil relative to its solubility in water. The higher the partition coefficient of a solute, the higher its oil or lipid solubility and the more readily it dissolves in a lipid bilayer. The relationship between the oil–water partition coefficient and permeability is described in the equation for permeability (see Question 2): the higher the partition coefficient of the solute, the higher its permeability in a lipid bilayer.

The partition coefficient is a dimensionless number (meaning that it has no units). It is measured by determining the concentration of solute in an oil phase relative to its concentration in an aqueous phase and expressing the two values as a ratio. When expressed as a ratio, the units of concentration cancel each other.

One potential point of confusion is that in the equation for permeability, K represents the partition coefficient (discussed in Question 4); in the equation for diffusion coefficient, K represents the Boltzmann constant.

4. As already discussed, permeability in a lipid bilayer is inversely correlated with molecular size and directly correlated with partition coefficient. Thus, a small solute with a high partition coefficient (i.e., high lipid solubility) has the highest permeability, and a large solute with a low partition coefficient has the lowest permeability.

Table 1–1 shows that among the four solutes, Solute B has the highest permeability because it has the smallest size and the highest partition coefficient. Solutes C and D have lower permeabilities than Solute A based on their larger molecular radii and their equal or lower partition coefficients.

5. Of the four solutes, Solute D has the lowest permeability because it has a large molecular size and the lowest partition coefficient.

6. This question asked you to calculate the net rate of diffusion of Solute A, which is described by the **Fick law of diffusion:**

$$J = P\,A\,(C_1 - C_2)$$

where

> J = net rate of diffusion (mmol/sec)
> P = permeability (cm/sec)
> A = surface area (cm^2)
> C_1 = concentration in solution 1 (mmol/mL)
> C_2 = concentration in solution 2 (mmol/mL)

In words, the equation states that the net rate of diffusion (also called **flux**, or **flow**) is directly correlated with the permeability of the solute in the membrane, the surface area available for diffusion, and the difference in concentration across the membrane. The net rate of diffusion of Solute A is:

$$
\begin{aligned}
J &= 5 \times 10^{-5}\text{ cm/sec} \times 1\text{ cm}^2 \times (20\text{ mmol/mL} - 10\text{ mmol/mL})\\
&= 5 \times 10^{-5}\text{ cm/sec} \times 1\text{ cm}^2 \times (10\text{ mmol/mL})\\
&= 5 \times 10^{-5}\text{ cm/sec} \times 1\text{ cm}^2 \times (10\text{ mmol/cm}^3)\\
&= 5 \times 10^{-4}\text{ mmol/sec, from high to low concentration}
\end{aligned}
$$

Note that there is one very useful trick in this calculation: 1 mL ≈ 1 cm^3.

7. If the surface area doubles, and all other conditions are unchanged, the net rate of diffusion of Solute A doubles (i.e., to 1×10^{-3} mmol/sec).

8. Because Solute B has the same molecular radius as Solute A, but twice the oil–water partition coefficient, the permeability and the net rate of diffusion of Solute B must be twice those of Solute A. Therefore, the permeability of Solute B is 1×10^{-4} cm/sec, and the net rate of diffusion of Solute B is 1×10^{-3} mmol/sec.

9. If the higher concentration of Solute B is doubled, then the net rate of diffusion increases to 3×10^{-3} mmol/sec, or threefold, as shown in the following calculation:

$$
\begin{aligned}
J &= 1 \times 10^{-4}\text{ cm/sec} \times 1\text{ cm}^2 \times (40\text{ mmol/mL} - 10\text{ mmol/mL})\\
&= 1 \times 10^{-4}\text{ cm/sec} \times 1\text{ cm}^2 \times (30\text{ mmol/mL})\\
&= 1 \times 10^{-4}\text{ cm/sec} \times 1\text{ cm}^2 \times (30\text{ mmol/cm}^3)\\
&= 3 \times 10^{-3}\text{ mmol/sec}
\end{aligned}
$$

If you thought that the diffusion rate would double (rather than triple), remember that the net rate of diffusion is directly related to the *difference* in concentration across the membrane; the *difference* in concentration is tripled.

Key topics

Diffusion coefficient

Fick law of diffusion

Flux, or flow

Partition coefficient

Permeability

Stokes–Einstein equation

Case 2

Osmolarity, Osmotic Pressure, and Osmosis

The information shown in Table 1–2 pertains to six different solutions.

TABLE 1–2	Comparison of Six Solutions			
Solution	Solute	Concentration	g	σ
1	Urea	1 mmol/L	1.0	0
2	NaCl	1 mmol/L	1.85	0.5
3	NaCl	2 mmol/L	1.85	0.5
4	KCl	1 mmol/L	1.85	0.4
5	Sucrose	1 mmol/L	1.0	0.8
6	Albumin	1 mmol/L	1.0	1.0

g, osmotic coefficient; σ, reflection coefficient.

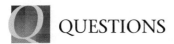 QUESTIONS

1. What is osmolarity, and how is it calculated?

2. What is osmosis? What is the driving force for osmosis?

3. What is osmotic pressure, and how is it calculated? What is effective osmotic pressure, and how is it calculated?

4. Calculate the osmolarity and effective osmotic pressure of each solution listed in Table 1–2 at 37°C. For 37°C, RT = 25.45 L-atm/mol, or 0.0245 L-atm/mmol.

5. Which, if any, of the solutions are isosmotic?

6. Which solution is hyperosmotic with respect to all of the other solutions?

7. Which solution is hypotonic with respect to all of the other solutions?

8. A semipermeable membrane is placed between Solution 1 and Solution 6. What is the difference in effective osmotic pressure between the two solutions? Draw a diagram that shows how water will flow between the two solutions and how the volume of each solution will change with time.

9. If the hydraulic conductance, or filtration coefficient (K_f), of the membrane in Question 8 is 0.01 mL/min-atm, what is the rate of water flow across the membrane?

10. Mannitol is a large sugar that does not dissociate in solution. A semipermeable membrane separates two solutions of mannitol. One solution has a mannitol concentration of 10 mmol/L, and the other has a mannitol concentration of 1 mmol/L. The filtration coefficient of the membrane is 0.5 mL/min-atm, and water flow across the membrane is measured as 0.1 mL/min. What is the reflection coefficient of mannitol for this membrane?

ANSWERS AND EXPLANATIONS

1. **Osmolarity** is the concentration of osmotically active particles in a solution. It is calculated as the product of solute concentration (e.g., in mmol/L) times the number of particles per mole in solution (i.e., whether the solute dissociates in solution). The extent of this dissociation is described by an **osmotic coefficient** called "**g**." If the solute does not dissociate, g = 1.0. If the solute dissociates into two particles, g = 2.0, and so forth. For example, for solutes such as urea or sucrose, g = 1.0 because these solutes do not dissociate in solution. On the other hand, for NaCl, g ≈ 2.0 because NaCl dissociates into two particles in solution, Na^+ and Cl^-. With this last example, it is important to note that Na^+ and Cl^- ions may interact in solution, making g slightly less than the theoretical, ideal value of 2.0.

   Osmolarity = g C

   where

   g = number of particles/mol in solution
   C = concentration (e.g., mmol/L)

   Two solutions that have the same calculated osmolarity are called **isosmotic.** If the calculated osmolarity of two solutions is different, then the solution with the higher osmolarity is **hyperosmotic** and the solution with the lower osmolarity is **hyposmotic.**

2. **Osmosis** is the flow of water between two solutions separated by a semipermeable membrane caused by a difference in solute concentration. The driving force for osmosis is a difference in **osmotic pressure** caused by the presence of solute. Initially, it may be surprising that the presence of solute can cause a pressure, which is explained as follows. Solute particles in a solution interact with pores in the membrane, and in so doing lower the hydrostatic pressure of the solution. The higher the solute concentration, the higher the osmotic pressure (see Question 3) and the lower the hydrostatic pressure (because of the interaction of solute with pores in the membrane). Thus, if two solutions have different solute concentrations (Fig. 1–1), then their osmotic and hydrostatic pressures are also different, and the difference in pressure causes water flow across the membrane (i.e., osmosis).

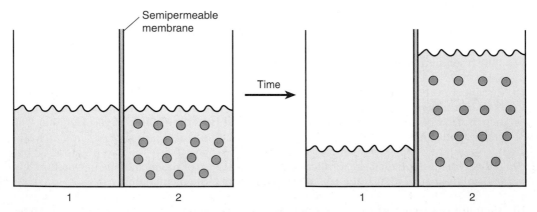

Figure 1–1   Osmosis of water across a semipermeable membrane.

3. The **osmotic pressure** of a solution is described by the **van't Hoff equation:**

$$\pi = g \, C \, RT$$

where

π = osmotic pressure [atmospheres (atm)]
g = number of particles/mol in solution
C = concentration (e.g., mmol/L)
R = gas constant (0.082 L-atm/mol-K)
T = absolute temperature (K)

In words, the van't Hoff equation states that the osmotic pressure of a solution depends on the concentration of osmotically active solute particles. The concentration of solute particles is converted to a pressure by multiplying it by the gas constant and the absolute temperature.

The concept of **"effective" osmotic pressure** involves a slight modification of the van't Hoff equation. Effective osmotic pressure depends on *both* the concentration of solute particles *and* the extent to which the solute crosses the membrane. The extent to which a particular solute crosses a particular membrane is expressed by a dimensionless factor called the **reflection coefficient (σ).** The value of the reflection coefficient can vary from 0 to 1.0 (Fig. 1–2). When $\sigma = 1.0$, the membrane is completely impermeable to the solute; the solute remains in the original solution and exerts its full osmotic pressure. When $\sigma = 0$, the membrane is freely permeable to the solute; solute diffuses across the membrane and down its concentration gradient until the concentrations in both solutions are equal. In this case, where $\sigma = 0$, the solutions on either side of the membrane have the same osmotic pressure because they have the same solute concentration; there is no difference in effective osmotic pressure across the membrane, and no osmosis of water occurs. When σ is between 0 and 1, the membrane is somewhat permeable to the solute; the effective osmotic pressure lies somewhere between its maximal value and 0.

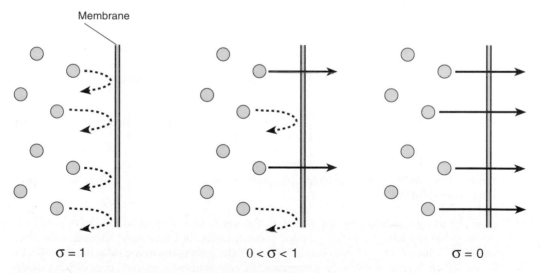

Figure 1–2   Reflection coefficient. (σ, reflection coefficient.)

Thus, to calculate the **effective osmotic pressure (π_{eff})**, the van't Hoff equation for osmotic pressure is modified by the value for σ, as follows:

$$\pi_{eff} = g\ C\ \sigma\ RT$$

where

π_{eff} = effective osmotic pressure (atm)
  g = number of particles/mol in solution
  C = concentration (e.g., mmol/L)
  R = gas constant (0.082 L-atm/mol-K)
  T = absolute temperature (K)
  σ = reflection coefficient (no units; varies from 0 to 1)

Isotonic solutions have the same effective osmotic pressure. When isotonic solutions are placed on either side of a semipermeable membrane, there is no difference in effective osmotic pressure across the membrane, no driving force for osmosis, and no water flow.

If two solutions have different effective osmotic pressures, then the one with the higher effective osmotic pressure is **hypertonic**, and the one with the lower effective osmotic pressure is **hypotonic**. If these solutions are placed on either side of a semipermeable membrane, then an osmotic pressure difference is present. This osmotic pressure difference is the driving force for water flow. Water flows from the hypotonic solution (with the lower effective osmotic pressure) into the hypertonic solution (with the higher effective osmotic pressure).

4. See Table 1–3.

TABLE 1–3	Calculated Values of Osmolarity and Effective Osmotic Pressure of Six Solutions	
Solution	**Osmolarity (mOsm/L)**	**Effective Osmotic Pressure (atm)**
1	1	0
2	1.85	0.0227
3	3.7	0.0453
4	1.85	0.0181
5	1	0.0196
6	1	0.0245

5. Solutions with the same calculated osmolarity are **isosmotic**. Therefore, Solutions 1, 5, and 6 are isosmotic with respect to each other. Solutions 2 and 4 are isosmotic with respect to each other.

6. Solution 3 has the highest calculated osmolarity. Therefore, it is hyperosmotic with respect to the other solutions.

7. According to our calculations, Solution 1 is hypotonic with respect to the other solutions because it has the lowest effective osmotic pressure (zero). But why zero? Shouldn't the urea particles in Solution 1 exert *some* osmotic pressure? The answer lies in the reflection coefficient of urea, which is zero: because the membrane is freely permeable to urea, urea diffuses down its concentration gradient until the concentrations of urea on both sides of the membrane are equal. At this point of equal concentration, urea exerts no "effective" osmotic pressure.

8. Solution 1 is 1 mmol/L urea, with an osmolarity of 1 mOsm/L and an effective osmotic pressure of 0. Solution 6 is 1 mmol/L albumin, with an osmolarity of 1 mOsm/L and an effective osmotic pressure of 0.0245 atm. According to the previous discussion, these two solutions are

isosmotic because they have the same osmolarity. However, they are *not isotonic* because they have different effective osmotic pressures. Solution 1 (urea) has the lower effective osmotic pressure and is hypotonic. Solution 6 (albumin) has the higher effective osmotic pressure and is hypertonic. The effective osmotic pressure difference ($\Delta\pi_{eff}$) is the difference between the effective osmotic pressure of Solution 6 and that of Solution 1:

$$\Delta\pi_{eff} = \pi_{eff} \text{ (Solution 6)} - \pi_{eff} \text{ (Solution 1)}$$
$$= 0.0245 \text{ atm} - 0 \text{ atm}$$
$$= 0.0245 \text{ atm}$$

If the two solutions are separated by a semipermeable membrane, water flows by osmosis from the hypotonic urea solution into the hypertonic albumin solution. With time, as a result of this water flow, the volume of the urea solution decreases and the volume of the albumin solution increases, as shown in Figure 1–3.

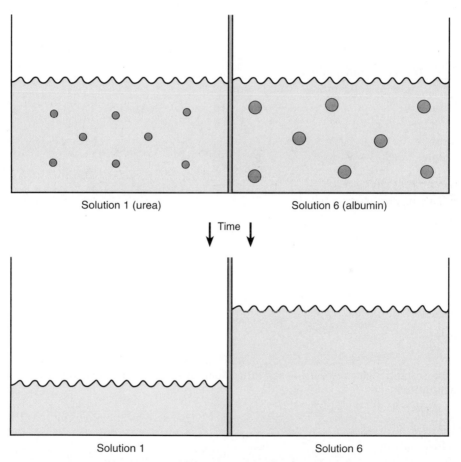

Figure 1–3 Osmotic water flow between a 1 mmol/L solution of urea and a 1 mmol/L solution of albumin. Water flows from the hypotonic urea solution into the hypertonic albumin solution.

9. **Osmotic water flow** across a membrane is the product of the osmotic driving force ($\Delta\pi_{eff}$) and the water permeability of the membrane, which is called the hydraulic conductance, or **filtration coefficient (K_f)**. In this question, K_f is given as 0.01 mL/min-atm, and $\Delta\pi_{eff}$ was calculated in Question 8 as 0.0245 atm.

$$\text{Water flow} = K_f \times \Delta\pi_{eff}$$
$$= 0.01 \text{ mL/min-atm} \times 0.0245 \text{ atm}$$
$$= 0.000245 \text{ mL/min}$$

10. This question is approached by using the relationship between water flow, hydraulic conductance (K_f), and difference in effective osmotic pressure that was introduced in Question 9. For each mannitol solution, $\pi_{eff} = \sigma \text{ g C RT}$. Therefore, the difference in effective osmotic pressure between the two mannitol solutions ($\Delta\pi_{eff}$) is:

$$\Delta\pi_{eff} = \sigma \text{ g } \Delta C \text{ RT}$$
$$\Delta\pi_{eff} = \sigma \times 1 \times (10 \text{ mmol/L} - 1 \text{ mmol/L}) \times 0.0245 \text{ L-atm/mmol}$$
$$= \sigma \times 0.2205 \text{ atm}$$

Now, substituting this value for $\Delta\pi_{eff}$ into the expression for water flow:

$$\text{Water flow} = K_f \times \Delta\pi_{eff}$$
$$= K_f \times \sigma \times 0.2205 \text{ atm}$$

Rearranging, substituting the value for water flow (0.1 mL/min), and solving for σ:

$$\sigma = \frac{0.1 \text{ mL}}{\text{min}} \times \frac{\text{min} - \text{atm}}{0.5 \text{ mL}} \times \frac{}{0.2205 \text{ atm}}$$
$$= 0.91$$

Key topics

Effective osmotic pressure (π_{eff})

Filtration coefficient (K_f)

Hyperosmotic

Hypertonic

Hyposmotic

Hypotonic

Isosmotic

Isotonic

Osmolarity

Osmosis

Osmotic coefficient (g)

Osmotic pressure (π)

Osmotic water flow

Reflection coefficient (σ)

van't Hoff equation

Case 3

Nernst Equation and Equilibrium Potentials

This case will guide you through the principles underlying diffusion potentials and electrochemical equilibrium.

 QUESTIONS

1. A solution of 100 mmol/L KCl is separated from a solution of 10 mmol/L KCl by a membrane that is very permeable to K^+ ions, but impermeable to Cl^- ions. What are the magnitude and the direction (sign) of the potential difference that will be generated across this membrane? (Assume that 2.3 RT/F = 60 mV.) Will the concentration of K^+ in either solution change as a result of the process that generates this potential difference?

2. If the same solutions of KCl described in Question 1 are now separated by a membrane that is very permeable to Cl^- ions, but impermeable to K^+ ions, what are the magnitude and the sign of the potential difference that is generated across the membrane?

3. A solution of 5 mmol/L $CaCl_2$ is separated from a solution of 1 µmol/L $CaCl_2$ by a membrane that is selectively permeable to Ca^{2+}, but is impermeable to Cl^-. What are the magnitude and the sign of the potential difference that is generated across the membrane?

4. A nerve fiber is placed in a bathing solution whose composition is similar to extracellular fluid. After the preparation equilibrates at 37°C, a microelectrode inserted into the nerve fiber records a potential difference across the nerve membrane as 70 mV, cell interior negative with respect to the bathing solution. The composition of the intracellular fluid and the extracellular fluid (bathing solution) is shown in Table 1–4. Assuming that 2.3 RT/F = 60 mV at 37°C, which ion is closest to electrochemical equilibrium? What can be concluded about the relative conductance of the nerve membrane to Na^+, K^+, and Cl^- under these conditions?

TABLE 1–4	Intracellular and Extracellular Concentrations of Na⁺, K⁺, and Cl⁻ in a Nerve Fiber	
Ion	**Intracellular Fluid**	**Extracellular Fluid**
Na^+	30 mmol/L	140 mmol/L
K^+	100 mmol/L	4 mmol/L
Cl^-	5 mmol/L	100 mmol/L

ANSWERS AND EXPLANATIONS

1. Two solutions that have different concentrations of KCl are separated by a membrane that is permeable to K+, but not to Cl−. Since in solution, KCl dissociates into K+ and Cl− ions, there is also a concentration gradient for K+ and Cl− across the membrane. Each ion would "like" to diffuse down its concentration gradient. However, the membrane is permeable only to K+. Thus, K+ ions diffuse across the membrane from high concentration to low concentration, but Cl− ions do not follow. As a result of this diffusion, net positive charge is carried across the membrane, creating a potential difference (**K+ diffusion potential**), as shown in Figure 1–4. The buildup of positive charge at the membrane retards further diffusion of K+ (positive is repelled by positive). Eventually, sufficient positive charge builds up at the membrane to exactly counterbalance the tendency of K+ to diffuse down its concentration gradient. This condition, called **electrochemical equilibrium**, occurs when the chemical and electrical driving forces on an ion (in this case, K+) are equal and opposite and no further net diffusion of the ion occurs.

Very few K+ ions need to diffuse to establish electrochemical equilibrium. Because very few K+ ions are involved, the process does not change the concentration of K+ in the bulk solutions. Stated differently, because of the prompt generation of the K+ diffusion potential, K+ does *not* diffuse until the two solutions have equal concentrations of K+ (as would occur with diffusion of an uncharged solute).

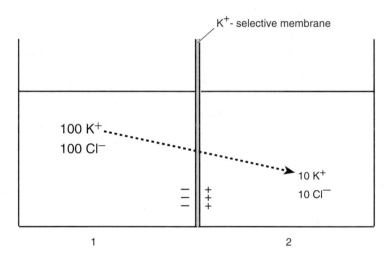

Figure 1–4   K+ diffusion potential.

The **Nernst equation** is used to calculate the magnitude of the potential difference generated by the diffusion of a single permeant ion (in this case, K+). Thus, the Nernst equation is used to calculate the **equilibrium potential** of an ion for a given concentration difference across the membrane, assuming that the membrane is permeable only to that ion.

$$E = -\frac{2.3\ RT}{z\ F}\ \log_{10}\frac{[C_1]}{[C_2]}$$

where

$$
\begin{aligned}
E &= \text{equilibrium potential (mV)} \\
2.3\ RT/F &= \text{constants (60 mV at 37°C)} \\
z &= \text{charge on diffusing ion (including sign)} \\
C_1 &= \text{concentration of the diffusing ion in one solution (mmol/L)} \\
C_2 &= \text{concentration of the diffusing ion in the other solution (mmol/L)}
\end{aligned}
$$

Now, to answer the question, what are the magnitude and the direction (sign) of the potential difference that is generated by the diffusion of K^+ ions down a concentration gradient of this magnitude? Stated differently, what is the K^+ equilibrium potential for this concentration difference? In practice, calculations involving the Nernst equation can be streamlined. Because these problems involve a logarithmic function, all signs in the calculation can be omitted, and the equation can be solved for the *absolute value* of the potential difference. For convenience, always put the higher concentration in the numerator and the lower concentration in the denominator. The correct sign of the potential difference is then determined intuitively, as illustrated in this question.

The higher K^+ concentration is 100 mmol/L, the lower K^+ concentration is 10 mmol/L, 2.3 RT/F is 60 mV at 37°C, and z for K^+ is +1. Because we are determining the **K^+ equilibrium potential** in this problem, "E" is denoted as E_{K^+}. Remember, that we agreed to omit all signs in the calculation and to determine the final sign intuitively later.

$$E_{K^+} = \frac{60 \text{ mV}}{1} \times \log_{10} \frac{100 \text{ mmol/L}}{10 \text{ mmol/L}}$$

$$= 60 \text{ mV} \times \log_{10} 10$$

$$= 60 \text{ mV} \times 1$$

$$= 60 \text{ mV (absolute value of the equilibrium potential)}$$

To determine the direction (sign) of the equilibrium potential, see Figure 1–4. Ask: Which way does K^+ diffuse to create this potential difference? It diffuses from high concentration (Solution 1) to low concentration (Solution 2). Positive charge accumulates near the membrane in Solution 2; negative charge remains behind at the membrane in Solution 1. Thus, the potential difference (or the K^+ equilibrium potential) is 60 mV, with Solution 1 negative with respect to Solution 2. (Or stated differently, the potential difference is 60 mV, with Solution 2 positive with respect to Solution 1.)

2. All conditions are the same as for Question 1, except that the membrane is permeable to Cl^- and impermeable to K^+. Again, both K^+ and Cl^- ions have a large concentration gradient across the membrane, and both ions would "like" to diffuse down that concentration gradient. However, now only Cl^- can diffuse. Cl^- diffuses from the solution that has the higher concentration to the solution that has the lower concentration, carrying a net negative charge across the membrane and generating a **Cl^- diffusion potential**, as shown in Figure 1–5. As negative charge builds up at the membrane, it prevents further net diffusion of Cl^- (negative repels negative).

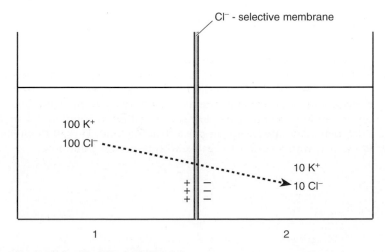

Figure 1–5 Cl^- diffusion potential.

At electrochemical equilibrium, the tendency for Cl⁻ to diffuse down its concentration gradient is exactly counterbalanced by the potential difference that is generated. In other words, the chemical and electrical driving forces on Cl⁻ are equal and opposite. Again, very few Cl⁻ ions need to diffuse to create this potential difference; therefore, the process does not change the Cl⁻ concentrations of the bulk solutions.

This time, we are using the Nernst equation to calculate the **Cl⁻ equilibrium potential (E_{Cl^-})**. The absolute value of the equilibrium potential is calculated by placing the higher Cl⁻ concentration in the numerator, the lower Cl⁻ concentration in the denominator, and ignoring all signs.

$$E_{Cl^-} = \frac{60 \text{ mV}}{1} \times \log_{10} \frac{100 \text{ mmol/L}}{10 \text{ mmol/L}}$$

$$= 60 \text{ mV} \times \log_{10} 10$$

$$= 60 \text{ mV} \times 1$$

$$= 60 \text{ mV (absolute value of the equilibrium potential)}$$

The sign of the potential difference is determined intuitively from Figure 1–5. Cl⁻ diffuses from high concentration in Solution 1 to low concentration in Solution 2. As a result, negative charge accumulates near the membrane in Solution 2, and positive charge remains behind at the membrane in Solution 1. Thus, the Cl⁻ equilibrium potential (E_{Cl^-}) is 60 mV, with Solution 2 negative with respect to Solution 1.

3. This problem is a variation on those you solved in Questions 1 and 2. There is a concentration gradient for $CaCl_2$ across a membrane that is selectively permeable to Ca^{2+} ions. You are asked to calculate the **Ca^{2+} equilibrium potential** for the stated concentration gradient (i.e., the potential difference that would exactly counterbalance the tendency for Ca^{2+} to diffuse down its concentration gradient). Ca^{2+} ions diffuse from high concentration to low concentration, and each ion carries two positive charges. Again, the absolute value of the equilibrium potential is calculated by placing the higher Ca^{2+} concentration in the numerator, the lower Ca^{2+} concentration in the denominator, and ignoring all signs. Remember that for Ca^{2+}, z is +2.

$$E_{Ca^{2+}} = \frac{60 \text{ mV}}{2} \times \log_{10} \frac{5 \text{ mmol/L}}{1 \text{ }\mu\text{mol/L}}$$

$$= 30 \text{ mV} \times \log_{10} \frac{5 \times 10^{-3} \text{ mol/L}}{1 \times 10^{-6} \text{ mol/L}}$$

$$= 30 \text{ mV} \times \log_{10} 5 \times 10^3 \text{ mol/L}$$

$$= 30 \text{ mV} \times 3.699$$

$$= 111 \text{ mV}$$

The sign of the equilibrium potential is determined intuitively from Figure 1–6. Ca^{2+} diffuses from high concentration in Solution 1 to low concentration in Solution 2, carrying positive charge across the membrane and leaving negative charge behind. Thus, the equilibrium potential for Ca^{2+} is 111 mV, with Solution 1 negative with respect to Solution 2.

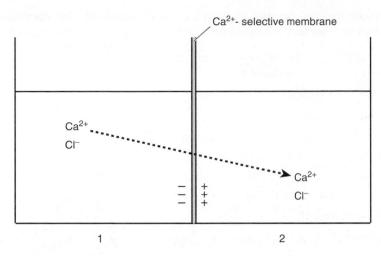

Figure 1–6 Ca^{2+} diffusion potential.

4. The problem gives the intracellular and extracellular concentrations of Na^+, K^+, and Cl^- and the measured **membrane potential** of a nerve fiber. The question asks which ion is closest to electrochemical equilibrium under these conditions. Indirectly, you are being asked which ion has the highest **permeability** or **conductance** in the membrane. The approach is to first calculate the equilibrium potential for each ion at the stated concentration gradient. (As before, use the Nernst equation to calculate the absolute value of the equilibrium potential, and determine the sign intuitively). Then, compare the *calculated* equilibrium potentials with the *actual* measured membrane potential. If the calculated equilibrium potential for an ion is close or equal to the measured membrane potential, then that ion is close to (or at) electrochemical equilibrium; that ion must have a high permeability or conductance. If the equilibrium potential for an ion is far from the measured membrane potential, then that ion is far from electrochemical equilibrium and must have a low permeability or conductance.

Figure 1–7 shows the nerve fiber and the concentrations of the three ions in the intracellular fluid and extracellular fluid. The sign of the equilibrium potential for each ion (determined intuitively) is superimposed on the nerve membrane in its correct orientation. It is important to know that membrane potentials and equilibrium potentials are always expressed as intracellular potential with respect to extracellular potential. For example, in this question, the membrane potential is 70 mV, cell interior negative; by convention, that is called –70 mV.

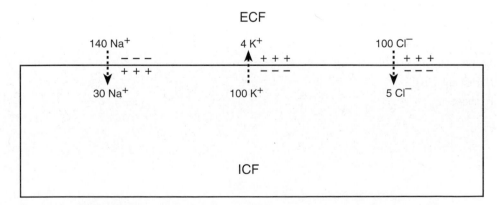

Figure 1–7 Orientation of equilibrium potentials for Na^+, K^+, and Cl^- in a nerve fiber.

Now the equilibrium potential for each ion can be calculated with the Nernst equation. Figure 1–7 can be referenced for the signs.

$$E_{Na^+} = \frac{60 \text{ mV}}{1} \times \log_{10} \frac{140 \text{ mmol/L}}{30 \text{ mmol/L}}$$

$$= 60 \text{ mV} \times \log_{10} 4.67$$

$$= 60 \text{ mV} \times 0.669$$

$$= 40 \text{ mV (or +40 mV, cell interior positive)}$$

$$E_{K^+} = \frac{60 \text{ mV}}{1} \times \log_{10} \frac{100 \text{ mmol/L}}{4 \text{ mmol/L}}$$

$$= 60 \text{ mV} \times \log_{10} 25$$

$$= 60 \text{ mV} \times 1.40$$

$$= 84 \text{ mV (or } -84 \text{ mV, cell interior negative)}$$

$$E_{Cl^-} = \frac{60 \text{ mV}}{1} \times \log_{10} \frac{100 \text{ mmol/L}}{5 \text{ mmol/L}}$$

$$= 60 \text{ mV} \times \log_{10} 20$$

$$= 60 \text{ mV} \times 1.3$$

$$= 78 \text{ mV (or } -78 \text{ mV, cell interior negative)}$$

These calculations are interpreted as follows. The equilibrium potential for Na^+ at the stated concentration gradient is +40 mV. In other words, for Na^+ to be at electrochemical equilibrium, the membrane potential must be +40 mV. However, the actual membrane potential of –70 mV is far from that value. Thus, we can conclude that Na^+, because it is far from electrochemical equilibrium, must have a low conductance or permeability. For K^+ to be at electrochemical equilibrium, the membrane potential must be –84 mV. The actual membrane potential is reasonably close, at –70 mV. Thus, we can conclude that K^+ is close to electrochemical equilibrium. The ion closest to electrochemical equilibrium is Cl^-; its calculated equilibrium potential of –78 mV is closest to the measured membrane potential of –70 mV. Thus, the conductance of the nerve cell membrane to Cl^- is highest, the conductance to K^+ is next highest, and the conductance to Na^+ is the lowest.

Key topics

Conductance

Diffusion potential

Electrochemical equilibrium

Equilibrium potential

Membrane potential

Nernst equation

Permeability

Case 4

Primary Hypokalemic Periodic Paralysis

Jimmy Jaworski is a 16-year-old sprinter on the high school track team. Recently, after he completed his events, he felt extremely weak, and his legs became "like rubber." Eating, especially carbohydrates, made him feel worse. After the most recent meet, he was unable to walk and had to be carried from the track on a stretcher. His parents were very alarmed and made an appointment for Jimmy to be evaluated by his pediatrician. As part of the workup, the pediatrician measured Jimmy's serum K^+ concentration, which was normal (4.5 mEq/L). However, because the pediatrician suspected a connection with K^+, the measurement was repeated immediately after a strenuous exercise treadmill test. After the treadmill test, Jimmy's serum K^+ was alarmingly low (2.2 mEq/L). Jimmy was diagnosed as having an inherited disorder called primary hypokalemic periodic paralysis and subsequently was treated with K^+ supplementation.

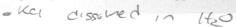

 QUESTIONS

1. What is the normal K^+ distribution between intracellular fluid and extracellular fluid? Where is most of the K^+ located?

2. What major factors can alter the distribution of K^+ between intracellular fluid and extracellular fluid?

3. What is the relationship between the serum K^+ concentration and the resting membrane potential of excitable cells (e.g., nerve, skeletal muscle)?

4. How does a decrease in serum K^+ concentration alter the resting membrane potential of skeletal muscle?

5. Propose a mechanism whereby a decrease in the serum K^+ concentration could lead to skeletal muscle weakness.

6. Why did Jimmy's weakness occur *after* exercise? Why did eating carbohydrates exacerbate (worsen) the weakness?

7. How would K^+ supplementation be expected to improve Jimmy's condition?

8. Another inherited disorder, called primary *hyper*kalemic periodic paralysis, involves an initial period of spontaneous muscle contractions (spasms), followed by prolonged muscle weakness. Using your knowledge of the ionic basis for the skeletal muscle action potential, propose a mechanism whereby an *increase* in the serum K^+ concentration could lead to spontaneous contractions followed by prolonged weakness.

ANSWERS AND EXPLANATIONS

1. Most of the body's K^+ is located in the intracellular fluid; K^+ is the major intracellular cation. The intracellular concentration of K^+ is more than 20 times that of extracellular K^+. This asymmetrical distribution of K^+ is maintained by the Na^+-K^+ adenosine triphosphatase (ATPase) that is present in all cell membranes. The Na^+-K^+ ATPase, using ATP as its energy source, actively transports K^+ from extracellular fluid to intracellular fluid against an electrochemical gradient, thus maintaining the high intracellular K^+ concentration.

2. Several factors, including hormones and drugs, can alter the **K^+ distribution** between intracellular fluid and extracellular fluid (Fig. 1–8). Such a redistribution is called a **K^+ shift** to signify that K^+ has *shifted* from extracellular fluid to intracellular fluid or from intracellular fluid to extracellular fluid. Because the normal concentration of K^+ in the extracellular fluid is low, K^+ shifts can cause profound changes in the concentration of K^+ in the extracellular fluid or in the serum.

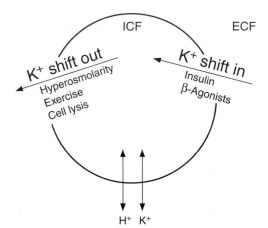

Figure 1–8 Internal K^+ balance. (ICF, intracellular fluid; ECF, extracellular fluid.)

The major factors that cause K^+ to shift *into* cells (from extracellular fluid to intracellular fluid) are **insulin, β-adrenergic agonists** (e.g., epinephrine, norepinephrine), and alkalemia. The major factors that cause K^+ to shift *out* of cells (from intracellular fluid to extracellular fluid) are lack of insulin, β-adrenergic antagonists, **exercise**, hyperosmolarity, cell lysis, and acidemia. Therefore, insulin and β-adrenergic agonists cause K^+ to shift from extracellular fluid to intracellular fluid and may cause a decrease in serum K^+ concentration (hypokalemia). Conversely, lack of insulin, β-adrenergic antagonists, exercise, hyperosmolarity, or cell lysis cause K^+ to shift from intracellular fluid to extracellular fluid and may cause an increase in serum K^+ concentration (hyperkalemia).

3. At rest (i.e., between action potentials), nerve and skeletal muscle membranes have a high permeability or conductance to K^+. There is also a large concentration gradient for K^+ across cell membranes created by the Na^+-K^+ ATPase (i.e., high K^+ concentration in intracellular fluid and low K^+ concentration in extracellular fluid). The large chemical driving force, coupled with the high conductance to K^+, causes K^+ to diffuse from intracellular fluid to extracellular fluid. As discussed in Case 3, this process generates an inside-negative potential difference, or K^+ diffusion potential, which is the basis for the **resting membrane potential.** The resting membrane potential approaches the **K^+ equilibrium potential** (calculated with the Nernst equation for a given K^+ concentration gradient) because the resting K^+ conductance is very high.

Changes in the serum (extracellular fluid) K⁺ concentration alter the K⁺ equilibrium potential, and consequently the resting membrane potential. The lower the serum K⁺ concentration, the greater the K⁺ concentration gradient across the membrane, and the more negative (hyperpolarized) the K⁺ equilibrium potential. The more negative the K⁺ equilibrium potential, the more negative the resting membrane potential. Conversely, the higher the serum K⁺ concentration, the smaller the K⁺ concentration gradient, and the less negative the K⁺ equilibrium potential and the resting membrane potential.

4. Essentially, this question has been answered: as the concentration of K⁺ in the serum decreases **(hypokalemia)**, the resting membrane potential of skeletal muscle becomes more negative (hyperpolarized). Thus, the lower the serum K⁺ concentration, the larger the K⁺ concentration gradient across the cell membrane, and the larger and more negative the K⁺ equilibrium potential. Because the K⁺ conductance of skeletal muscle is very high at rest, the membrane potential is driven toward this more negative K⁺ equilibrium potential. *more(→) ⇒ ie.. wonts to leave the cell even more.*

5. To answer this question about why Jimmy was weak, it is necessary to understand the events *more.* that are responsible for action potentials in skeletal muscle. Figure 1–9 shows a single action potential superimposed by the relative conductances to K⁺ and Na⁺.

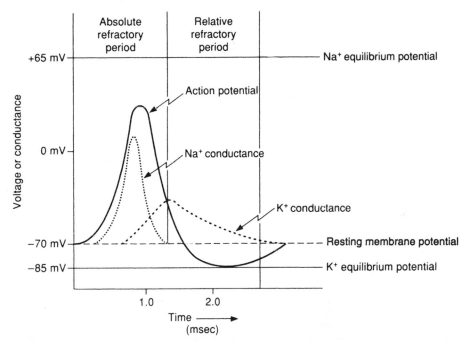

Figure 1–9 Nerve and skeletal muscle action potential and associated changes in Na⁺ and K⁺ conductance. (Reprinted, with permission, from Costanzo LS. *BRS Physiology*. 4th ed. Baltimore: Lippincott Williams & Wilkins; 2007:11.)

The **action potential** in skeletal muscle is a very rapid event (lasting approximately 1 msec) and is composed of **depolarization** (the upstroke) followed by **repolarization.** The resting membrane potential is approximately –70 mV (cell negative). Because of the high conductance to K⁺, the resting membrane potential approaches the K⁺ equilibrium potential, as described earlier. At rest, the conductance to Na⁺ is low; therefore, the resting membrane potential is far from the Na⁺ equilibrium potential. The action potential is initiated when **inward current** (positive charge entering the muscle cell) depolarizes the muscle cell membrane. This inward current is usually the result of current spread from action potentials at neighboring sites. If there is sufficient inward current to depolarize the muscle membrane to the **threshold potential** (to approximately –60 mV), **activation gates** on voltage-gated Na⁺ channels rapidly open.

As a result, the Na^+ conductance increases and becomes even higher than the K^+ conductance. This rapid increase in Na^+ conductance produces an inward Na^+ current that further depolarizes the membrane potential toward the Na^+ equilibrium potential, which constitutes the **upstroke of the action potential.** The upstroke is followed by repolarization to the resting membrane potential. Repolarization is caused by two slower events: closure of **inactivation gates** on the Na^+ channels (leading to closure of the Na^+ channels and decreased Na^+ conductance) and increased K^+ conductance, which drives the membrane potential back toward the K^+ equilibrium potential. → makes sense b/c usually it is always diffusing out!

Now, we can use these concepts and answer the question of why Jimmy's decreased serum K^+ concentration led to his skeletal muscle weakness. Decreased serum K^+ concentration increased the negativity of both the K^+ equilibrium potential and the resting membrane potential, as already discussed. Because the resting membrane potential was further from the threshold potential, more inward current was required to depolarize the membrane to threshold to initiate the upstroke of the action potential. In other words, firing action potentials became more difficult. Without action potentials, Jimmy's skeletal muscle could not contract, and as a result, his muscles felt weak and "rubbery."

6. We can speculate about why Jimmy's periodic paralysis occurred *after* extreme exercise, and why it was exacerbated by eating carbohydrates. By mechanisms that are not completely understood, exercise causes K^+ to shift from intracellular fluid to extracellular fluid. It may also lead to a transient local increase in the K^+ concentration of extracellular fluid. (Incidentally, this local increase in K^+ concentration is one of the factors that causes an increase in muscle blood flow during exercise). Normally, after exercise, K^+ is reaccumulated in skeletal muscle cells. Because of his inherited disorder, in Jimmy this reaccumulation of K^+ was exaggerated and led to hypokalemia.

Ingestion of carbohydrates exacerbated his muscle weakness because glucose stimulates insulin secretion. Insulin is a major factor that causes uptake of K^+ into cells. This insulin-dependent K^+ uptake augmented the postexercise K^+ uptake and caused further hypokalemia.

7. K^+ supplementation provided more K^+ to the extracellular fluid, which offset the exaggerated uptake of K^+ into muscle cells that occurred after exercise. Once the pediatrician understood the physiologic basis for Jimmy's problem (too much K^+ shifting into cells after exercise), sufficient K^+ could be supplemented to prevent the serum K^+ from decreasing.

8. Another disorder, primary *hyper*kalemic periodic paralysis, also leads to skeletal muscle weakness. However, in this disorder, the weakness is preceded by muscle spasms. This pattern is also explained by events of the muscle action potential.

The initial muscle spasms (hyperactivity) can be understood from our earlier discussion. When the serum K^+ concentration increases **(hyperkalemia)**, the K^+ equilibrium potential and the resting membrane potential become less negative (depolarized). The resting membrane potential is moved closer to threshold potential, and as a result, less inward current is required to initiate the upstroke of the action potential.

It is more difficult to understand why the initial phase of muscle hyperactivity is followed by prolonged weakness. If the muscle membrane potential is closer to threshold, won't it continue to fire away? Actually, no. The explanation lies in the behavior of the two sets of gates on the **Na^+ channels.** Activation gates on Na^+ channels *open* in response to depolarization; these gates are responsible for the upstroke of the action potential. However, inactivation gates on the Na^+ channel *close* in response to depolarization, albeit more slowly than the activation gates open. Therefore, in response to prolonged depolarization (as in hyperkalemia), the inactivation gates close and remain closed. When the inactivation gates are closed, the Na^+ channels are closed, regardless of the position of the activation gates. For the upstroke of the action potential to occur, both sets of gates on the Na^+ channels must be open; if the inactivation gates are closed, no action potentials can occur.

Key topics

Action potential

Activation gates

β-Adrenergic agonists (epinephrine, norepinephrine)

Depolarization

Exercise

Hyperkalemia

Hypokalemia

Inactivation gates

Insulin

Inward current

K^+ distribution

K^+ equilibrium potential

K^+ shifts

Na^+ channels

Repolarization

Resting membrane potential

Threshold potential

Upstroke

Case 5

Epidural Anesthesia: Effect of Lidocaine on Nerve Action Potentials

Sue McKnight, a healthy 27-year-old woman, was pregnant with her first child. The pregnancy was completely normal. However, as the delivery date approached, Sue became increasingly fearful of the pain associated with a vaginal delivery. Her mother and five sisters had told her horror stories about their experiences with labor and delivery. Sue discussed these fears with her obstetrician, who reassured her that she would be a good candidate for epidural anesthesia. The obstetrician explained that during this procedure, lidocaine, a local anesthetic, is injected into the epidural space around the lumbar spinal cord. The anesthetic drug prevents pain by blocking action potentials in the sensory nerve fibers that serve the pelvis and perineum. Sue was comforted by this information and decided to politely excuse herself from further conversations with "helpful" relatives. Sue went into labor on her due date. She received an epidural anesthetic midway through her 10-hour labor and delivered an 8 lb 10 oz boy with virtually no pain. She reported to her mother and sisters that epidural anesthesia is "the greatest thing since sliced bread."

 QUESTIONS

1. Lidocaine and other local anesthetic agents block action potentials in nerve fibers by binding to specific ion channels. At low concentration, these drugs decrease the rate of rise of the upstroke of the action potential. At higher concentrations, they prevent the occurrence of action potentials altogether. Based on this information and your knowledge of the ionic basis of the action potential, which ion channel would you conclude is blocked by lidocaine?

2. Lidocaine is a weak base with a pK of 7.9. At physiologic pH, is lidocaine primarily in its charged or uncharged form?

3. Lidocaine blocks ion channels by binding to receptors from the *intracellular* side of the channel. Therefore, to act, lidocaine must cross the nerve cell membrane. Using this information, if the pH of the epidural space were to decrease from 7.4 to 7.0 (becomes more acidic), would drug activity increase, decrease, or be unchanged?

4. Based on your knowledge of how nerve action potentials are propagated, how would you expect lidocaine to alter the conduction of the action potential along a nerve fiber?

ANSWERS ON NEXT PAGE

ANSWERS AND EXPLANATIONS

1. To determine which ion channel is blocked by lidocaine, it is necessary to review which ion channels are important in **action potentials.** At **rest** (i.e., between action potentials), the conductance to K^+ and Cl^- is high, mediated respectively by K^+ and Cl^- channels in the nerve membrane. Thus, the resting membrane potential is driven toward the K^+ and Cl^- equilibrium potentials. During the **upstroke** of the nerve action potential, **voltage-gated Na^+ channels** are most important. These channels open in response to depolarization, and this opening leads to further depolarization toward the Na^+ equilibrium potential. During **repolarization,** the voltage-gated Na^+ channels close and K^+ channels open; as a result, the nerve membrane is repolarized back toward the resting membrane potential.

   Lidocaine and other **local anesthetic agents** block voltage-gated Na^+ channels in the nerve membrane. At low concentrations, this blockade results in a slower rate of rise (dV/dt) of the upstroke of the action potential. At higher concentrations, the upstroke is prevented altogether, and no action potentials can occur.

2. According to the Brønsted–Lowry nomenclature for **weak acids,** the proton donor is called HA and the proton acceptor is called A^-. With **weak bases** (e.g., lidocaine), the proton donor has a net positive charge and is called BH^+; the proton acceptor is called B. Because the pK of lidocaine (a weak base) is 7.9, the predominant form of lidocaine at physiologic pH (7.4) is BH^+, with its net positive charge. This can be confirmed with the **Henderson–Hasselbalch equation,** which is used to calculate the relative concentrations of BH^+ and B at a given pH as follows:

$$pH = pK + \log \frac{B}{BH^+}$$

Physiologic pH is 7.4, and the pK of lidocaine is 7.9. Thus:

$$7.4 = 7.9 + \log \frac{B}{BH^+}$$

$$-0.5 = \log \frac{B}{BH^+}$$

$$0.316 = B/BH^+$$

or

$$BH^+/B = 3.16$$

In words, at physiologic pH, the concentration of BH^+ (with its net positive charge) is approximately three times the concentration of B (uncharged).

3. As discussed in Question 2, the BH^+ form of lidocaine has a net positive charge, and the B form of lidocaine is uncharged. You were told that lidocaine must cross the lipid bilayer of the nerve membrane to act from the intracellular side of the Na^+ channel. Because the uncharged (B) form of lidocaine is more lipophilic (i.e., **high lipid solubility**) than the positively charged (BH^+) form, it crosses the nerve cell membrane more readily. Thus, at physiologic pH, although the positively charged (BH^+) form is predominant (see Question 2), it is the uncharged form that enters the nerve fiber.

If the pH of the epidural space decreases to 7.0, the equilibrium shifts toward the BH^+ form, again demonstrated by the Henderson–Hasselbalch equation.

$$pH = pK + \log \frac{B}{BH^+}$$

$$7.0 = 7.9 + \log \frac{B}{BH^+}$$

$$-0.9 = \log \frac{B}{BH^+}$$

$$0.126 = B/BH^+$$

or

$$BH^+/B = 7.94$$

At this more acidic pH, the amount of the charged form of lidocaine is now approximately eight times that of the uncharged form. When the pH is more acidic, *less* of the permeant, uncharged form of the drug is present. Thus, access of the drug to its intracellular site of action is impaired, and the drug is *less* effective.

4. **Propagation of action potentials** (e.g., along sensory nerve axons) occurs by the spread of local currents from active depolarized regions (i.e., regions that are firing action potentials) to adjacent inactive regions. These local depolarizing currents are caused by the **inward Na^+ current** of the upstroke of the action potential. When lidocaine blocks voltage-gated Na^+ channels, the inward Na^+ current of the upstroke of the action potential does not occur. Thus, propagation of the action potential, which depends on this depolarizing inward current, is also prevented.

Key topics

Action potentials

Henderson–Hasselbalch equation

Inward Na^+ current

Lidocaine

Lipid solubility

Local anesthetics

Local currents

Propagation of action potentials

Repolarization

Upstroke

Voltage-gated Na^+ channels

Weak acids

Weak bases

Case 6

Multiple Sclerosis: Myelin and Conduction Velocity

Meg Newton is a 32-year-old assistant at a horse-breeding farm in Virginia. She feeds, grooms, and exercises the horses. At age 27, she had her first episode of blurred vision. She was having trouble reading the newspaper and the fine print on labels. She had made an appointment with an optometrist, but when her vision cleared on its own, she was relieved and canceled the appointment. Ten months later, the blurred vision returned, this time with other symptoms that could not be ignored. She had double vision and a "pins and needles" feeling and severe weakness in her legs. She was even too weak to walk the horses to pasture.

Meg was referred to a neurologist, who ordered a series of tests. Magnetic resonance imaging (MRI) of the brain showed lesions typical of multiple sclerosis. Visual evoked potentials had a prolonged latency that was consistent with decreased nerve conduction velocity. Since the diagnosis, Meg has had two relapses, and she is currently being treated with interferon beta.

 QUESTIONS

1. How is the action potential propagated in nerves (such as sensory nerves of the visual system)?

2. What is a length constant, and what factors increase it?

3. Why is it said that action potentials propagate "nondecrementally?"

4. What is the effect of nerve diameter on conduction velocity, and why?

5. What is the effect of myelination on conduction velocity, and why?

6. In myelinated nerves, why must there be periodic breaks in the myelin sheath (nodes of Ranvier)?

7. Meg was diagnosed with multiple sclerosis, a disease of the central nervous system, in which axons lose their myelin sheath. How does the loss of the myelin sheath alter nerve conduction velocity?

ANSWERS ON NEXT PAGE

ANSWERS AND EXPLANATIONS

1. Propagation of action potentials occurs along nerve fibers by **spread of local currents.** At rest, the nerve fiber is polarized (i.e., inside negative with respect to outside). When an action potential occurs, the inward current of the upstroke of the action potential depolarizes the membrane and reverses the polarity at that site (i.e., that site briefly becomes inside positive). The depolarization then spreads to adjacent sites along the nerve fiber by local current flow, or **electrotonic conduction,** as shown in Figure 1–10. As the depolarization spreads electrotonically to adjacent areas, it decays. Thus, local currents are conducted **decrementally,** and as a consequence, the further from the site of the action potential, the smaller the local depolarization. Importantly, though, if these local currents depolarize an adjacent region to threshold, it will fire an action potential (i.e., the action potential is propagated).

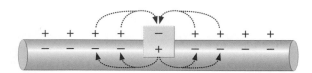

Figure 1–10 Unmyelinated axon showing spread of depolarization by local current flow. Box shows active zone where action potential has reversed the polarity across the membrane.

2. Length constant is defined as the distance from the original site of depolarization (the site of the action potential) where the potential has fallen, or decayed, to 63% of its original value; the longer the length constant, the less the decay, and the further local current spread occurs along the axon. Length constant can be increased in two ways: **increasing *membrane* resistance** (such that current is forced to flow down the axon interior rather than leaking out across the membrane) and **decreasing *internal* resistance** of the axon (such that current flows more readily along the axon interior).

3. As described before, local currents are conducted along axons *decrementally.* Why, then, is it said that **action potentials propagate *nondecrementally?*** In the process of local current spread, if a neighboring site is depolarized to threshold, *it* fires an action potential. This regenerative process, by creating a new action potential at a site further along the axon, restores the full extent of depolarization. Depolarization now spreads from this new site and depolarizes neighboring sites to threshold; those neighboring sites fire action potentials, continuing the process along the axon. The restorative function that periodically creates new action potentials ensures that the depolarization does not die out along the length of the axon.

4. **Increased diameter** is associated with decreased internal resistance of the nerve fiber, which increases the length constant. Increased length constant leads to increased **conduction velocity,** because the local currents will spread further down the axon.

5. **Myelination** increases conduction velocity. Myelin is an insulator of axons, increasing membrane resistance and decreasing membrane capacitance. By **increasing membrane resistance,** current is forced to flow down the axon interior and less current is lost across the cell membrane (increased **length constant**); because more current flows down the axon, conduction velocity is increased. By **decreasing membrane capacitance,** local currents depolarize the membrane more rapidly, which also increases conduction velocity.

6. In order for action potentials to be conducted in myelinated nerves, there must be periodic breaks in the myelin sheath (at the **nodes of Ranvier**). The nerve action potential consists of depolarization (due to opening of cell membrane Na^+ channels), followed by repolarization

(due to opening of cell membrane K⁺ channels). Opening of these channels permits the flow of ions across the membrane that produces the characteristic depolarization and repolarization of the action potential. In myelinated nerves, these Na⁺ and K⁺ channels are not distributed along the entire axon membrane, but are concentrated at nodes of Ranvier. Thus, at the nodes, the ionic currents, necessary for the action potential, can flow across the membrane. Between nodes, membrane resistance is very high and current is forced to flow rapidly down the nerve axon to the next node, where the next action potential can be generated. Thus, the action potential appears to "jump" from one node of Ranvier to the next, which is called **saltatory conduction** (Fig. 1–11). If there were no breaks in the myelin sheath, there would be no regions of ion channel density (e.g., Na⁺ channels) where action potentials could occur to restore the full level of depolarization.

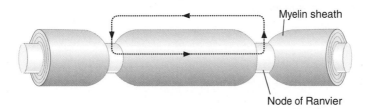

Myelin sheath

Node of Ranvier

Figure 1–11   Myelinated axon. Action potentials can occur at nodes of Ranvier.

7. **Multiple sclerosis** is the most common demyelinating disease of the central nervous system. Loss of the myelin sheath around nerves causes a **decrease in membrane resistance**, which means that current "leaks out" across the membrane during electrotonic conduction. In other words, current decays more rapidly (**decreased length constant**) as it flows down the axon, and because of this decay, may be insufficient to generate an action potential when it reaches the next node of Ranvier.

Key topics

Capacitance (or membrane capacitance)

Conduction velocity (of action potential)

Electrotonic conduction

Length constant

Local currents

Multiple sclerosis

Myelin

Nodes of Ranvier

Propagation of action potentials

Resistance (or membrane resistance)

Saltatory conduction

Case 7

Myasthenia Gravis: Neuromuscular Transmission

Wendy Chu is a 23-year-old photographer for a busy local newspaper. Over the last 8 months, she experienced "strange" symptoms. She had severe eyestrain when she read for longer than 15 minutes. She became tired when she chewed her food, brushed her teeth, or dried her hair; and she had extreme fatigue on the job. Despite her strong work ethic, Wendy had to excuse herself from several "shoots" because she simply could not carry the heavy equipment. Wendy is not a complainer, but she began to worry about these vague symptoms.

  She was evaluated by her physician, who suspected myasthenia gravis. While awaiting the results of a serum antibody test, the physician initiated a trial of pyridostigmine, an acetylcholinesterase inhibitor. Wendy immediately felt better while taking the drug; her strength returned to almost normal. Meanwhile, the results of the antibody test were positive, confirming the diagnosis of myasthenia gravis.

 QUESTIONS

1. What steps are involved in neuromuscular transmission?

2. What antibody was measured in Wendy's serum? Against what protein is this antibody directed?

3. Using your description of neuromuscular transmission, explain why severe muscle weakness (e.g., ocular, jaw) occurs in myasthenia gravis.

4. Why does pyridostigmine, an acetylcholinesterase inhibitor, improve muscle strength in myasthenia gravis?

5. Consider the following drugs that act at various steps in neuromuscular transmission. What is the action of each drug, and which drugs are *contraindicated* in myasthenia gravis?

   Botulinus toxin
   Curare
   Neostigmine
   Hemicholinium

ANSWERS ON NEXT PAGE

ANSWERS AND EXPLANATIONS

1. **Neuromuscular transmission** is the process whereby an action potential in a motoneuron produces an action potential in the muscle fibers that it innervates. The steps in neuromuscular transmission, shown in Figure 1–12, are as follows: (i) An action potential is propagated down the motoneuron until the presynaptic terminal is depolarized. (ii) Depolarization of the presynaptic terminal causes voltage-gated Ca^{2+} channels to open, and Ca^{2+} flows into the nerve terminal. (iii) Uptake of Ca^{2+} into the nerve terminal causes exocytosis of stored **acetylcholine (ACh)** into the synaptic cleft. (iv) ACh diffuses across the synaptic cleft to the **muscle end-plate,** where it binds to **nicotinic ACh receptors (AChRs).** (v) The nicotinic AChR is also an ion channel for Na^+ and K^+. When ACh binds to the receptor, the channel opens. (vi) Opening of the channel causes both Na^+ and K^+ to flow down their respective electrochemical gradients. As a result, depolarization occurs. (vii) This depolarization, called the **end-plate potential,** spreads to neighboring regions of the muscle fiber. (viii) Finally, the muscle fibers are depolarized to threshold and fire action potentials. Through this elaborate sequence of events, an action potential in the motoneuron causes an action potential in the muscle fibers that it innervates.

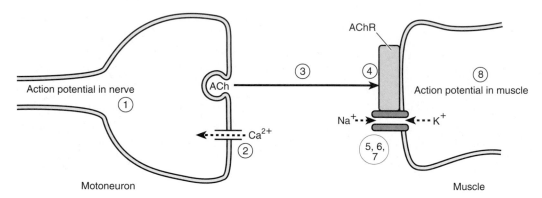

Figure 1–12 Steps in neuromuscular transmission. The numbers correspond to the steps discussed in the text. (ACh, acetylcholine; AChR, ACh receptor.)

2. Wendy's physician suspected myasthenia gravis and measured serum levels of an antibody to the **nicotinic AChR.** Accordingly, the antibody is called AChR-ab.

3. In **myasthenia gravis,** abnormal antibodies to AChR (AChR-ab) are produced, circulate in the blood, and bind to nicotinic receptors on the muscle end-plates. When antibodies are bound to AChR, the receptors are not available to be activated by the ACh that is released physiologically from motoneurons. Thus, while normal action potentials occur in the motoneurons and ACh is released normally, the ACh cannot cause depolarization of muscle end-plates. Without depolarization of muscle end-plates, there can be no action potentials or contraction in the muscle.

4. After ACh binds to and activates AChR on the muscle end-plate, it is degraded by **acetylcholinesterase,** an enzyme that is also present on the muscle end-plate. This degradative step, whose byproducts are choline and acetate, terminates the action of ACh on the muscle fiber. Choline is taken up into the motoneuron terminal and recycled into the synthesis of more ACh.

   Pyridostigmine is an **acetylcholinesterase inhibitor** that binds to acetylcholinesterase and thereby reduces binding and degradation of ACh at the muscle end-plate. In the treatment of myasthenia gravis, pyridostigmine prevents degradation of ACh, increasing its synaptic concentration and prolonging its action. The longer the muscle end-plate is exposed to high concentrations of ACh, the greater the likelihood that action potentials and contraction in the muscle will occur.

5. In principle, any drug that interferes with any step in neuromuscular transmission is contraindicated in myasthenia gravis. **Botulinus toxin** blocks the release of ACh from motoneuron terminals, and therefore causes total blockade of neuromuscular transmission; it is contraindicated in myasthenia gravis. **Curare**, a competitive inhibitor of ACh for the AChR on the muscle end plate, prevents depolarization of the muscle fiber; it is contraindicated. **Neostigmine** is an acetylcholinesterase inhibitor that is related to pyridostigmine and is used to *treat* myasthenia gravis by preventing ACh degradation. **Hemicholinium** blocks the reuptake of choline into motoneuron terminals, thereby depleting stores of ACh; it is contraindicated.

Key topics

Acetylcholine (ACh)

Acetylcholine receptor (AChR)

Acetylcholinesterase

Acetylcholinesterase inhibitor

Botulinus toxin

Curare

End-plate potential

Hemicholinium

Muscle (motor) end-plate

Myasthenia gravis

Neostigmine

Neuromuscular transmission

Nicotinic receptor

Pyridostigmine

Case 8

Pheochromocytoma: Effects of Catecholamines

Helen Ames is a 51-year-old homemaker who experienced what she thought were severe menopausal symptoms. These awful "attacks" were becoming more frequent. Her heart raced and pounded; she had a throbbing headache and visual disturbances; she felt hot, but her hands and feet were cold; and she was nauseated, sometimes to the point of vomiting. Mrs. Ames called her physician, who agreed that the symptoms were probably menopausal and pre-scribed hormone replacement therapy over the phone. Mrs. Ames took the hormones (a com-bination of estrogen and progesterone), but they did not relieve her symptoms. The attacks were occurring almost daily. She made an appointment with her physician.

In the physician's office, Mrs. Ames' blood pressure was severely elevated at 200/110, and her heart rate was increased at 110 beats/min. To rule out a pheochromocytoma (a rare tumor of the adrenal medulla), the physician ordered a 24-hour urine measurement of 3-methoxy-4-hydroxymandelic acid (VMA). To his surprise, the results of the 24-hour urinary VMA test were positive, a finding that provided nearly conclusive evidence of a pheochromocytoma. A computed tomographic scan confirmed that Mrs. Ames had a 3-cm mass on her right adrenal gland. While awaiting surgery to remove the tumor, she was given phenoxybenzamine, an α_1-adrenergic antagonist. After an appropriate dosage of phenoxybenzamine was estab-lished, she was also given a low dose of propranolol, a β-adrenergic antagonist. She was cleared for surgery when the medications had decreased her blood pressure to 140/90.

 QUESTIONS

1. What is the relationship of the adrenal medulla to the autonomic nervous system?

2. What hormones are secreted by a pheochromocytoma?

3. Why does an elevated urinary level of VMA (a metabolite of epinephrine and norepinephrine) suggest the presence of a pheochromocytoma? Why is it necessary to do a 24-hour measure-ment of VMA, rather than a spot-urine test?

4. In view of the pathophysiology of pheochromocytoma, explain Mrs. Ames' symptoms, specif-ically her increased heart rate, pounding heart, cold hands and feet, visual disturbances, and nausea and vomiting. What receptors are involved in each of these symptoms?

5. Why are two values reported for arterial pressure, and what is the significance of each value? Why were both the systolic and diastolic blood pressures elevated?

6. Is there a plausible explanation for the fact that Mrs. Ames felt hot, even though her hands and feet were cold?

7. How did phenoxybenzamine lower Mrs. Ames' blood pressure?

8. After the dosage of phenoxybenzamine was established, what was the goal of adding a low dose of propranolol?

9. What might have happened if Mrs. Ames had been given propranolol alone?

ANSWERS ON NEXT PAGE

ANSWERS AND EXPLANATIONS

1. The **adrenal medulla** is a specialized ganglion of the **sympathetic division** of the autonomic nervous system. The preganglionic neurons have their cell bodies in the thoracic spinal cord. Axons of these preganglionic neurons travel in the greater splanchnic nerve to the adrenal medulla, where they synapse on **chromaffin cells** and release the neurotransmitter acetylcholine. When stimulated, chromaffin cells (the postsynaptic unit) secrete catecholamines (epinephrine and norepinephrine) into the circulation (Fig. 1–13).

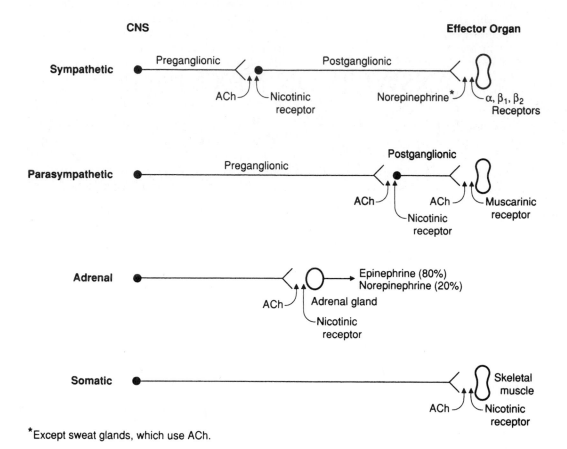

*Except sweat glands, which use ACh.

Figure 1–13 Organization of the autonomic nervous system. The somatic nervous system is included for reference only. (ACh, acetylcholine; CNS, central nervous system.) (Reprinted, with permission, from Costanzo LS. *BRS Physiology.* 4th ed. Baltimore: Lippincott Williams & Wilkins; 2007:34.)

2. **A pheochromocytoma** is a tumor of the adrenal medulla gland that secretes large quantities of **epinephrine** and **norepinephrine.** As with the normal adrenal medulla, the greater secretory component is epinephrine (80%) and the lesser component is norepinephrine (20%), although the percentage of norepinephrine is higher than that in the normal adrenal.

3. **3-Methoxy-4-hydroxymandelic acid (VMA)** is a major metabolite of both epinephrine and norepinephrine. When epinephrine and norepinephrine are degraded by the enzymes **catechol-*O*-methyltransferase (COMT)** and **monoamine oxidase (MAO)**, the final metabolic product is VMA, which is excreted in urine. Thus, when a pheochromocytoma produces large quantities of epinephrine and norepinephrine, urinary excretion of VMA is increased.

A 24-hour urine sample is necessary because the tumor secretes its hormones in bursts, or pulses; a single spot-urine sample might "miss" large secretory bursts of the hormones.

4. All of Mrs. Ames' symptoms can be explained in terms of the actions of catecholamines on the various organ systems (Table 1–5). In the **heart**, catecholamines have three major effects, each mediated by a β_1 **receptor**: increased heart rate; increased contractility, or force of contraction; and increased conduction velocity through the atrioventricular node. In Mrs. Ames, excess amounts of catecholamines caused the sensation that her heart was racing (increased heart rate) and pounding (increased contractility). In **blood vessels**, primarily arterioles, catecholamines cause vasoconstriction in most vascular beds (e.g., cutaneous and splanchnic) through α_1 **receptors.** Vasoconstriction of cutaneous blood vessels leads to decreased cutaneous blood flow and cold skin, especially in the feet and hands. In blood vessels of skeletal muscle, however, catecholamines cause the opposite effect (vasodilation) through β_2 **receptors.** The effects on vision are explained by sympathetic effects on the **eye muscles.** In the radial muscle of the iris, catecholamines cause contraction (α_1 receptor); in the ciliary muscle, catecholamines cause dilation (β_2 receptor). The **gastrointestinal** effects of catecholamines include relaxation of the smooth muscle wall of the gastrointestinal tract (α_2 and β_2 receptors); contraction of the gastrointestinal sphincters (α_1 receptors); and increased production of saliva (β_1 receptors). The coordinated actions on the muscle wall and sphincters slow the motility of chyme through the gastrointestinal tract, and may lead to nausea and even vomiting.

TABLE 1–5 *Effect of the Autonomic Nervous System on Organ Systems*

Organ	Sympathetic Action	Sympathetic Receptor	Parasympathetic Action (receptors are muscarinic)
Heart	↑ Heart rate	β_1	↓ Heart rate
	↑ Contractility	β_1	↓ Contractility (atria)
	↑ AV node conduction	β_1	↓ AV node conduction
Vascular smooth muscle	Constricts blood vessels in skin; splanchnic	α_1	—
	Dilates blood vessels in skeletal muscle	β_2	—
Gastrointestinal tract	↓ Motility	α_2, β_2	↑ Motility
	Constricts sphincters	α_1	Relaxes sphincters
Bronchioles	Dilates bronchiolar smooth muscle	β_2	Constricts bronchiolar smooth muscle
Male sex organs	Ejaculation	α	Erection
Bladder	Relaxes bladder wall	β_2	Contracts bladder wall
	Constricts sphincter	α_1	Relaxes sphincter
Sweat glands	↑ Sweating	Muscarinic (sympathetic cholinergic)	—
Kidney	↑ renin secretion	β_1	—
Fat cells	↑ lipolysis	β_1	—

AV, atrioventricular. (Reprinted, with permission, from Costanzo LS. *BRS Physiology*. 4th ed. Baltimore: Lippincott Williams & Wilkins; 2007:37.)

5. Mrs. Ames' blood pressure was reported as 200/110. (Normal blood pressure is 120/80.) The two numbers refer, respectively, to systolic arterial pressure and diastolic arterial pressure. Arterial pressure is not expressed as a single value because systemic arterial pressure changes over the course of the cardiac cycle. **Systolic pressure** is the highest value for arterial pressure and is measured just after blood is ejected from the left ventricle into the large arteries (i.e., systole). **Diastolic pressure** is the lowest value for arterial pressure and is measured when the ventricle is relaxed and blood is flowing from the arteries to the veins and back to the heart (i.e., diastole).

In Mrs. Ames' case, both systolic and diastolic pressures were significantly elevated. These elevations are explained by the effects of excess catecholamines on the heart and blood vessels that have already been discussed. Catecholamines increase both heart rate and contractility. These two effects combine to produce an increase in cardiac output (the volume of blood ejected from the ventricle per minute). An increase in cardiac output means that, during systole, a greater blood volume is ejected into the arteries. This increase in arterial volume is reflected in a higher systolic pressure. In addition, catecholamines cause constriction of arterioles in many vascular beds. This constriction has the effect of "holding" more blood on the arterial side of the circulation, which increases both systolic and diastolic pressures.

The preceding explanation of the effects of catecholamines on the heart and blood vessels may be somewhat misleading because it suggests that these effects are entirely independent. They are not independent, but interact as follows. As described earlier, the vasoconstrictor effect of catecholamines in several vascular beds causes an increase in **total peripheral resistance (TPR)**, which increases systemic arterial pressure. Systemic arterial pressure is the **afterload** of the left ventricle (i.e., the pressure against which the left ventricle must eject blood). An increase in systemic arterial pressure, or afterload, means that the left ventricle must work harder to eject blood. As a result, the effects of catecholamines to increase cardiac output are partially, or even completely, offset by the increase in afterload.

6. As already discussed, Mrs. Ames' hands and feet were cold because catecholamines cause arteriolar vasoconstriction in the cutaneous circulation. However, why would she *feel* hot? The answer lies in the role of the cutaneous circulation in dissipating the heat generated by metabolism. Normally, heat is removed from the body through responses directed by the hypothalamus. These responses include *decreased* sympathetic outflow to the cutaneous blood vessels, resulting in vasodilation. Warm blood from the body core is shunted to the skin surface, where heat is then dissipated by convection and radiation. When a pheochromocytoma is present, the large quantities of circulating catecholamines cancel or override this cutaneous vasodilatory response. As a result, the body retains heat from metabolism that should have been dissipated.

7. **Phenoxybenzamine, an α_1-adrenergic antagonist,** inhibits all effects of catecholamines that are mediated through α_1 receptors. These effects include vasoconstriction of cutaneous and splanchnic blood vessels; contraction of the sphincters of the gastrointestinal tract; and contraction of the radial muscle of the iris. As discussed earlier, one of the major reasons that Mrs. Ames' systolic and diastolic blood pressures were so high was that excess catecholamines caused vasoconstriction of arterioles (increased TPR). When this vasoconstriction was blocked by an α_1-adrenergic antagonist, TPR was decreased, and both diastolic and systolic blood pressures were decreased.

8. Once treatment with the α_1-adrenergic antagonist was established, low doses of **propranolol, a β-adrenergic antagonist,** could be safely administered to reduce blood pressure further. The drugs were intentionally given in this sequence because of the effects of high levels of catecholamines on the heart and blood vessels. Recall that constriction of arterioles by catecholamines increases arterial pressure (afterload). One effect of this increased afterload is that it is more difficult for the left ventricle to eject blood. Thus, increased afterload offsets the other effects of catecholamines to increase cardiac output.

Once Mrs. Ames' afterload was reduced by the α_1-adrenergic antagonist, the work of the left ventricle was reduced, and it was easier for the ventricle to eject blood. At this point, the effects of excess catecholamines to increase cardiac output (through increased heart rate and contractility) would have become evident. In other words, Mrs. Ames' blood pressure may have remained elevated, even in the presence of an α_1-adrenergic antagonist. Addition of propranolol, a β-adrenergic antagonist, blocked the effects of excess catecholamines on heart rate and contractility and further reduced her blood pressure.

9. It would have been dangerous to give Mrs. Ames a β-adrenergic antagonist (e.g., propranolol) without also giving her an α_1-adrenergic antagonist. As we have already discussed, excess circulating catecholamines caused vasoconstriction of her arterioles and increased her arterial pressure (afterload). Increased afterload made it more difficult for the ventricles to eject blood. The action of catecholamines to increase contractility through cardiac β_1 receptors partially offset this difficulty. If Mrs. Ames' cardiac β_1 receptors had been blocked by propranolol (without the assistance of phenoxybenzamine to lower TPR and afterload), her heart might not have been able to eject enough blood to serve the metabolic needs of her tissues (cardiac failure).

Key topics

Adrenal medulla

Afterload

Catechol-*O*-methyltransferase (COMT)

Chromaffin cells

Diastolic pressure

Epinephrine

3-methoxy-4-hydroxymandelic acid (VMA)

Monoamine oxidase (MAO)

Norepinephrine

Phenoxybenzamine

Pheochromocytoma

Propranolol

α_1-adrenergic antagonist

β-adrenergic antasgonist

α_1 receptors

α_2 receptors

β_1 receptors

β_2 receptors

Systolic pressure

Total peripheral resistance (TPR)

Case 9

Shy–Drager Syndrome: Central Autonomic Failure

Ben Garcia was a 54-year-old executive with a large, thriving investment company. He was well regarded among his clients as the consummate professional. He and his wife of 32 years had two children, both of whom were college graduates. Life was great until Mr. Garcia found, to his embarrassment, that he was occasionally impotent. His wife teased him gently about "getting old." However, his impotence rapidly progressed from "occasional" to "frequent" to "every time." Additionally, Mr. Garcia was experiencing urinary problems. He felt enormous urgency to urinate, but had difficulty producing a urinary stream. His embarrassment (because of the nature of his symptoms), combined with his busy schedule, kept him from seeking medical attention. It wasn't until he arose from bed one morning and fainted that he made an appointment with his physician. By the time he saw his physician, he had been feeling dizzy every morning for a month and had an array of symptoms that convinced him that something was terribly wrong. In addition to impotence, urinary difficulties, and dizziness when he stood up, he had double vision, indigestion, diarrhea, and heat intolerance.

Mr. Garcia was referred to a neurologist who, based on the global nature of his symptoms and the results of a specific ocular test, diagnosed him as having Shy–Drager syndrome, a rare, progressive disease of the central autonomic nervous system. Shy–Drager syndrome is associated with degeneration of preganglionic neurons of the intermediolateral cell column of the spinal cord, autonomic ganglia in the periphery, and autonomic centers in the hypothalamus. As a result, both the sympathetic and parasympathetic divisions of the autonomic nervous system are profoundly impaired.

As part of his treatment, Mr. Garcia was instructed to elevate his head during sleep and to wear support stockings to prevent blood from pooling in his veins. He also took an aldosterone analogue to increase his blood volume. Each of these measures was an attempt to ameliorate the dizziness and fainting that he experienced when he stood up. Mr. Garcia and his family understood that the treatments were palliative and that there was no cure for his degenerative disease. He died at home at 58 years of age, 4 years after the onset of his symptoms.

 QUESTIONS

1. Which organ systems or bodily functions would you expect to be adversely affected by degeneration of the central autonomic nervous system?

2. As experienced by Mr. Garcia, often the earliest symptom of Shy–Drager syndrome is impotence. Describe the normal autonomic control of male sexual response, and explain why it is impaired in patients who have central autonomic failure.

3. Describe the autonomic control of micturition, including the functions of the detrusor muscle and the sphincters of the bladder. Why did Mr. Garcia experience urinary urgency, but was then unable to void normally?

4. Why was Mr. Garcia heat-intolerant?

5. The ocular test involved instilling methacholine (a cholinergic muscarinic agonist) into the conjunctival sac. In Mr. Garcia, methacholine caused exaggerated miosis (constriction of the pupil caused by contraction of the circular muscle of the iris). Is there a plausible explanation for why his response to methacholine was greater than that of a healthy person?

6. The hallmark of Shy–Drager syndrome is orthostatic hypotension (a decrease in blood pressure that occurs when a person stands up). When a healthy person stands up, orthostatic hypotension does not occur because autonomic reflexes operate to maintain a constant arterial pressure. What are the reflex responses that prevent orthostatic hypotension in healthy individuals, and why were these responses impaired in Mr. Garcia?

7. Support stockings prevent blood from pooling in the leg veins. How would these stockings have been helpful in alleviating Mr. Garcia's orthostatic hypotension?

8. Aldosterone and its analogues produce an increase in extracellular fluid volume. How did the aldosterone analogue help to alleviate Mr. Garcia's orthostatic hypotension?

9. Name three classes of drugs that would have been *absolutely contraindicated* in Mr. Garcia's case.

ANSWERS AND EXPLANATIONS

1. The **autonomic nervous system** controls the function of virtually every organ system and every bodily function, usually as a result of an interplay between the sympathetic and parasympathetic divisions. (See Table 1–5 in Case 8 to review autonomic control of organ system functions.) Central failure of the autonomic nervous system, as seen in Shy–Drager syndrome, would be predicted to adversely affect every organ system. This failure affects control of arterial blood pressure; function of the bronchioles, which regulate the flow of air into the lungs; motility, secretion, digestive, and absorptive functions of the gastrointestinal tract; filling and emptying of the bladder; male sexual response, including erection and ejaculation; function of the eye muscles that control near and far vision; activity of the sweat glands involved in thermoregulation; and metabolic functions of the liver and adipose tissue. It is difficult to imagine a more comprehensive list of bodily functions, and it is easy to appreciate why Mr. Garcia was so sick.

2. The male sexual response consists of erection and ejaculation. **Erection** is under parasympathetic control (**muscarinic receptors**), which causes the venous sinuses of the corpus cavernosa to fill with blood and the penis to become erect. **Ejaculation** is under sympathetic control (a receptors), which causes the ischiocavernosa and bulbocavernosa muscles to contract.

3. The detrusor muscle of the bladder wall is composed of smooth muscle that has both sympathetic (β_2 receptors) and parasympathetic (muscarinic receptors) innervation. The internal sphincter of the bladder is also composed of smooth muscle, with both sympathetic (a_1 receptors) and parasympathetic (muscarinic receptors) innervation. The external sphincter is skeletal muscle, which is under trained voluntary control.

   Normal bladder function has two phases: filling and emptying (micturition). When the **bladder is filling** with urine, **sympathetic** control dominates. The detrusor muscle relaxes (sympathetic β_2 receptors), and the internal sphincter contracts (sympathetic α_1 receptors). When the bladder is full, mechanoreceptors in the wall sense the fullness and relay this information to the spinal cord and then to the brainstem, where the micturition reflex is coordinated. During **micturition**, or emptying, **parasympathetic** control dominates. The detrusor muscle contracts (parasympathetic muscarinic receptors), and the internal sphincter relaxes (parasympathetic muscarinic receptors), allowing the bladder to empty.

   In Mr. Garcia, both sympathetic control (filling) and parasympathetic control (emptying) of the bladder were impaired. Because of the loss of sympathetic control, his bladder did not fill normally, and he felt urinary urgency when his bladder contained a small amount of urine. Because of the loss of parasympathetic control, his bladder could not contract forcefully enough to produce a normal urinary stream.

4. **Thermoregulatory sweat glands** are controlled by the sympathetic nervous system. This sympathetic innervation is unusual in that postganglionic neurons innervating the sweat glands release acetylcholine (i.e., they are sympathetic *cholinergic* fibers). (In contrast, most sympathetic postganglionic neurons release norepinephrine—that is, they are sympathetic *adrenergic* fibers). In keeping with this unusual feature, the receptors on sweat glands are the *cholinergic* muscarinic type. As the name suggests, thermoregulatory sweating is important for dissipation of the heat generated by metabolism, especially when the ambient temperature is high. Loss of sympathetic innervation in Shy–Drager syndrome led to impairment of thermoregulatory sweating and caused heat intolerance.

5. The ocular test involved instilling a cholinergic muscarinic agonist into the eye. In healthy persons, the cholinergic agonist methacholine produces **miosis** (constriction of the pupil) by causing the circular muscle of the iris to contract. In Mr. Garcia, the miosis response was exaggerated. Why would he have an *exaggerated* parasympathetic cholinergic response when his central parasympathetic nervous system was impaired? The answer involves the sensitivity of

cholinergic receptors on the circular muscle of the iris. Without normal parasympathetic innervation, the receptors are up-regulated (i.e., increased number of receptors), a condition called **denervation hypersensitivity.** Thus, when an exogenous cholinergic agonist (e.g., methacholine) was instilled in Mr. Garcia's eyes, it caused a larger than usual miosis response.

6. When a healthy person stands up suddenly, blood pools in the veins of the legs, and there is a transient decrease in arterial blood pressure. This decrease is only transient because it is detected and immediately corrected by reflexes involving the sympathetic and parasympathetic nervous systems **(baroreceptor reflex).** For this reflex to occur, information about blood pressure must be relayed from baroreceptors in the carotid sinus to specific brainstem centers. These brainstem centers orchestrate an increase in sympathetic outflow to the heart and blood vessels and a decrease in parasympathetic outflow to the heart (Fig. 1–14). The sympathetic and parasympathetic effects include an increase in heart rate and contractility, which combine to produce an increase in cardiac output; constriction of arterioles, with a resultant increase in total peripheral resistance; and venoconstriction, which increases venous return to the heart. These effects, in combination, restore arterial pressure to its normal set-point value. The responses occur so quickly that healthy persons are unaware of them, or may be briefly aware of an increase in heart rate.

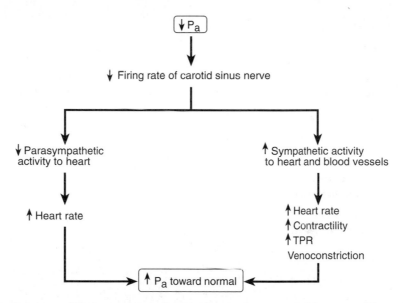

Figure 1–14   Responses of the baroreceptor reflex to a decrease in mean arterial pressure. (P_a, arterial pressure; TPR, total peripheral resistance.)

   In Mr. Garcia, the baroreceptor reflex was severely impaired because of central damage to the sympathetic and parasympathetic nervous systems. When he stood up, his arterial pressure fell **(orthostatic hypotension)** and could not be corrected by autonomic reflexes. He felt dizzy and fainted because the sustained decrease in arterial pressure caused a decrease in cerebral blood flow.

7. Support stockings constrict the veins in the legs and prevent the venous pooling of blood that initiates an orthostatic decrease in blood pressure.

8. **Aldosterone** (secreted by the adrenal cortex) and its analogues increase the reabsorption of Na^+ in the kidney and thereby increase both extracellular fluid volume and blood volume. Because most of the blood volume is contained in the veins, an increase in total blood volume leads to an increase in venous blood volume and venous return, which produces an increase in cardiac output and arterial pressure.

9. Mr. Garcia's disease involved loss of both sympathetic and parasympathetic control of his organ systems. Any drug that would further antagonize either sympathetic or parasympathetic activity (e.g., inhibition of autonomic receptors on the end organs) would have exacerbated his problems. Your list might include α-adrenergic receptor antagonists (e.g., phenoxybenzamine), β-adrenergic receptor antagonists (e.g., propranolol), muscarinic receptor antagonists (e.g., atropine), and nicotinic receptor antagonists (e.g., hexamethonium). (Recall that nicotinic receptors are present on postsynaptic neurons in both sympathetic and parasympathetic ganglia.)

Key topics

α-adrenergic receptors

β-adrenergic receptors

Aldosterone

Autonomic nervous system

Baroreceptor reflex

Denervation hypersensitivity

Ejaculation

Erection

Micturition

Miosis

Muscarinic receptors

Nicotinic receptors

Orthostatic hypotension

Parasympathetic nervous system

Regulation of arterial pressure

Sympathetic nervous system

Thermoregulatory sweat glands

Cardiovascular Physiology

Case 10

Essential Cardiovascular Calculations

This case is designed to take you through important basic calculations involving the cardiovascular system. Use the information provided in Table 2–1 to answer the questions. Part of the challenge in answering these questions will be in deciding which information you need in order to perform each calculation. Good luck!

TABLE 2–1	Cardiovascular Values for Case 10
Parameter	**Value**
Systolic pressure (aorta)	124 mm Hg
Diastolic pressure (aorta)	82 mm Hg
R-R interval	800 msec
Left ventricular end-diastolic volume	140 mL
Left ventricular end-systolic volume	70 mL
Mean pulmonary artery pressure	15 mm Hg
Right atrial pressure	2 mm Hg
Left atrial pressure	5 mm Hg
O_2 consumption (whole body)	250 mL/min
O_2 content of systemic arterial blood	0.20 mL O_2/mL blood
O_2 content of pulmonary arterial blood	0.152 mL O_2/mL blood

R-R interval, time between R-waves on the electrocardiogram.

 QUESTIONS

1. Mean arterial pressure is not the simple average of systolic and diastolic pressures. Why not? How is mean arterial pressure estimated? From the information given in Table 2–1, calculate the mean arterial pressure in this case.

2. Calculate the stroke volume, cardiac output, and ejection fraction of the left ventricle.

3. Calculate cardiac output using the Fick principle.

4. What is the definition of total peripheral resistance (TPR)? What equation describes the relationship between TPR, arterial pressure, and cardiac output? What is the value of TPR in this case?

5. How is pulmonary vascular resistance calculated? What is the value of pulmonary vascular resistance in this case? Compare the calculated values for pulmonary vascular resistance and TPR, and explain any difference in the two values.

6. What is total blood flow (in mL/min) through *all* of the pulmonary capillaries?

7. What is total blood flow (in mL/min) through *all* of the systemic arteries?

8. What information, in addition to that provided in Table 2–1, is needed to calculate the resistance of the renal vasculature?

9. If the diameter of the aorta is 20 mm, what is the velocity of aortic blood flow? Would you expect the velocity of blood flow in systemic capillaries to be higher, lower, or the same as the velocity of blood flow in the aorta?

ANSWERS ON NEXT PAGE

ANSWERS AND EXPLANATIONS

1. Systemic arterial pressure is not a single value because arterial pressure varies over the course of each cardiac cycle. Its highest value is **systolic pressure**, which is measured just after blood is ejected from the left ventricle into the aorta (i.e., systole). Its lowest value is **diastolic pressure**, which is measured as blood flows from the arteries into the veins and back to the heart (i.e., diastole).

Mean arterial pressure cannot be calculated as the simple average of systolic and diastolic pressures because averaging does not take into account the fact that a greater fraction of each cardiac cycle is spent in diastole (approximately two-thirds) than in systole (approximately one-third). Thus, *mean* arterial pressure is closer to diastolic pressure than to systolic pressure. Figure 2–1 shows an arterial pressure tracing over a single cardiac cycle. The difference between systolic pressure and diastolic pressure is called **pulse pressure.**

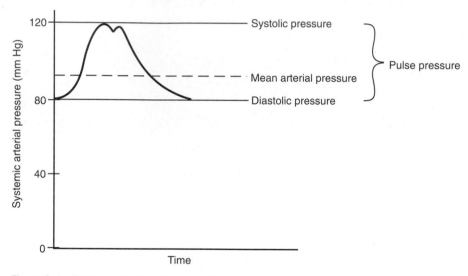

Figure 2–1 Systemic arterial pressure during the cardiac cycle.

Although this approach is impractical, mean arterial pressure can be determined by measuring the area under the arterial pressure curve. Alternatively, mean arterial pressure can be estimated as follows:

Mean arterial pressure = diastolic pressure + 1/3 pulse pressure

= diastolic pressure + 1/3 (systolic pressure – diastolic pressure)

where

Diastolic pressure = lowest value for arterial pressure in a cardiac cycle

Systolic pressure = highest value for arterial pressure in a cardiac cycle

Pulse pressure = systolic pressure – diastolic pressure

Therefore, in this case:

Mean arterial pressure = 82 mm Hg + 1/3 (124 mm Hg – 82 mm Hg)

= 82 mm Hg + 1/3 (42 mm Hg)

= 82 mm Hg + 14 mm Hg

= 96 mm

2. These calculations concern the cardiac output of the left ventricle. The basic relationships are as follows:

Stroke volume = end-diastolic volume – end-systolic volume

where

Stroke volume = volume ejected by the ventricle during systole (mL)

End-diastolic volume = volume in the ventricle before ejection (mL)

End-systolic volume = volume in the ventricle after ejection (mL)

Cardiac output = stroke volume × heart rate

where

Cardiac output = volume ejected by the ventricle per minute (mL/min)

Stroke volume = volume ejected by the ventricle (mL)

Heart rate = beats/min

Ejection fraction = stroke volume/end-diastolic volume

where

Ejection fraction = fraction of the end-diastolic volume ejected in one stroke

Now we can use these basic equations to calculate stroke volume, cardiac output, and ejection fraction in this case.

Stroke volume = left ventricular end-diastolic volume
– left ventricular end-systolic volume

= 140 mL – 70 mL

= 70 mL

Cardiac output is the volume ejected by the left ventricle per minute. It is calculated as the product of stroke volume (determined to be 70 mL) and heart rate. Heart rate is not given in Table 2–1, but it can be calculated from the **R-R interval.** "R" is the R-wave on the electrocardiogram and represents electrical activation of the ventricles. The R-R interval is the time elapsed from one R-wave to the next (Fig. 2–2). It is also called **cycle length** (i.e., time elapsed in one cardiac cycle).

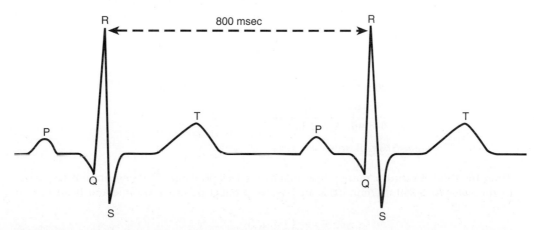

Figure 2–2 Electrocardiogram measured from lead II. The interval between R-waves is the cycle length.

Cycle length can be used to calculate heart rate as follows:

Heart rate = 1/cycle length

$$= 1/800 \text{ msec}$$
$$= 1/0.8 \text{ sec}$$
$$= 1.25 \text{ beats/sec}$$
$$= 75 \text{ beats/min}$$

Cardiac output = stroke volume × heart rate

$$= 70 \text{ mL} \times 75 \text{ beats/min}$$
$$= 5,250 \text{ mL/min}$$

Ejection fraction = stroke volume / end-diastolic volume

$$= 70 \text{ mL/140 mL}$$
$$= 0.5, \text{ or } 50\%$$

3. As shown in Question 2, we *calculate* cardiac output as the product of stroke volume and heart rate. However, we *measure* cardiac output by the **Fick principle of conservation of mass.** The Fick principle for measuring cardiac output employs two basic assumptions: (i) pulmonary blood flow (the cardiac output of the right ventricle) equals systemic blood flow (the cardiac output of the left ventricle) in the steady state, and (ii) the rate of O_2 utilization by the body is equal to the difference between the amount of O_2 leaving the lungs in pulmonary venous blood and the amount of O_2 returning to the lungs in pulmonary arterial blood. This relationship can be stated mathematically as follows:

$$O_2 \text{ consumption} = \text{cardiac output} \times [O_2]_{\text{pulmonary vein}} - \text{cardiac output} \times [O_2]_{\text{pulmonary artery}}$$

Rearranging to solve for cardiac output:

$$\textbf{Cardiac output } = \frac{\textbf{O}_2 \textbf{ consumption}}{[\textbf{O}_2]_{\textbf{pulmonary vein}} - [\textbf{O}_2]_{\textbf{pulmonary artery}}}$$

where

Cardiac output = cardiac output (mL/min)
O_2 consumption = O_2 consumption by the body (mL O_2/min)
$[O_2]_{\text{pulmonary vein}}$ = O_2 content of pulmonary venous blood (mL O_2/mL blood)
$[O_2]_{\text{pulmonary artery}}$ = O_2 content of pulmonary arterial blood (mL O_2/mL blood)

In this case, cardiac output can be calculated by substituting values from Table 2–1. To find the appropriate values in the table, recall that systemic arterial blood is equivalent to pulmonary venous blood.

$$\text{Cardiac output } = \frac{250 \text{ (mL/min)}}{0.20 \text{ mL } O_2/\text{mL blood} - 0.152 \text{ mL } O_2/\text{mL blood}}$$

$$= \frac{250 \text{ mL/min}}{0.048 \text{ mL } O_2/\text{mL blood}}$$

$$= 5208 \text{ mL/min}$$

Thus, the value for cardiac output measured by the Fick principle (5,208 mL/min) is very close to the value of 5,250 mL/min calculated as the product of stroke volume and heart rate in Question 2.

4. Total peripheral resistance (TPR) is the collective resistance to blood flow that is provided by all of the blood vessels on the *systemic* side of the circulation. These blood vessels include the aorta, large and small arteries, arterioles, capillaries, venules, veins, and vena cava. Most of this resistance resides in the **arterioles.**

The fundamental equation of the cardiovascular system relates blood flow, blood pressure, and resistance. The relationship is analogous to the one that relates current (I), voltage (V), and resistance (R) in electrical circuits as expressed by the **Ohm's law** ($I = \Delta V/R$). Blood flow is analogous to current flow, blood pressure is analogous to voltage, and hemodynamic resistance is analogous to electrical resistance. Thus, the equation for blood flow is:

$$Q = \Delta P/R$$

or, rearranging and solving for R,

$$R = \Delta P/Q$$

where

Q = blood flow (mL/min)
ΔP = pressure difference (mm Hg)
R = resistance (mm Hg/mL per min)

Therefore, to calculate *total* peripheral resistance (TPR), it is necessary to know the *total* blood flow through the systemic circulation (i.e., cardiac output of the left ventricle) and the pressure difference across the *entire* systemic circulation. In solving this problem, it may be helpful to visualize the organization and circuitry of the cardiovascular system (Fig. 2–3).

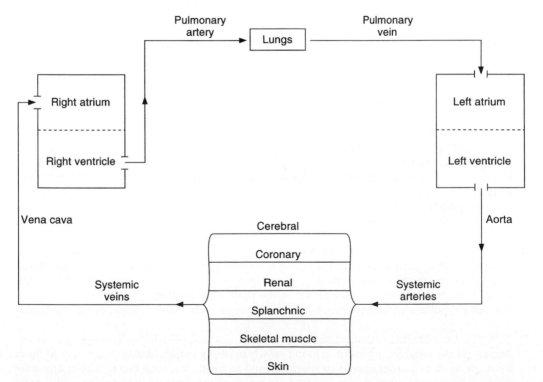

Figure 2–3 Circuitry of the cardiovascular system. (Reprinted, with permission, from Costanzo LS. *BRS Physiology.* 4th ed. Baltimore: Lippincott Williams & Wilkins; 2007:69.)

Cardiac output was calculated by different methods in Questions 2 and 3 as 5,250 mL/min and 5,208 mL/min, respectively. These values are similar, and we can (arbitrarily) take the average value (5,229 mL/min) to represent cardiac output. The pressure difference across the systemic circulation (ΔP) is the difference in pressure at the inflow and outflow points. Inflow pressure is aortic pressure, and outflow pressure is right atrial pressure. In Question 1, mean aortic pressure was calculated as 96 mm Hg. Right atrial pressure is given in Table 2–1 as 2 mm Hg. Thus, ΔP across the systemic circulation is 96 mm Hg – 2 mm Hg, or 94 mm Hg. Resistance (R), which represents TPR, is:

$$R = \Delta P/Q$$

or

TPR = (mean arterial pressure – right atrial pressure)/cardiac output
    = (96 mm Hg – 2 mm Hg)/5,229 mL/min
    = 94 mm Hg/5,229 mL/min
    = 0.018 mm Hg/mL per min

5. Pulmonary vascular resistance is calculated in the same way that TPR was calculated in Question 4. We need to know the values for pulmonary blood flow (cardiac output of the right ventricle) and the pressure difference across the pulmonary circulation. To determine pulmonary blood flow, it is necessary to understand that the left and right sides of the heart operate in series (i.e., blood flows sequentially from the left heart to the right heart and back to the left heart). Thus, in the steady state, the cardiac output of the right ventricle (pulmonary blood flow) equals the cardiac output of the left ventricle, or 5,229 mL/min. The pressure difference across the pulmonary circulation is inflow pressure minus outflow pressure. The inflow pressure is mean pulmonary artery pressure (15 mm Hg), and the outflow pressure is left atrial pressure (5 mm Hg). Thus, **pulmonary vascular resistance** is:

R = ΔP/Q
  = (mean pulmonary artery pressure – left atrial pressure) / cardiac output
  = (15 mm Hg – 5 mm Hg) / 5,229 mL/min
  = 10 mm Hg / 5,229 mL/min
  = 0.0019 mm Hg/mL per min

Although pulmonary blood flow is equal to systemic blood flow, pulmonary vascular resistance is only one-tenth the value of systemic vascular resistances. How is this possible? Since pulmonary resistance is lower than systemic resistance, shouldn't pulmonary blood flow be higher than systemic blood flow? No, because pulmonary pressures are also much lower than systemic pressures. Thus, pulmonary blood flow can be exactly equal to systemic blood flow because pulmonary vascular resistance and pressures are proportionately lower than systemic vascular resistance and pressures.

6. Because of the serial arrangement of blood vessels within the lungs (i.e., blood flows from the pulmonary artery to smaller arteries to arterioles to capillaries to veins), the total blood flow at any level of the pulmonary vasculature (e.g., at the level of all of the pulmonary capillaries) is the same. Thus, total blood flow through *all* of the pulmonary capillaries equals total blood flow through the pulmonary artery, which is the cardiac output of the right ventricle, or 5,229 mL/min.

7. This question addresses the same issue as Question 6, but as applied to the systemic circulation. Because of the serial arrangement of blood vessels in the systemic circulation (i.e., blood flows from the aorta to smaller arteries to arterioles, and so forth), the total blood flow at any level of the systemic vasculature (e.g., at the level of all of the arteries) is the same. Thus, total blood flow through *all* of the systemic arteries equals the cardiac output of the left ventricle, or 5,229 mL/min.

8. The principles that were used to determine TPR (or to determine pulmonary vascular resistance) can also be used to calculate the vascular resistance of individual organs (e.g., kidney). Recall how the **pressure, flow, resistance relationship** was rearranged to solve for resistance: $R = \Delta P/Q$. R can also represent the resistance of the blood vessels in an individual organ (e.g., kidney), ΔP can represent the pressure difference across the organ's vasculature (e.g., for the kidney, the pressure in the renal artery minus the pressure in the renal vein), and Q can represent the organ's blood flow (e.g., renal blood flow).

Actually, none of the exact information needed to calculate renal vascular resistance is available in Table 2–1 or from the previous calculations. Renal arterial pressure is close, but not exactly equal, to mean arterial pressure that was calculated for the aorta in Question 1. The mean pressure in large "downstream" arteries is slightly lower than the pressure in the aorta. (It must be lower in order for blood to flow in the right direction, that is, from the aorta to the distal arteries.) Like the pressure in any large vein, renal venous pressure must be slightly higher than right atrial pressure. Because of the parallel arrangement of arteries off the aorta, renal blood flow is only a fraction of total systemic blood flow.

9. The **velocity of blood flow** is the rate of linear displacement of blood per unit time:

$$v = Q/A$$

where

v = linear velocity of blood (cm/min)
Q = blood flow (mL/min)
A = cross-sectional area of a blood vessel (cm^2)

In words, velocity is proportional to blood flow and is inversely proportional to the cross-sectional area of the blood vessel. Blood flow through the aorta is total systemic blood flow, or cardiac output, which is 5,229 mL/min. The cross-sectional area can be calculated from the diameter of the aorta, which is 20 mm (radius, 10 mm).

$$v = \frac{Q}{\pi r^2}$$

$$= \frac{5229 \text{ mL/min}}{3.14 \times (10 \text{ mm})^2}$$

$$= \frac{5229 \text{ mL/min}}{3.14 \times 1 \text{ cm}^2}$$

$$= \frac{5229 \text{ cm}^3/\text{min}}{3.14 \text{ cm}^2}$$

$$= 1665 \text{ cm/min}$$

Based on the inverse relationship between velocity and radius of blood vessels, the velocity of blood flow should be lower in *all* of the capillaries than in the aorta. (Of course, a single capillary has a smaller radius than the aorta, but *all* of the capillaries have a larger collective radius and cross-sectional area than the aorta.)

Key topics

Cardiac output

Cycle length

Diastolic pressure

Ejection fraction

Electrocardiogram (ECG)

Fick principle of conservation of mass

Heart rate

Mean arterial pressure

Ohm's law

Pressure, blood flow, resistance relationship

Pulmonary vascular resistance

Pulse pressure

R-R interval

Stroke volume

Systolic pressure

Total peripheral resistance (TPR) or systemic vascular resistance

Velocity of blood flow

Case 11

Ventricular Pressure–Volume Loops

Figure 2–4 shows a pressure–volume loop for the left ventricle. This loop shows the relationship between left ventricular pressure (in mm Hg) and left ventricular volume (in mL) over a single cardiac cycle. Use Figure 2–4 to answer the following questions.

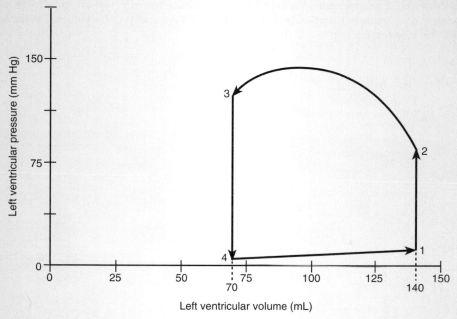

Figure 2–4 Left ventricular pressure–volume loop. (Adapted, with permission, from Costanzo LS. *BRS Physiology.* 4th ed. Baltimore: Lippincott Williams & Wilkins; 2007:82.)

 QUESTIONS

1. Describe the events that occur in the four segments between numbered points on the pressure–volume loop (e.g., 1 → 2, 2 → 3). Correlate each segment with events in the cardiac cycle.

2. According to Figure 2–4, what is the value for left ventricular end-diastolic volume? What is the value for end-systolic volume?

3. What is the approximate value for stroke volume? What is the approximate value for ejection fraction?

4. Which portion, or portions, of the pressure–volume loop correspond to diastole? To systole?

5. Which portions of the pressure–volume loop are isovolumetric?

6. At which numbered point does the aortic valve open? At which numbered point does the aortic valve close? At which numbered point does the mitral valve open?

7. At which numbered point, or during which segment, would the first heart sound be heard?

8. At which numbered point, or during which segment, would the second heart sound be heard?

9. Superimpose a new pressure–volume loop to illustrate the effect of an increase in left ventricular end-diastolic volume (i.e., increased preload). What is the effect on stroke volume?

10. Superimpose a new pressure–volume loop to illustrate the effect of an increase in contractility. What is the effect on end-systolic volume? What is the effect on ejection fraction?

11. Superimpose a new pressure–volume loop to illustrate the effect of an increase in aortic pressure (i.e., increased afterload). What is the effect on end-systolic volume? What is the effect on ejection fraction?

ANSWERS ON NEXT PAGE

ANSWERS AND EXPLANATIONS

1. Figure 2–4 shows a single left ventricular cycle of contraction, ejection of blood, relaxation, and filling (to begin another cycle). This figure can be used to describe the events as follows. **1 → 2 is isovolumetric contraction.** During this phase, the ventricle (which was previously filled from the atrium) is contracting. Contraction causes a steep increase in ventricular pressure. However, because the aortic valve is closed, no blood is ejected and left ventricular volume remains constant (i.e., is isovolumetric). **2 → 3 is ventricular ejection.** The ventricle is still contracting, causing ventricular pressure to increase further. The aortic valve is now open, and blood is ejected from the left ventricle, which causes ventricular volume to decrease. **3 → 4 is isovolumetric relaxation.** The left ventricle relaxes, and ventricular pressure decreases. Both the aortic and the mitral valves are closed, and ventricular volume remains constant. **4 → 1 is ventricular filling.** The left ventricle is still relaxed, but now the mitral valve is open and the ventricle is filling with blood from the atrium. Because the ventricle is relaxed, the increase in ventricular volume causes only a small increase in ventricular pressure.

2. **End-diastolic volume** is the volume present in the ventricle after filling is complete, but before any blood is ejected into the aorta. Therefore, end-diastolic volume is present at points 1 and 2 (approximately 140 mL). **End-systolic volume** is the volume that remains in the left ventricle after ejection is complete, but before the ventricle fills again (i.e., the volume at points 3 and 4, which is approximately 70 mL).

3. **Stroke volume** is the volume ejected during systole (ventricular ejection). Thus, stroke volume is represented by the *width of the pressure–volume loop*, or approximately 70 mL (140 mL – 70 mL). **Ejection fraction** is stroke volume expressed as a fraction of end-diastolic volume (i.e., stroke volume/end-diastolic volume), or 70 mL/140 mL, or 0.5 (50%).

4. **Diastole** is the portion of the **cardiac cycle** when the ventricle is relaxed (i.e., is not contracting). Diastole corresponds to segments 3 → 4 (isovolumetric relaxation) and 4 → 1 (ventricular filling). **Systole** is the portion of the cardiac cycle when the ventricle is contracting. Thus, systole corresponds to segments 1 → 2 (isovolumetric contraction) and 2 → 3 (ventricular ejection).

5. By definition, **isovolumetric** portions of the ventricular cycle are those in which ventricular volume is constant (i.e., the ventricle is neither filling with blood nor ejecting blood). Isovolumetric segments are 1 → 2 and 3 → 4.

6. The **aortic valve** opens at point 2, when ventricular pressure exceeds aortic pressure. Opening of the aortic valve is followed immediately by ejection of blood and a decrease in ventricular volume. The aortic valve closes at point 3, and ejection of blood ceases. The **mitral valve** (the atrioventricular valve of the left heart) opens at point 4, and ventricular filling begins.

7. The **first heart sound** corresponds to closure of the **atrioventricular valves.** This closure occurs at the end of ventricular filling, at the beginning of isovolumetric contraction. Thus, the first heart sound occurs at point 1.

8. The **second heart** sound corresponds to closure of the aortic valve, at point 3.

9. End-diastolic volume **(preload)** is the volume of blood contained in the ventricle just before contraction. Therefore, an increase in ventricular end-diastolic volume (e.g., produced by an infusion of saline) means the ventricle has filled to a greater volume during diastole. In Figure 2–5, point 1 shifts to the right to represent the increased end-diastolic volume. The **Frank–Starling relationship** for the ventricle states that the greater the end-diastolic volume, the greater the stroke volume. Therefore, without any change in contractility, an increase in end-diastolic volume causes an increase in stroke volume, as evidenced by increased width of the pressure–volume loop.

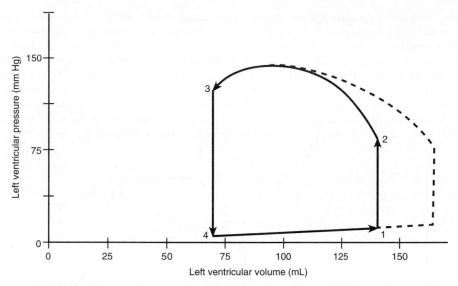

Figure 2–5   Effect of an increase in preload on the left ventricular pressure–volume loop. (Adapted, with permission, from Costanzo LS. *BRS Physiology.* 4th ed. Baltimore: Lippincott Williams & Wilkins; 2007:83.)

10. **Contractility (inotropy)** is the intrinsic ability of myocardial fibers to develop tension at a given muscle length (i.e., at a given end-diastolic volume). Contractility is directly correlated with the **intracellular Ca^{2+} concentration,** which dictates how many cross-bridges cycle and, therefore, how much tension is generated. When contractility is increased (e.g., by positive inotropic agents, such as norepinephrine or digitalis), the ventricle can develop greater tension and pressure during systole. As a result, stroke volume increases (Fig. 2–6), less blood remains in the ventricle after ejection, and, therefore, end-systolic volume decreases. Because ejection fraction is stroke volume expressed as a fraction of end-diastolic volume, if stroke volume increases and end-diastolic volume is unchanged, ejection fraction must have increased.

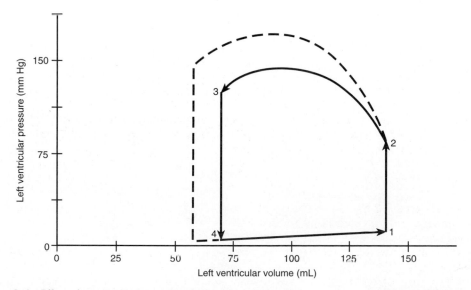

Figure 2–6   Effect of an increase in contractility on the left ventricular pressure–volume loop. (Adapted, with permission, from Costanzo LS. *BRS Physiology.* 4th ed. Baltimore: Lippincott Williams & Wilkins; 2007:83.)

11. **Afterload** is the pressure against which the ventricles must eject blood. Afterload of the left ventricle is aortic pressure. To open the aortic valve and eject blood, left ventricular pressure must increase to a level greater than aortic pressure. Thus, if afterload increases, the left ventricle must work harder than usual to overcome this higher pressure. Figure 2–7 shows the consequences of an increase in afterload. During isovolumetric contraction (1 → 2) and ventricular ejection (2 → 3), ventricular pressure increases to a higher level than normal. Because of the increased afterload, stroke volume is compromised, more blood remains in the left ventricle after ejection, and end-systolic volume is increased. Because stroke volume decreases and end-diastolic volume is unchanged, ejection fraction must have decreased.

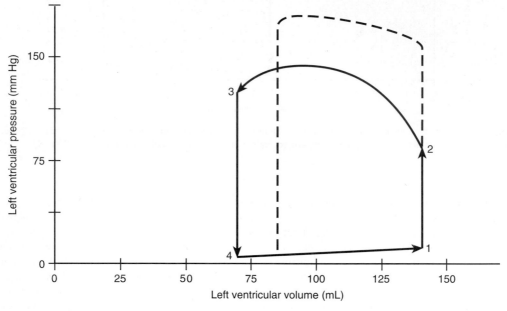

Figure 2–7 Effect of an increase in afterload on the left ventricular pressure–volume loop. (Adapted, with permission, from Costanzo LS. *BRS Physiology.* 4th ed. Baltimore: Lippincott Williams & Wilkins; 2007:83.)

Key topics

Afterload

Aortic valve

Atrioventricular valves

Cardiac cycle

Contractility (inotrophy)

Diastole

Ejection fraction

End-diastolic volume

End-systolic volume

Frank-Starling relationship

Heart sounds

Mitral valve

Preload

Stroke volume

Systole

Ventricular pressure–volume loops

Case 12

Responses to Changes in Posture

Joslin Chambers is a 27-year-old assistant manager at a discount department store. One morning, she awakened from a deep sleep and realized that she was more than an hour late for work. She panicked, momentarily regretting her late-night socializing, and then jumped out of bed. Briefly, she felt light-headed and thought she might faint. She had the sensation that her heart was "racing." Had she not been so late for work, she would have returned to bed. As she walked toward the bathroom, she noticed that her light-headedness dissipated. The rest of her day was uneventful.

 QUESTIONS

1. When Joslin moved rapidly from a supine (lying) position to a standing position, there was a brief, initial decrease in arterial pressure that caused her light-headedness. Describe the sequence of events that produced this transient fall in arterial pressure.

2. Why did the decrease in arterial pressure cause Joslin to feel light-headed?

3. Joslin's light-headedness was only transient because a reflex was initiated that rapidly restored arterial pressure to normal. Describe the specific effects of this reflex on heart rate, myocardial contractility, total peripheral resistance (TPR), and capacitance of the veins. What receptors are involved in each of these responses?

4. How does each component of the reflex (e.g., the effect on heart rate) help to restore arterial pressure? (Hint: It may help to write the equation that relates arterial pressure, cardiac output, and TPR.)

5. In addition to the reflex correction of blood pressure, the fact that Joslin walked to the bathroom helped return her arterial pressure to normal. How did walking help?

ANSWERS ON NEXT PAGE

ANSWERS AND EXPLANATIONS

1. **Orthostatic hypotension** is the phenomenon whereby arterial pressure decreases when one stands up. When a person suddenly moves from a supine (lying) position to a standing position, blood pools in the veins of the legs. (Because the capacitance, or compliance, of the veins is high, they can hold large volumes of blood.) This pooling decreases venous return to the heart, which decreases cardiac output by the **Frank–Starling mechanism.** (The Frank–Starling mechanism describes the relationship between venous return and cardiac output. Increases in venous return lead to increases in end-diastolic volume. Up to a point, increases in end-diastolic volume lead to increases in cardiac output. Conversely, decreases in venous return lead to decreases in cardiac output.) Because arterial pressure is affected by the volume of blood in the arteries, a decrease in cardiac output (i.e., less blood is pumped into the arterial system) causes a decrease in arterial pressure.

2. When Joslin stood up quickly, she felt light-headed because a brief period of cerebral ischemia occurred as a result of the decrease in arterial pressure. The autoregulatory range for cerebral blood flow is 60 to 140 mm Hg. In other words, **cerebral blood flow** is maintained constant as long as arterial pressure is greater than 60 mm Hg and less than 140 mm Hg. When Joslin stood up, her arterial pressure briefly decreased below this critical autoregulatory range. As a result, cerebral blood flow decreased, and she felt light-headed.

3. **Baroreceptors located in the carotid sinus** and the aortic arch sensed the decrease in arterial pressure. The **baroreceptor reflex** then orchestrated a series of compensatory responses, including increased sympathetic outflow to the heart and blood vessels. There are four consequences of this increased sympathetic outflow:

   • Increased heart rate (the sensation of a racing heart), a **positive chronotropic effect** mediated by β_1-**adrenergic receptors** in the sinoatrial node.

   • Increased **contractility** of the ventricles, a **positive inotropic effect** mediated by β_1-**adrenergic receptors** in the ventricular muscle.

   • Increased **arteriolar constriction**, mediated by α_1-**adrenergic receptors** on vascular smooth muscle of the arterioles.

   • Increased **venoconstriction**, mediated by α_1-**adrenergic receptors** on vascular smooth muscle of the veins.

4. All of the components of the baroreceptor reflex contributed to the restoration of Joslin's arterial pressure (Fig. 2–8).

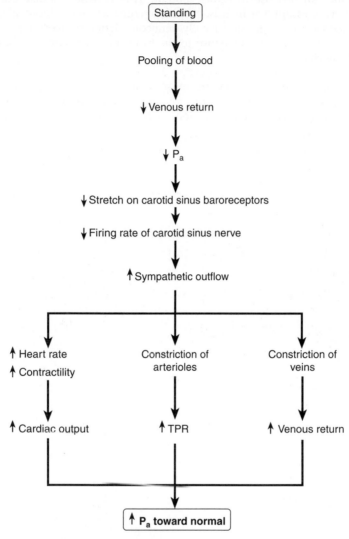

Figure 2–8 Cardiovascular responses in a person moving suddenly from a supine to a standing position. (P_a, arterial pressure; TPR, total peripheral resistance.)

These contributions can be appreciated by reviewing the relationship between arterial pressure, cardiac output, and TPR:

P_a = cardiac output × TPR

where

$$P_a = \text{mean arterial pressure}$$
$$\text{Cardiac output} = \text{volume of blood ejected from the left ventricle/min}$$
$$\text{TPR} = \text{total peripheral resistance}$$

In words, arterial pressure depends on the volume of blood pumped into the arteries from the left ventricle and the resistance of the arterioles. (It may be helpful to think of arteriolar resistance as "holding" blood on the arterial side of the circulation.)

Now, using the equation, consider how each portion of the baroreceptor reflex helped to restore Joslin's arterial pressure back to normal. The increased heart rate and contractility combined to produce an increase in cardiac output. The increased cardiac output caused an increase in arterial pressure. The increased arteriolar constriction produced an increase in TPR, which also increased arterial pressure. Finally, venoconstriction led to decreased capacitance of the veins, which increased venous return to the heart and increased cardiac output (by the Frank–Starling mechanism).

5. As Joslin walked toward the bathroom, the muscular activity compressed the veins in her legs and decreased venous capacitance (i.e., the volume of blood the veins can hold). This effect, combined with sympathetic venoconstriction, increased venous return to the heart and cardiac output.

Key topics

Arterial blood pressure (P_a)

Arteriolor constriction

Autoregulation

Baroreceptor reflex

Carotid sinus baroreceptors

Cardiac output

Cerebral blood flow

Chronotropic effects

Contractility

Frank–Starling mechanism

Inotropic effects

Orthostatic hypotension

Pressure, blood flow, resistance relationship

α or α_1 receptors

β or β_1 receptors

Sympathetic nervous system

Venoconstriction

Case 13

Cardiovascular Responses to Exercise

Cassandra Farias is a 34-year-old dietician at an academic medical center. She believes in the importance of a healthy lifestyle and was intrigued when the division of cardiology recruited healthy female volunteers for a study on the cardiovascular responses to exercise. Cassandra met the study criteria (i.e., 25–40 years old, no medications, normal weight for height, normal blood pressure), and she was selected for participation.

Control measurements were taken of Cassandra's blood pressure, heart rate, and arterial and venous P_{O_2}; her stroke volume was estimated. Cassandra then walked on the treadmill for 30 minutes at 3 miles per hour. Her blood pressure and heart rate were monitored continuously, and her arterial and venous P_{O_2} were measured at the end of the exercise period (Table 2–2).

TABLE 2–2	Cassandra's Cardiovascular Responses to Exercise	
Parameter	Control (Pre-exercise)	Exercise
Systolic blood pressure	110 mm Hg	145 mm Hg
Diastolic blood pressure	70 mm Hg	60 mm Hg
Heart rate	75 beats/min	130 beats/min
Stroke volume (estimated)	80 mL	110 mL
Arterial P_{O_2}	100 mm Hg	100 mm Hg
Venous P_{O_2}	40 mm Hg	25 mm Hg

 QUESTIONS

1. To set the stage for the following questions, describe the cardiovascular responses to moderate exercise, including the roles of the autonomic nervous system and local control of blood flow in skeletal muscle. What is the ultimate "purpose" of these cardiovascular responses?

2. What were Cassandra's mean arterial pressure and pulse pressure for the control and exercise periods, respectively?

3. What was her cardiac output for the control and exercise periods, respectively? Of the two factors that contribute to cardiac output (stroke volume and heart rate), which factor made the greater contribution to the increase in cardiac output that was seen when Cassandra exercised, or do these factors have equal weight?

4. What is the significance of the observed change in pulse pressure?

5. Why was systolic pressure increased during exercise? Why did diastolic pressure remain unchanged?

6. If Cassandra had been taking propranolol (a β-adrenergic antagonist), how might the responses to exercise have been different? Would her "exercise tolerance" have increased, decreased, or remained the same?

7. Early in the exercise period, Cassandra's skin was cool to the touch. However, at the peak of exercise, her skin was flushed and very warm to the touch. What mechanisms were responsible for these changes in skin color and temperature as the exercise progressed?

8. Arterial and venous P_{O_2} were measured before and after exercise. Explain why venous P_{O_2} decreased but arterial P_{O_2} did not.

ANSWERS AND EXPLANATIONS

1. The "goal" of the cardiovascular responses to **exercise** is to **increase O$_2$ delivery** to muscles that are working harder (skeletal and cardiac muscle). The major mechanism for providing this additional O$_2$ is increased blood flow to the exercising skeletal muscle and the myocardium.

In principle, blood flow in an organ can be increased in two ways: (i) total blood flow (cardiac output) can increase, which also increases blood flow to individual organs; or (ii) blood flow can be redistributed so that the percentage of total flow to some organs is increased at the expense of other organs. During exercise, both of these mechanisms are utilized: cardiac output increases significantly (through increases in heart rate and stroke volume), *and* blood flow is redistributed to skeletal muscle and myocardium, so that these tissues receive a greater percentage of the (increased) cardiac output. Figure 2–9 summarizes these responses.

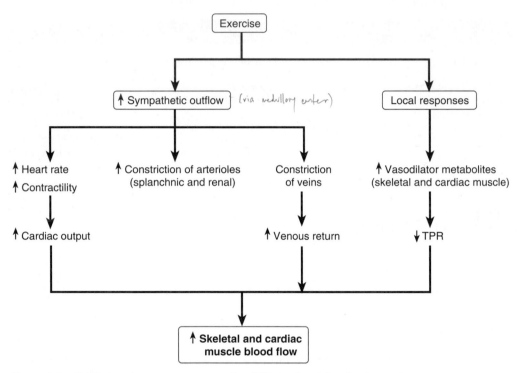

Figure 2–9 Cardiovascular responses to exercise. (TPR, total peripheral resistance.)

At the initiation of exercise, muscle mechanoreceptors and chemoreceptors trigger reflexes that send afferent signals to the cerebral motor cortex. The cerebral cortex then directs responses that include **increased sympathetic outflow** to the heart and blood vessels. (i) In the heart, increased sympathetic activity, through activation of **β$_1$ receptors**, produces an **increase in heart rate** and an **increase in contractility.** The increase in contractility results in increased stroke volume. Together with increased heart rate, this increased stroke volume produces an increase in cardiac output. (Recall that cardiac output = stroke volume × heart rate.) (ii) In addition, increased sympathetic activity, through **α$_1$ receptors**, produces **arteriolar constriction** in some vascular beds (e.g., splanchnic, renal) and venoconstriction. (iii) **Venoconstriction** (combined with compression of the veins by the squeezing action of skeletal muscle) increases venous return to the heart. Increased venous return is an essential component of the response to exercise; it provides the increased end-diastolic volume that is needed to produce the increase in cardiac output (**Frank–Starling mechanism**).

In addition to these central responses that are orchestrated by the sympathetic nervous system, **local responses** occur in skeletal and cardiac muscle to increase their blood flow. In skeletal muscle, as the metabolic rate increases, **metabolites** such as lactate, K^+, **nitric oxide**, and **adenosine** are generated. These metabolites produce vasodilation of skeletal muscle arterioles, thereby increasing local blood flow. This local vasodilation in skeletal muscle is so prominent that it is responsible for an overall *decrease* **in total peripheral resistance (TPR)**. (If these local responses in skeletal muscle did not occur, TPR would have *increased* as a result of sympathetic vasoconstriction.) Local responses also dominate in the myocardium, where they are primarily mediated by adenosine and decreased P_{O_2} and cause vasodilation and increased coronary blood flow.

2. Recall the calculations of pulse pressure and mean arterial pressure from Case 10:

> Pulse pressure = systolic pressure – diastolic pressure
> Mean arterial pressure = diastolic pressure + 1/3 pulse pressure

During the control period, Cassandra's **pulse pressure** was *40 mm Hg* (110 mm Hg – 70 mm Hg). During exercise, her pulse pressure increased to *85 mm Hg* (145 mm Hg – 60 mm Hg). During the control period, **mean arterial pressure** was *83 mm Hg* [70 mm Hg + 1/3 (40 mm Hg)]. During the exercise period, mean arterial pressure increased to *88 mm Hg* [60 mm Hg + 1/3 (85 mm Hg)]. You may wish to add this data on pulse pressure and mean arterial pressure to the data provided in Table 2–2.

3. Cardiac output is the product of stroke volume and heart rate, as discussed in Case 10:

Cardiac output = stroke volume × heart rate

Thus, in the control period, Cassandra's cardiac output was *6 L/min* (80 mL/beat × 75 beats/min = 6,000 mL/min, or 6 L/min). During exercise, her cardiac output increased dramatically to *14.3 L/min* (110 mL/beat × 130 beats/min = 14,300 mL/min, or 14.3 L/min). Again, you may wish to add these values to the data in Table 2–2.

To determine whether stroke volume or heart rate made the greater contribution to the increase in cardiac output, it is helpful to evaluate the observed changes on a percentage basis. In other words, during exercise, how much did cardiac output, stroke volume, and heart rate change as a percentage of their control values? Cardiac output increased from a control value of 6 L/min to 14.3 L/min during exercise. Thus, cardiac output increased by 8.3 L (14.3 L/min – 6 L/min = 8.3 L/min), or 138% above the control value (8.3 L/min ÷ 6 L/min = 1.38). Stroke volume increased from 80 mL/beat to 110 mL/beat, an increase of 30 mL/beat, or 38% above the control value. Heart rate increased from 75 beats/min to 130 beats/min, or 73% above the control value. Thus, the dramatic increase in cardiac output has two components, increased stroke volume and increased heart rate, and the increase in heart rate is the more significant factor.

4. Cassandra's **pulse pressure**, the difference between systolic and diastolic pressures, increased from a control value of 40 mm Hg to 85 mm Hg during exercise. To understand what this change means, consider what the pulse pressure represents. Because of the large amount of elastic tissue in the arterial walls, they are relatively stiff and noncompliant. (Yes! Compliance is the inverse of elastance.) Therefore, during systole, when blood is rapidly ejected from the left ventricle into the systemic arteries, arterial pressure increases rapidly from its lowest value (diastolic pressure) to its highest value (systolic pressure). The magnitude of this increase in pressure (i.e., pulse pressure) depends on the volume of blood ejected from the ventricle **(stroke volume)** and the compliance of the arteries. Cassandra's pulse pressure increased during exercise because her stroke volume increased.

5. The explanation for the increase in **systolic pressure** is the same as the explanation for the increase in pulse pressure: a larger stroke volume was ejected into the arteries during systole.

    On the other hand, **diastolic pressure** was *decreased*, which may be surprising. However, think about what diastolic pressure represents: it is the pressure in the arteries while the heart is relaxed (in diastole) and blood is flowing from the arteries to the veins and back to the heart. Because of the decrease in TPR during exercise, diastolic pressure can decrease.

6. **Propranolol** is a β-adrenergic receptor antagonist. Propranolol blocks β_1 receptors that mediate the sympathetic increases in heart rate and contractility. Recall that these effects on heart rate and contractility were the major mechanisms underlying Cassandra's increased cardiac output. Furthermore, increased cardiac output was a major mechanism for increasing O_2 delivery during exercise. Therefore, had Cassandra been taking propranolol, her exercise tolerance would have been significantly reduced.

7. **Cutaneous blood flow** exhibits a biphasic response to exercise. Early in exercise, vasoconstriction of cutaneous arterioles occurs as a result of the activation of sympathetic α_1 receptors. Blood flow is shunted away from the skin, and the skin is cool. As exercise progresses, body temperature increases secondary to increased O_2 consumption, and sympathetic centers controlling cutaneous blood flow in the anterior hypothalamus are inhibited. This selective inhibition of sympathetic activity produces vasodilation in cutaneous arterioles. As a result, warmed blood is shunted from the body core to venous plexus near the skin surface, as evidenced by redness and warmth of the skin.

8. Cassandra's skeletal and cardiac muscle performed increased work and used more O_2 during exercise than at rest. To help meet the increased demand for O_2, her skeletal and cardiac muscles extracted more O_2 from arterial blood. As a result, the P_{O_2} of venous blood was lower than normal; the normal P_{O_2} of venous blood is 40 mm Hg, and Cassandra's venous P_{O_2} was 25 mm Hg. (In the respiratory portion of your course, you will appreciate that this increased O_2 **extraction** is accomplished by a **right shift of the O_2–hemoglobin dissociation curve.** Right shifts of this curve are produced by increased temperature, increased P_{CO_2}, and decreased pH, all of which are consequences of an increased metabolic rate.) Thus, in addition to increased blood flow, which delivered more O_2 to the exercising muscles, more O_2 was extracted from the blood.

    Now for a puzzling question. If Cassandra's venous P_{O_2} was decreased, shouldn't her arterial P_{O_2} also have been decreased? No, not if O_2 exchange in the lungs restored the P_{O_2} of the blood to its normal arterial value of 100 mm Hg. Mixed venous blood enters the right side of the heart and is pumped to the lungs for oxygenation. In Cassandra's case, even though this venous blood had a lower P_{O_2} than normal, the diffusion of O_2 from alveolar gas was rapid enough to raise P_{O_2} to its normal arterial value (100 mm Hg). This blood then left the lungs through the pulmonary veins, entered the left side of the heart, and became systemic arterial blood. (You may be correctly thinking that people with lung diseases that interfere with O_2 diffusion might not be able to restore their arterial P_{O_2} to the normal value of 100 mm Hg, especially during exercise, when more O_2 is extracted by the exercising tissues.)

Key topics

Adenosine

Cardiac output

Cutaneous blood flow

Exercise

Frank–Starling mechanism

Local control of muscle blood flow

Local metabolites

Mean arterial pressure

Nitric oxide

O_2 delivery

O_2 extraction

O_2–hemoglobin dissociation curve

Propranolol

Pulse pressure

α_1 receptors

β_1 receptors

Right shift of the O_2–hemoglobin dissociation curve

Total peripheral resistance (TPR)

Case 14

Renovascular Hypertension: The Renin–Angiotensin–Aldosterone System

Stewart Hanna is a 58-year-old partner in a real estate firm. Over the years, the pressures of the job have taken their toll. Mr. Hanna has smoked two packs of filtered cigarettes a day for 40 years. He tries to watch his diet, but "required" business lunches and cocktail hours have driven his weight up to 210 lb. (He is 5 feet, 9 inches tall.) He recently separated from his wife of 35 years and is dating a much younger woman. Suddenly realizing how out of shape he had become, he made an appointment for a physical examination.

In his physician's office, Mr. Hanna's blood pressure was 180/125 (normal, 120/80). The physician heard a continuous abdominal bruit (sound). Because of Mr. Hanna's elevated blood pressure and the bruit, the physician drew a venous blood sample to determine plasma renin levels. After receiving the results, the physician ordered an additional test called a differential renal vein renin. Mr. Hanna's plasma renin activity was 10 ng/mL per hr (normal, 0.9–3.3 ng/mL per hr). His differential renal vein renin (left to right) was 1.6 (normal is 1.0).

The test results were consistent with left renal artery stenosis. Mr. Hanna was scheduled for a renal arteriogram, which showed 80% occlusion of the left renal artery as a result of severe atherosclerotic disease. A balloon angioplasty was performed immediately to clear the occlusion. Mr. Hanna's blood pressure was expected to return to normal after the procedure. He was ordered to stop smoking, follow a low-fat diet, exercise regularly, and undergo periodic physical examinations.

 QUESTIONS

1. How did occlusion of Mr. Hanna's left renal artery lead to an increase in plasma renin activity?

2. How did the increase in plasma renin activity cause an elevation in Mr. Hanna's arterial blood pressure (called renovascular hypertension)?

3. The differential renal vein renin measurement involves determining the renin level in venous blood from each kidney. In healthy persons, the renal vein renin level from each kidney is approximately the same; therefore, the ratio of left to right renin is 1.0. In Mr. Hanna, this ratio was elevated to 1.6. Although it is not apparent, the elevation of the ratio actually had two components: (i) his left renal vein renin was increased and (ii) his right renal vein renin was decreased. Why was renin secretion increased in the left kidney and decreased in the right kidney?

4. The abdominal bruit was caused by turbulent blood flow through the stenosed (narrowed) left renal artery. Why did narrowing of the artery cause renal blood flow to become turbulent?

5. If the balloon angioplasty was not successful, Mr. Hanna would be treated with an angiotensin-converting enzyme (ACE) inhibitor (e.g., captopril). What is the rationale for using ACE inhibitors to treat hypertension caused by renal artery stenosis?

ANSWERS ON NEXT PAGE

ANSWERS AND EXPLANATIONS

1. Atherosclerotic disease caused occlusion (narrowing) of Mr. Hanna's left renal artery. This occlusion caused a **decrease in renal perfusion pressure**, which then stimulated renin secretion from the kidney's **juxtaglomerular cells** (Fig. 2–10). Increased quantities of renin, secreted by Mr. Hanna's left kidney, entered renal venous blood and then the systemic circulation (increased **plasma renin activity**).

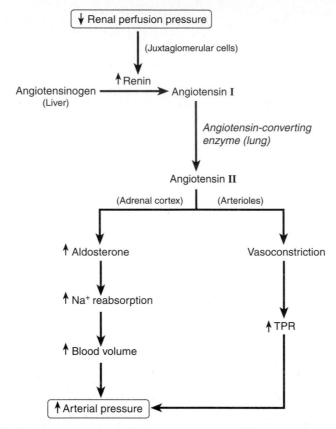

Figure 2–10   The renin–angiotensin II–aldosterone system. (TPR, total peripheral resistance.)

2. Renin is an enzyme that catalyzes the conversion of angiotensinogen (renin substrate) to angiotensin I. **Angiotensin I** is then converted, primarily in the lungs, to **angiotensin II**, which has several biologic actions. The first action of angiotensin II is to stimulate the synthesis and secretion of **aldosterone** by the adrenal cortex; aldosterone increases renal Na$^+$ reabsorption, extracellular fluid volume, and blood volume. The second action of angiotensin II is to cause vasoconstriction of arterioles; this vasoconstriction increases total peripheral resistance (TPR). In Mr. Hanna, the increase in blood volume (which increased venous return and cardiac output) combined with the increase in TPR to produce an increase in his arterial pressure. (Recall from Case 10 that P$_a$ = cardiac output × TPR.)

   Mr. Hanna had **renovascular hypertension,** in which his left kidney incorrectly sensed low **arterial pressure.** Because his left renal artery was stenosed, there was a decrease in left renal perfusion pressure that activated the renin–angiotensin II–aldosterone system and produced an increase in arterial pressure above normal.

3. In the question, you were told that the ratio of left to right renin was elevated for two reasons: (i) increased renin secretion by the left kidney and (ii) decreased renin secretion by the right kidney.

   Based on the earlier discussion, it is relatively easy to state why left renal renin secretion was increased: narrowing of the *left* renal artery led to decreased *left* renal perfusion pressure and increased *left* renal renin secretion.

   But how can we explain *decreased* renin secretion by the right kidney? The answer lies in the response of the normal right kidney to the increased arterial pressure (that resulted from stenosis of the left renal artery). The right kidney sensed increased arterial pressure, and responded appropriately by decreasing its renin secretion.

4. Narrowing of the left renal artery resulted in **turbulent blood flow**, which made a sound called a **bruit.** The probability of turbulence is given by the **Reynolds number:**

   $$\text{Reynolds number} = \frac{\rho dv}{\eta}$$

   where

   ρ = density of blood
   d = diameter of the blood vessel
   v = velocity of blood flow
   η = viscosity of blood

   The higher the Reynolds number, the higher the probability of turbulent blood flow. In general, a Reynolds number greater than 2,000 predicts turbulence. Initially, the relationship between blood vessel size and turbulence is puzzling. Diameter (d) is in the numerator. If a blood vessel narrows and its diameter decreases, shouldn't the Reynolds number also decrease, making turbulence *less* likely? No, because what is "hidden" in the Reynolds number equation is the relationship between velocity of blood flow and radius of the blood vessel. Recall the equation for **velocity of blood flow** from Case 10:

   $$v = Q/A$$

   where v is velocity, Q is blood flow, and A is area, or πr^2. Thus, velocity, which appears in the numerator of the Reynolds number equation, is *inversely correlated* with radius to the second power (r^2). Diameter, which also appears in the numerator, is *directly correlated* with radius to the first power. In other words, because of the greater second-power dependence on velocity, the Reynolds number increases as vessel radius decreases.

5. The reason why **angiotensin-converting enzyme (ACE) inhibitors** such as **captopril** successfully lower arterial pressure in renovascular hypertension should be evident from the pathogenesis of the elevated blood pressure. In Mr. Hanna's case, unilateral renal artery stenosis led to increased plasma renin activity, which led to increased levels of angiotensin II. Angiotensin II caused the increase in arterial pressure, both directly by vasoconstriction, and indirectly through the actions of aldosterone. Blocking the production of angiotensin II by inhibiting ACE activity interrupts this sequence of events.

Key topics

Aldosterone

Angiotensin II

Angiotensin-converting enzyme (ACE) inhibitors

Arterial blood pressure

Bruit

Captopril

Juxtaglomerular cells

Plasma renin activity

Renal perfusion pressure

Renin-angiotensin II-aldosterone system

Renovascular hypertension

Reynolds number

Turbulent blood flow

Velocity of blood flow

Case 15

Hypovolemic Shock: Regulation of Blood Pressure

Mavis Byrne is a 78-year-old widow who was brought to the emergency room one evening by her sister. Early in the day, Mrs. Byrne had seen bright red blood in her stool, which she attributed to hemorrhoids. She continued with her daily activities: she cleaned her house in the morning, had lunch with friends, and volunteered in the afternoon as a "hugger" in the newborn intensive care unit. However, the bleeding continued all day, and by dinnertime, she could no longer ignore it. Mrs. Byrne does not smoke or drink alcoholic beverages. She takes aspirin, as needed, for arthritis, sometimes up to 10 tablets daily.

In the emergency room, Mrs. Byrne was light-headed, pale, cold, and very anxious. Her hematocrit was 29% (normal for women, 36–46%). Table 2–3 shows her blood pressure and heart rate in the lying (supine) and upright (standing) positions.

TABLE 2–3	*Mrs. Byrne's Blood Pressure and Heart Rate*	
Parameter	Lying Down (Supine)	Upright (Standing)
Blood pressure	90/60	75/45
Heart rate	105 beats/min	135 beats/min

An infusion of normal saline was started, and a blood sample was drawn to be typed and cross-matched to prepare for a blood transfusion. A colonoscopy showed that the bleeding came from herniations in the colonic wall, called diverticula. (When arteries in the colon wall rupture, bleeding can be quite vigorous.) By the time of the colonoscopy, the bleeding had stopped spontaneously. Because of the quantity of blood lost, Mrs. Byrne received two units of whole blood and was admitted for observation. The physicians were prepared to insert a bladder catheter to allow continuous monitoring of urine output. However, by the next morning, her normal color had returned, she was no longer light-headed, and her blood pressure, both lying and standing, had returned to normal. No additional treatment or monitoring was needed. Mrs. Byrne was discharged to the care of her sister and advised to "take it easy."

 QUESTIONS

1. What is the definition of circulatory shock? What are the major causes?

2. After the gastrointestinal blood loss, what sequence of events led to Mrs. Byrne's decreased arterial pressure?

3. Why was Mrs. Byrne's arterial pressure lower in the upright position than in the lying (supine) position?

4. Mrs. Byrne's heart rate was elevated (105 beats/min) when she was supine. Why? Why was her heart rate even more elevated (135 beats/min) when she was upright?

5. If central venous pressure and pulmonary capillary wedge pressure had been measured, would you expect their values to have been increased, decreased, or the same as in a healthy person?

6. What is hematocrit? Why was Mrs. Byrne's hematocrit decreased, and why was this decrease potentially dangerous?

7. Why was her skin pale and cold?

8. If Mrs. Byrne's urinary Na^+ excretion had been measured, would you expect it to be higher, lower, or the same as that of a healthy person? Why?

9. How was the saline infusion expected to help her condition?

10. Why did the physicians consider monitoring her urine output? How do prostaglandins "protect" renal blood flow after a hemorrhage? In this regard, why was it dangerous that Mrs. Byrne had been taking aspirin?

11. Had her blood loss been more severe, Mrs. Byrne might have received a low dose of dopamine, which has selective actions in various vascular beds. In cerebral, cardiac, renal, and mesenteric vascular beds, dopamine is a vasodilator; in muscle and cutaneous vascular beds, dopamine is a vasoconstrictor. Why is low-dose dopamine helpful in the treatment of hypovolemic shock?

ANSWERS ON NEXT PAGE

ANSWERS AND EXPLANATIONS

1. **Shock (or circulatory shock)** is a condition in which decreased blood flow causes decreased tissue perfusion and O_2 delivery. Untreated, shock can lead to impaired tissue and cellular metabolism and, ultimately, death.

   In categorizing the causes of shock, it is helpful to consider the components of the cardiovascular system that determine blood flow to the tissues: the heart (the pump), the blood vessels, and the volume of blood in the system. Shock can be caused by a failure of, or deficit in, any of these components. **Hypovolemic shock** occurs when circulating blood volume is decreased because of loss of whole blood (hemorrhagic shock), loss of plasma volume (e.g., burn), or loss of fluid and electrolytes (e.g., vomiting, diarrhea). **Cardiogenic shock** is caused by myocardial impairment (e.g., myocardial infarction, congestive heart failure). **Mechanical obstruction to blood flow** can occur anywhere in the circulatory system and cause a local decrease in blood flow. **Neurogenic shock** (e.g., deep general anesthesia, spinal anesthesia, spinal cord injury) involves loss of vasomotor tone, which leads to venous pooling of blood. **Septic or anaphylactic shock** involves increased filtration across capillary walls, which leads to decreased circulating blood volume.

2. Mrs. Byrne had a gastrointestinal **hemorrhage** and lost a significant volume of whole blood. How did this blood loss lead to decreased arterial pressure? Although it is tempting to picture blood pouring out of the arteries as the direct cause of her decreased arterial pressure, this explanation is an oversimplification. A number of intervening steps are involved. Recall that because the capacitance of the veins is high, most of the blood volume is contained in the veins, not in the arteries. Therefore, when a hemorrhage occurs, most of the blood volume that is lost comes from the veins. A decrease in venous volume leads to a decrease in venous return to the heart and a decrease in **end-diastolic volume** (preload). A decrease in end-diastolic volume leads to a decrease in cardiac output by the **Frank–Starling mechanism** (the length–tension relationship for the ventricles). A decrease in cardiac output leads to a decrease in arterial pressure, as expressed by the familiar relationship: Arterial pressure = cardiac output × total peripheral resistance (symbolically, P_a = cardiac output × TPR). Thus, after blood loss, the fundamental problem is decreased venous volume and venous return, leading to decreased cardiac output. In textbooks, you will see references to **filling pressure**, venous filling pressure, or cardiac filling pressure. All of these terms refer to the relationships between venous volume, venous return, cardiac output, and (ultimately) arterial pressure.

3. Mrs. Byrne's arterial pressure was lower in the upright position than in the supine position **(orthostatic hypotension)** because when she was upright, blood pooled in the veins of her legs and her venous return was further compromised. As a result, end-diastolic volume was further reduced, which led to further reductions in cardiac output and arterial pressure.

4. Asking why Mrs. Byrne's heart rate was elevated brings us to the larger issues of **compensatory responses to hemorrhage**. Essentially, decreased arterial pressure triggers several compensatory mechanisms, including an increase in heart rate, that attempt to restore blood pressure to normal (Fig. 2–11).

   Two major mechanisms are activated in response to decreased arterial pressure: (i) the baroreceptor reflex and (ii) the renin–angiotensin II–aldosterone system (discussed in Question 8).

   In the **baroreceptor reflex**, sympathetic outflow to the heart and blood vessels is increased. As a result, heart rate and contractility increase and cause an increase in cardiac output. There is arteriolar constriction, which increases TPR, and there is venoconstriction, which increases venous return. Looking once again at the equation for arterial pressure (P_a = cardiac output × TPR), you can appreciate how each of these changes works to restore arterial pressure toward normal.

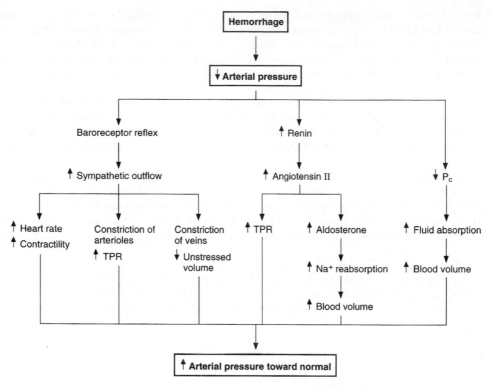

Figure 2–11 Cardiovascular responses to hemorrhage. (P_c, capillary hydrostatic pressure; TPR, total peripheral resistance.) (Reprinted, with permission, from Costanzo LS. *BRS Physiology.* 4th ed. Baltimore: Lippincott Williams & Wilkins; 2007:104.)

Mrs. Byrne's heart rate was more elevated in the upright position than in the supine position because her arterial blood pressure was lower when she was upright (venous pooling). Therefore, the baroreceptor mechanism was more strongly stimulated, and sympathetic stimulation of the heart and blood vessels (including the increase in heart rate) was exaggerated.

5. **Central venous pressure** is measured in the vena cava. Its value is related to the volume of blood in the veins and is approximately equal to right atrial pressure. **Pulmonary capillary wedge pressure** is measured by advancing a catheter through the pulmonary artery until it "wedges" in the artery's smallest branch. At that point, the catheter senses pulmonary capillary pressure, which is nearly equal to left atrial pressure.

Thus, central venous pressure estimates right atrial pressure, and pulmonary capillary wedge pressure estimates left atrial pressure. The values reflect end-diastolic volume, or preload, of the right and left ventricles, respectively. Had they been measured, Mrs. Byrne's central venous pressure and pulmonary capillary wedge pressure both would have been *decreased* because of the loss of blood volume from the venous side of the circulation.

6. **Hematocrit** is the fraction (or percentage) of blood volume occupied by red blood cells; the remaining fraction of whole blood is plasma, which is mostly water. A decrease in hematocrit can be caused by any number of factors, including blood loss, decreased red blood cell production, increased red blood cell destruction, or an increase in plasma volume without an accompanying increase in red blood cell volume.

In Mrs. Byrne's case, the decreased hematocrit was probably secondary to hemorrhage of whole blood. But, wait a minute! You may be asking: If *whole* blood was lost from the gastrointestinal tract, why would hematocrit be changed (reasoning that red blood cells and plasma were lost proportionately)? In the first hours after hemorrhage, it is true that hematocrit is unchanged. However, as plasma volume is restored (as a result of increased aldosterone levels [see the answer to Question 8], increased capillary absorption of fluid, and the infusion of saline), plasma volume increases, but red blood cell volume does not. (It takes about 7 days for stem cells to become mature red blood cells.) Therefore, Mrs. Byrne's hematocrit was decreased by *dilution.*

A decrease in hematocrit is dangerous because red blood cells contain **hemoglobin,** the O_2-carrying protein of blood. Thus, after a hemorrhage, there are two potentially lethal consequences for O_2 **delivery** to the tissues: the decrease in blood flow to the tissues (i.e., decreased cardiac output) and the decreased O_2-carrying capacity of the blood (decreased hematocrit).

7. Mrs. Byrne's pale, cold skin is typical of the response to hemorrhage, reflecting vasoconstriction of cutaneous arterioles. As the baroreceptor reflex was initiated in response to decreased arterial pressure (see Question 4), sympathetic vasoconstriction of arterioles occurred in many vascular beds, including the skin. Cutaneous vasoconstriction particularly makes sense as it allows the body to increase arterial pressure and redirect blood flow to more vital organs, (e.g., brain, heart).

8. If **urinary Na^+ excretion** had been measured, it likely would have been *decreased.* The reason for this decreased Na^+ excretion is activation of the **renin–angiotensin II–aldosterone system** in response to decreased arterial pressure. Increased levels of aldosterone cause increased Na^+ reabsorption in the late distal tubule and collecting duct of the kidney (i.e., decreased Na^+ excretion). This mechanism is designed to increase the amount of Na^+ in extracellular fluid, which increases extracellular fluid volume and blood volume. Increased blood volume leads to increased venous return, increased cardiac output, and ultimately, increased arterial pressure.

9. In an attempt to restore venous return and cardiac output, Mrs. Byrne received an infusion of saline to increase her extracellular fluid volume and blood volume. The saline infusion accomplished a result similar to the body's endogenous aldosterone, only faster.

10. A critical element in the response to hemorrhage, and one that may determine the outcome for the patient, is the "balancing act" between vasoconstriction in some organs (e.g., kidney) and maintaining blood flow in those organs. Increased sympathetic activity and increased angiotensin II both produce vasoconstriction and an increase in TPR, which is important to the body's attempt to restore arterial pressure (recall that P_a = cardiac output × TPR). However, vasoconstriction, by increasing resistance, decreases blood flow in the involved organs.

Of particular note is the kidney, where both sympathetic activity and angiotensin II cause arteriolar vasoconstriction. If unopposed, this vasoconstriction can compromise **renal blood flow** and **glomerular filtration rate (GFR)**, producing renal failure and even death. Thus, had Mrs. Byrne not recovered quickly, it would have been important to monitor her urine output as an indicator of renal perfusion and renal function.

Notice the word "unopposed" in the previous paragraph. Perhaps this word led you to question whether there are endogenous "modulators" of the vasoconstricting effects of sympathetic activity and angiotensin II in the kidneys. Yes, there are! **Prostaglandins** serve this modulatory role. Both sympathetic activity and angiotensin II cause increased local production of prostaglandin E_2 and prostaglandin I_2, which are renal vasodilators. Thus, the vasoconstrictive effects of sympathetic activity and angiotensin II are offset by the vasodilatory effects of endogenous prostaglandins. Renal blood flow is thereby protected and maintained in high vasoconstrictor states, such as hemorrhage.

The confounding and potentially harmful issue with Mrs. Byrne was her use of large amounts of aspirin for her arthritis. Aspirin, a **nonsteroidal anti-inflammatory drug (NSAID),** is a cyclooxygenase inhibitor that blocks prostaglandin synthesis. Therefore, Mrs. Byrne was at risk for developing renal failure if her ingestion of aspirin prevented the protective, vasodilatory effects of prostaglandins.

11. Mrs. Byrne's physicians were prepared to administer a low dose of **dopamine** if her blood pressure and blood flow (as reflected in the color returning to her skin) had not been corrected. Dopamine, a precursor of norepinephrine, has its own vasoactive properties, as explained in the question. Low doses of dopamine selectively dilate arterioles in critical organs (i.e., heart, brain, kidney) and selectively constrict arterioles in less critical organs (e.g., skeletal muscle, skin), thus redirecting blood flow where it is most needed. In particular, the kidneys, which might otherwise be vasoconstricted as a result of increased sympathetic activity and angiotensin II, may be spared by the vasodilatory actions of dopamine.

Key topics

Aldosterone

Anaphylactic shock

Arterial pressure regulation

Baroreceptor reflex

Cardiac filling pressure, or filling pressure

Cardiogenic shock

Central venous pressure

Dopamine

End-diastolic volume

Frank–Starling mechanism

Glomerular filtration rate (GFR)

Hematocrit

Hemoglobin

Hemorrhage

Hypovolemic shock

Neurogenic shock

Nonsteroidal anti-inflammatory drug (NSAID)

O_2 delivery

Orthostatic fall in arterial pressure (orthostasis)

Prostaglandins

Pulmonary capillary wedge pressure

Renal blood flow

Renin–angiotensin II–aldosterone system

Septic shock

Shock, or circulatory shock

Case 16

Primary Pulmonary Hypertension: Right Ventricular Failure

At the time of her death, Celia Lukas was a 38-year-old homemaker and mother of three children, 15, 14, and 12 years of age. She had an associate's degree in computer programming from a community college, but had not worked outside the home since the birth of her first child. Keeping house and driving the children to activities kept her very busy. To stay in shape, she took aerobics classes at the local community center. The first sign that Celia was ill was vague: she fatigued easily. However, within 6 months, Celia was short of breath (dyspnea), both at rest and when she exercised, and she had swelling in her legs and feet. She made an appointment to see her physician.

On physical examination, Celia's jugular veins were distended, her liver was enlarged (hepatomegaly), and she had ascites in her peritoneal cavity and edema in her legs. A fourth heart sound was audible over her right ventricle. The physician was very concerned and immediately scheduled Celia for a chest x-ray, an electrocardiogram (ECG), and a cardiac catheterization.

The chest x-ray showed enlargement of the right ventricle and prominent pulmonary arteries. The ECG findings were consistent with right ventricular hypertrophy. The results of cardiac catheterization are shown in Table 2–4.

TABLE 2–4	Results of Celia's Cardiac Catheterization
Pressure	**Value**
Mean pulmonary artery pressure	35 mm Hg (normal, 15 mm Hg)
Right ventricular pressure	Increased
Right atrial pressure	Increased
Pulmonary capillary wedge pressure	Normal

Consulting physicians in cardiology and pulmonology concluded that Celia had primary pulmonary hypertension, a rare type of pulmonary hypertension that is caused by diffuse pathologic changes in the pulmonary arteries. These abnormalities lead to increased pulmonary vascular resistance and pulmonary hypertension, which causes right ventricular failure (cor pulmonale). Celia was treated with vasodilator drugs, but they were not effective. Her name was added to a list of patients awaiting a heart–lung transplant. However, she died of right heart failure before a transplant could be performed.

 QUESTIONS

1. Why did increased pulmonary vascular resistance cause an increase in pulmonary artery pressure (pulmonary hypertension)?

2. What values are needed to calculate pulmonary vascular resistance?

3. Discuss the concept of "afterload" of the ventricles. What is the afterload of the left ventricle? What is the afterload of the right ventricle? What is the effect of increased afterload on stroke volume, cardiac output, ejection fraction, and end-systolic volume? How did Celia's increased pulmonary artery pressure lead to right ventricular failure?

4. In the context of Celia's right ventricular failure, explain the data from the cardiac catheterization.

5. Why does right ventricular failure cause right ventricular hypertrophy? (Hint: Use the law of Laplace to answer this question.)

6. Increased systemic venous pressure and jugular vein distension are the sine qua non (defining characteristics) of right ventricular failure. Why were Celia's jugular veins distended?

7. During what portion of the cardiac cycle is the fourth heart sound heard? What is the meaning of an audible fourth heart sound?

8. Why did right ventricular failure lead to edema on the systemic side of the circulation (e.g., ascites, edema in the legs)? Discuss the Starling forces involved. Would you expect pulmonary edema to be present in right ventricular failure?

9. Celia very much wanted to attend a family reunion in Denver. Her physicians told her that the trip was *absolutely contraindicated* because of Denver's high altitude. Why is ascent to high altitude so dangerous in a person with pulmonary hypertension? (Knowledge of pulmonary physiology is necessary to answer this question.)

10. The physician hoped that vasodilator drugs would improve Celia's condition. What was the physician's reasoning?

ANSWERS AND EXPLANATIONS

1. To explain why **increased pulmonary vascular resistance** (caused by intrinsic pathology of the small pulmonary arteries) led to increased pulmonary artery pressure, it is necessary to think about the relationship between pressure, flow, and resistance. Recall this relationship from Case 10: ΔP = blood flow × resistance. Mathematically, it is easy to see that if blood flow (in this case, pulmonary blood flow) is constant and resistance of the blood vessels increases, then ΔP, the pressure difference between the pulmonary artery and the pulmonary vein, must increase. ΔP could increase because pressure in the pulmonary artery increases *or* because pressure in the pulmonary vein decreases. (Note, however, that a decrease in pulmonary vein pressure would have little impact on ΔP because its value is normally very low.)

   In Celia, ΔP increased because her pulmonary arterial pressure increased. As pulmonary vascular resistance increased, resistance to blood flow increased, and blood "backed up" proximal to the pulmonary microcirculation into the pulmonary arteries. Increased blood volume in the pulmonary arteries caused increased pressure.

2. **Pulmonary vascular resistance** is calculated by rearranging the equation for the pressure, flow, resistance relationship. ΔP = blood flow × resistance; thus, resistance = ΔP/blood flow. ΔP is the pressure difference between the pulmonary artery and the pulmonary vein. Pulmonary blood flow is equal to the cardiac output of the right ventricle, which in the steady state, is equal to the cardiac output of the left ventricle. Thus, the values needed to calculate pulmonary vascular resistance are: pulmonary artery pressure, pulmonary vein pressure (or left atrial pressure), and cardiac output.

3. Afterload of the ventricles is the pressure against which the ventricles must eject blood. **Afterload of the left ventricle** is aortic pressure. **Afterload of the right ventricle** is pulmonary artery pressure. For blood to be ejected during systole, left ventricular pressure must increase above aortic pressure, and right ventricular pressure must increase above pulmonary artery pressure.

   Celia's increased pulmonary artery pressure had a devastating effect on the function of her right ventricle. Much more work was required to develop the pressure required to open the pulmonic valve and eject blood into the pulmonary artery. As a result, right ventricular stroke volume, cardiac output, and ejection fraction were decreased. Right ventricular end-systolic volume was increased, as blood that should have been ejected into the pulmonary artery remained in the right ventricle. (Celia had **cor pulmonale**, or right ventricular failure secondary to pulmonary hypertension.)

4. Celia's **cardiac catheterization** showed that her pulmonary artery pressure was increased, her right ventricular pressure and right atrial pressure were increased, and her **pulmonary capillary wedge pressure** was normal. The increased pulmonary artery pressure (the cause of Celia's right ventricular failure) has already been discussed: pulmonary artery pressure increased secondary to increased pulmonary vascular resistance. Right ventricular pressure increased because more blood than usual remained in the ventricle after systolic ejection. As right ventricular pressure increased, it was more difficult for blood to move from the right atrium to the right ventricle; as a result, right atrial volume and pressure also increased. Pulmonary capillary wedge pressure (*left* atrial pressure) was normal, suggesting that there was no failure on the left side of the heart.

5. Right ventricular failure led to **right ventricular hypertrophy** (evident from Celia's chest x-ray and ECG) because her right ventricle was required to perform increased work against an increased afterload. The right ventricular wall thickens (hypertrophies) as an adaptive mechanism for performing more work. This adaptive response is explained by the **law of Laplace** for a sphere (a sphere being the approximate shape of the heart):

$$P = \frac{2HT}{r}$$

where

P = ventricular pressure
H = ventricular wall thickness (height)
T = wall tension
r = radius of the ventricle

Thus, ventricular pressure correlates directly with developed wall tension and wall thickness, and inversely with radius. The thicker the ventricular wall, the greater the pressure that can be developed at a given tension. Celia's right ventricle hypertrophied adaptively so that it could develop the higher pressures required to eject blood against the increased pulmonary artery pressure.

6. Celia's jugular veins were distended with blood because right ventricular failure caused blood to back up into the right ventricle, and then into the right atrium and the systemic veins.

7. A **fourth heart sound** is not normally audible in adults. However, it may occur in **ventricular hypertrophy,** where ventricular compliance is decreased. During filling of a less compliant ventricle, blood flow produces noise (the fourth heart sound). Thus, when it is present, the fourth heart sound is heard during atrial systole.

8. As already explained, right ventricular failure caused blood to back up into the systemic veins, which increased systemic venous pressure. The **Starling forces** that determine fluid movement across capillary walls can be used to explain why edema would form on the systemic side of the circulation (e.g., **ascites, edema** in the legs) when systemic venous pressure is increased (Fig. 2–12).

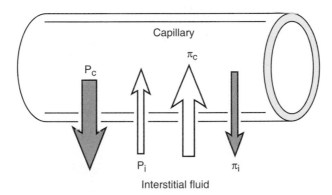

Figure 2–12   Starling pressures across the capillary wall. (P_c, capillary hydrostatic pressure; P_i, interstitial hydrostatic pressure; π_c, capillary oncotic pressure; π_i, interstitial oncotic pressure.)

There are four Starling pressures (or forces) across the capillary wall: capillary hydrostatic pressure (P_c), capillary oncotic pressure (π_c), interstitial hydrostatic pressure (P_i), and interstitial oncotic pressure (π_i). As shown in Figure 2–12, P_c and π_i favor filtration of fluid out of the capillary, and π_c and P_i favor absorption of fluid into the capillary. In most capillary beds, the Starling pressures are such that there is a small net filtration of fluid that is returned to the circulation by the **lymphatics.**

$$J_v = K_f[(P_c - P_i) - (\pi_c - \pi_i)]$$

where

J_v = fluid movement
K_f = hydraulic conductance
P_c = capillary hydrostatic pressure

P_i = interstitial hydrostatic pressure
π_c = capillary oncotic pressure
π_i = interstitial oncotic pressure

Edema occurs when filtration of fluid increases and exceeds the capacity of the lymphatics to return it to the circulation. The question, then, is why there was increased filtration of fluid in Celia's case (assuming that her lymphatic function was normal). The answer lies in her increased systemic venous pressure, which caused an increase in capillary hydrostatic pressure (P_c). Increases in P_c *favor* filtration.

Pulmonary edema would *not* be expected to occur in right ventricular failure. **Pulmonary edema** occurs in *left* ventricular failure, where blood backs up behind the left ventricle into the left atrium and pulmonary veins. An increase in pulmonary venous pressure then leads to increased pulmonary capillary hydrostatic pressure and increased filtration of fluid into the pulmonary interstitium. Celia's left atrial pressure (estimated by pulmonary capillary wedge pressure) was normal, suggesting that she did not have left ventricular failure; thus, pulmonary venous pressure is not expected to have been elevated and pulmonary edema is not expected to have occurred.

9. At **high altitude**, barometric pressure is decreased, resulting in decreased partial pressure of atmospheric gases, such as O_2. If Celia had traveled to Denver, she would have breathed air with a lower Po_2 than the air at sea level. Such **alveolar hypoxia** produces vasoconstriction in the pulmonary circulation (normally a protective mechanism in the lungs that diverts blood flow away from hypoxic areas). Celia's pulmonary vascular resistance was already abnormally elevated as a result of her intrinsic disease. So-called **hypoxic vasoconstriction** at high altitude would have further increased her pulmonary vascular resistance and pulmonary arterial pressure, and further increased the afterload on her right ventricle. (Incident-ally, hypoxic vasoconstriction is unique to the lungs. Other vascular beds *dilate* in response to hypoxia.)

10. The physician hoped that vasodilator drugs would dilate pulmonary arterioles and decrease Celia's pulmonary vascular resistance and pulmonary arterial pressure, thus lowering the afterload of the right ventricle.

Key topics

Afterload

Ascites

Cardiac catheterization

Cor pulmonale

Edema

Fourth heart sound

High altitude

Hypoxic vasoconstriction

Law of Laplace

Lymph, or lymphatic, vessels

Pulmonary capillary wedge pressure

Pulmonary edema

Pulmonary hypertension

Pulmonary vascular resistance

Right heart, or right ventricular, failure

Right ventricular hypertrophy

Starling forces or pressures

Case 17

Myocardial Infarction: Left Ventricular Failure

Marvin Zimmerman is a 52-year-old construction manager who is significantly overweight. Despite his physician's repeated admonitions, Marvin ate a rich diet that included red meats and high-calorie desserts. Marvin also enjoyed unwinding with a few beers each evening. He joked with the guys, "I guess I'm a heart attack waiting to happen." He had occasional chest pains (angina) that were relieved by nitroglycerin.

The evening of his myocardial infarction, Marvin went to bed early because he wasn't feeling well. He awakened at 2:00 A.M. with crushing pressure in his chest and pain radiating down his left arm that was not relieved by nitroglycerin. He was nauseated and sweating profusely. He also had difficulty breathing (dyspnea), especially when he was recumbent (orthopnea). His breathing was "noisy." Marvin's wife called 911, and paramedics arrived promptly and transported him to the nearest hospital.

In the emergency room, Marvin's blood pressure was 105/80. Inspiratory rales were present, consistent with pulmonary edema, and his skin was cold and clammy. Sequential electrocardiograms and serum levels of cardiac enzymes (creatine phosphokinase and lactate dehydrogenase) suggested a left ventricular wall myocardial infarction. Pulmonary capillary wedge pressure, obtained during cardiac catheterization, was 30 mm Hg (normal, 5 mm Hg). His ejection fraction, measured with two-dimensional echocardiography, was 0.35 (normal, 0.55).

Marvin was transferred to the coronary intensive care unit. He was treated with a thrombolytic agent to prevent another myocardial infarction, digitalis (a positive inotropic agent), and furosemide (a loop diuretic). After 7 days in the hospital, he was sent home on a strict, low-fat, low-Na⁺ diet.

 QUESTIONS

1. Marvin had a left ventricular wall infarction secondary to myocardial ischemia. This damage to the left ventricle compromised its function as a pump; the left ventricle could no longer generate enough pressure to eject blood normally. Draw the normal Frank–Starling relationship for the left ventricle. Superimpose a second curve showing the Frank–Starling relationship after the myocardial infarction, and use this relationship to predict changes in stroke volume and cardiac output.

2. Which information provided in the case tells you that Marvin's stroke volume was decreased?

3. What is the meaning of Marvin's decreased ejection fraction?

4. Why was Marvin's pulmonary capillary wedge pressure increased?

5. Why did pulmonary edema develop? (In your explanation, discuss the Starling forces involved.) Why is pulmonary edema so dangerous?

6. Why did Marvin have dyspnea and orthopnea?

7. Why was Marvin's skin cold and clammy?

8. What was the rationale for treating Marvin with a positive inotropic agent, such as digitalis? (Hint: See Figure 2–13, which shows the Frank–Starling relationship.)

9. What was the rationale for treating Marvin with furosemide (a loop diuretic)?

10. A medical student in the coronary intensive care unit asked whether Marvin should also be treated with propranolol (a β-adrenergic antagonist). The student reasoned that propranolol would reduce the myocardial O_2 requirement and possibly prevent another infarction. Why does propranolol decrease the myocardial O_2 requirement? The attending physician pointed out that there could be a risk associated with the use of propranolol. What is this risk?

11. Why was Marvin sent home on a low-Na^+ diet?

ANSWERS ON NEXT PAGE

ANSWERS AND EXPLANATIONS

1. The **Frank–Starling relationship** for the ventricle states that stroke volume and cardiac output increase with increased ventricular end-diastolic volume (Fig. 2–13). Applied to the left ventricle, the volume of blood ejected in systole depends on the volume present in the ventricle at the end of diastolic filling (i.e., preload).

   The underlying physiologic principle of the Frank–Starling relationship is the **length–tension relationship for ventricular muscle.** Analogous to the length–tension relationship in skeletal muscle, sarcomere length (which is set by end-diastolic volume) determines the degree of overlap of thick and thin filaments. The degree of overlap determines the *possibility* of cross-bridge formation and cycling. The number of cross-bridges that *actually* cycle then depends on the intracellular Ca^{2+} concentration. Thus, two factors determine how much tension is generated by the ventricle: muscle length (i.e., extent of overlap of thick and thin filaments) and intracellular Ca^{2+} concentration.

   In ventricular failure, contractility decreases and the intrinsic ability of the myocardial fibers to produce tension is impaired; thus, for a given end-diastolic volume, stroke volume and cardiac output are decreased.

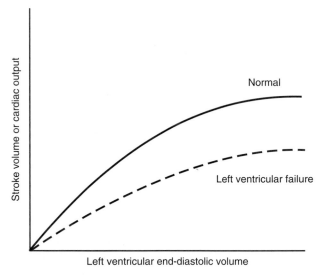

Figure 2–13   Effect of ventricular failure on the Frank–Starling relationship.

2. Several pieces of information are consistent with decreased left ventricular stroke volume, including increased pulmonary capillary wedge pressure (see answer to Question 4) and decreased ejection fraction (see answer to Question 3).

   However, the most specific information indicating that Marvin's stroke volume was decreased was his decreased pulse pressure. Recall that **pulse pressure** is the difference between systolic and diastolic blood pressure. Marvin's systolic pressure was 105 mm Hg, and his diastolic pressure was 80 mm Hg; therefore, his pulse pressure was only 25 mm Hg. (Normal arterial pressure is 120/80, with a pulse pressure of 40 mm Hg.) Stroke volume is an important determinant of pulse pressure: the blood volume ejected from the ventricle in systole causes arterial pressure to increase from its lowest value (diastolic pressure) to its highest value (systolic pressure). Thus, Marvin's decreased stroke volume resulted in a decreased pulse pressure.

3. Ejection fraction = stroke volume/end-diastolic volume; in other words, **ejection fraction** is the fraction of the end-diastolic volume that is ejected during systole. Ejection fraction

is related to **contractility,** which is decreased in ventricular failure. Marvin's stroke volume was only 0.35 (35%) compared with the normal value of 0.55 (55%).

4. **Pulmonary capillary wedge pressure** is an estimate of left atrial pressure. It is measured by advancing a cannula through the pulmonary artery until it lodges ("wedges") in its smallest branches. At that point, the cannula senses pulmonary capillary pressure, which is nearly equal to **left atrial pressure.**

   Marvin's pulmonary capillary wedge pressure was increased because his left atrial pressure was increased. His left atrial pressure was increased secondary to decreased left ventricular stroke volume and ejection fraction. Following ejection, more blood than normal remained behind in the left ventricle; as a result, left ventricular pressure and left atrial pressure both increased.

5. The decrease in left ventricular ejection fraction caused blood to "back up" in the left side of the heart, increasing left ventricular and left atrial pressures. The increase in left atrial pressure led to increased pulmonary venous pressure. The increase in pulmonary venous pressure led to increased pulmonary capillary hydrostatic pressure (P_c), which is the major **Starling force** favoring filtration of fluid into the pulmonary interstitium (see Case 16 and Figure 2–12).

   When the filtration of fluid exceeded the capacity of Marvin's pulmonary lymphatics to remove the fluid, **pulmonary edema** occurred. Initially, the excess fluid accumulated in the interstitial space, but eventually it also "flooded" the alveoli.

   Pulmonary edema is dangerous because it compromises gas exchange in the lungs. Although this discussion is more the venue of pulmonary physiology, briefly, pulmonary edema increases the diffusion distance for O_2. When the diffusion distance increases, there is decreased diffusion of O_2 from alveolar gas into pulmonary capillary blood. In addition, pulmonary blood flow is shunted away from alveoli that are filled with fluid rather than with air (i.e., hypoxic vasoconstriction). As a result, there is impaired oxygenation of pulmonary capillary blood, which causes **hypoxemia** (decreased Po_2 of arterial blood). Hypoxemia is an important cause of **hypoxia** (decreased O_2 delivery to the tissues).

6. If you are a first-year medical student, you may need help with the terms "dyspnea" and "orthopnea."

   Dyspnea is the sensation of difficult breathing. The etiology of dyspnea in pulmonary edema is not entirely clear, but the following factors play a role: (i) Juxtacapillary (J) receptors are stimulated by the accumulation of interstitial fluid, and trigger reflexes that stimulate rapid, shallow breathing. (ii) Bronchial congestion stimulates the production of mucus. As a result, resistance of the bronchi is increased, causing wheezing and respiratory distress (called "cardiac asthma," referring to the left ventricular failure that produced the pulmonary edema). (iii) Accumulation of edema fluid leads to decreased pulmonary compliance, which increases the work of breathing.

   Orthopnea is dyspnea that is precipitated by lying down. When a person lies down, venous return from the lower extremities back to the heart is increased. In left ventricular failure, increased venous return compounds the pulmonary venous congestion that is already present.

7. Marvin's skin was cold and clammy because the stress of the myocardial infarction produced a massive outpouring of **catecholamines** (epinephrine and norepinephrine) from the adrenal medulla. The circulating catecholamines activated α_1-**adrenergic receptors** in cutaneous vascular beds and reduced **cutaneous blood flow.**

8. As already discussed, damage to the left ventricle (secondary to the myocardial infarction) led to decreased contractility, decreased stroke volume, and decreased cardiac output for a given end-diastolic volume. Consider the Frank–Starling relationships that you constructed for Question 1. The curve for ventricular failure is lower than the curve for a normal ventricle,

reflecting decreased contractility, stroke volume, and cardiac output. **Positive inotropic agents,** such as **digitalis,** increase contractility by increasing intracellular Ca^{2+} concentration. Digitalis was expected to increase contractility and return the Frank–Starling relationship toward that seen in a normal ventricle.

9. One of the most dangerous aspects of Marvin's condition was the increased pulmonary venous pressure that caused his pulmonary edema. (As already discussed, the cardiac output of the left ventricle was impaired, and blood backed up into the pulmonary veins.) Therefore, one therapeutic strategy was to reduce venous blood volume by reducing extracellular fluid volume. **Loop diuretics,** such as **furosemide,** are potent inhibitors of Na^+ reabsorption in the renal thick ascending limb; when Na^+ reabsorption in the thick ascending limb is inhibited, Na^+ excretion increases. The resulting decrease in extracellular Na^+ content leads to decreased extracellular fluid volume and blood volume.

10. **Propranolol,** a **β-adrenergic antagonist,** reduces myocardial O_2 requirement by blocking β_1 receptors in the sinoatrial node and ventricular muscle. Normally, these β_1 receptors mediate increases in heart rate and contractility, which increase cardiac output. Cardiac output is part of the "work" of the heart, and this work requires O_2. Therefore, antagonizing β_1 receptors with propranolol decreases heart rate, contractility, cardiac output, and myocardial O_2 consumption.

    Perhaps you've anticipated a potential risk in treating Marvin with a β-adrenergic antagonist. Propranolol could further decrease his already compromised cardiac output, and thus should be given cautiously.

11. Extracellular fluid volume is determined by extracellular Na^+ content. A **low-Na^+ diet** was recommended to reduce extracellular fluid volume and blood volume, and to prevent subsequent episodes of pulmonary edema (similar to the idea of treating Marvin with a diuretic).

Key topics

β-adrenergic antagonist

Contractility

Cutaneous blood flow

Digitalis, or cardiac glycosides

Dyspnea

Ejection fraction

Frank–Starling relationship

Furosemide

Hypoxemia

Hypoxia

Left heart failure

Left ventricular failure

Loop diuretics

Orthopnea

Positive inotropism

Propranolol

Pulmonary capillary wedge pressure

Pulmonary edema

Pulse pressure

Starling force

Case 18

Ventricular Septal Defect

A wealthy Spanish businessman joined a humanitarian trip to a remote village in South America. While working in the village, he met a family whose 9-month old daughter, Paola, was failing to thrive. She was bright-eyed and eager to play with her older siblings, but she simply did not have the strength. The businessman arranged for Paola to be tested at an academic medical center in Spain.

Extensive medical testing revealed that Paola had a ventricular septal defect. She had a pansystolic murmur that was loudest at the left sternal border. Chest radiographs showed enlargement of the left atrium and ventricle, and echocardiography confirmed the presence of a ventricular shunt. On cardiac catheterization, P_{O_2} in the right atrium was 40 mm Hg, and P_{O_2} in the right ventricle was 70 mm Hg. Mixed venous P_{O_2} was 40 mm Hg, and systemic arterial P_{O_2} was 100 mm Hg.

Following surgery to correct the defect, Paola recovered quickly and returned home to her family. The businessman receives periodic updates and photographs, all of which show Paola "growing like a weed" and looking healthier and more robust every day.

 QUESTIONS

1. In children with ventricular septal defects, what is the path of blood flow during the cardiac cycle?

2. What is the direction of Paola's ventricular shunt, and what evidence supports your conclusion?

3. What caused Paola's murmur, and why was it described as "pansystolic"?

4. Explain the observed values for P_{O_2} in the right atrium and right ventricle.

5. Why did Paola have a normal value for systemic arterial P_{O_2}?

6. Paola's congenital ventricular septal defect resulted in a significant ventricular shunt at the time she was seen by physicians. However, if the shunt had been assessed before birth, it would have been very small. Why does a ventricular septal defect not cause a significant shunt in the prenatal period?

ANSWERS AND EXPLANATIONS

1. **Ventricular septal defects** provide an abnormal route for blood flow between the ventricles. Typically, in children, because systolic pressure is higher in the left ventricle than the right ventricle, blood flows from the left side to the right side; the blood that flows through the ventricular septal defect is called a **shunt**.

   During normal systole, all of the cardiac output of the left ventricle flows into the aorta. When a ventricular septal defect is present, a portion of the output of the left ventricle flows through the shunt to the right ventricle (Fig. 2–14). This shunted blood is added to the blood already in the right ventricle, increasing right ventricular end-diastolic volume. On the next beat, because there is increased right ventricular end-diastolic volume, there is increased right heart cardiac output **(Frank–Starling mechanism)**, increased pulmonary artery blood flow, increased venous return to the left atrium, and increased filling of the left ventricle.

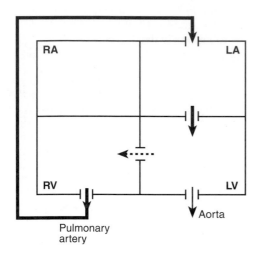

Figure 2–14 Blood flow through ventricular septal defect. The dashed arrow shows the left-to-right shunt through a ventricular septal defect. The heavy arrow shows the path of increased blood flow. The thin, solid arrow shows blood flow through the aortic valve. (LA, left atrium; LV, left ventricle; RA, right atrium; RV, right ventricle.)

2. Paola has a **left-to-right shunt**, a conclusion that is supported by the following observations: (i) there was enlargement of the left atrium and ventricle due to increased venous return to the left side of the heart; (ii) Po_2 was higher in the right ventricle than the right atrium (see Question 4); and (iii) systemic arterial Po_2 was normal (see Question 5).

3. A **pansystolic murmur** exhibits uniform intensity and is heard throughout systole. Paola's murmur was caused by turbulent blood flow through the ventricular septal defect (Fig. 2–15). The murmur began at the onset of ventricular systole, which is marked by closure of the mitral valve (S_1); at this point, although both ventricles are contracting, left ventricular pressure was raised to a higher value than was right ventricular pressure. The difference in left and right ventricular pressures caused blood to flow through the intraventricular defect, from left to right. The murmur ceases at the end of ventricular systole, which is marked by closure of the aortic valve (S_2); at this point, the ventricles relaxed, left ventricular pressure no longer exceeded right ventricular pressure, and flow through the septal defect stopped.

S_1 S_2 **Figure 2–15**   Systolic murmur due to ventricular septal defect.

4. The P_{O_2} of right ventricular blood was higher than the P_{O_2} of right atrial blood, which is a classic observation in persons with a left-to-right ventricular shunt. The reason for this observation is best understood by considering the cardiac circuitry as follows. Mixed venous blood from the systemic tissues has a relatively low P_{O_2} (40 mm Hg) and fills the right heart. "Arterialized" blood that has undergone gas exchange in the lungs has a relatively high P_{O_2} (100 mm Hg) and fills the left heart. In the presence of a left-to-right ventricular shunt, a portion of this arterialized blood flows through the ventricular septal defect into the right ventricle; the arterialized blood mixes with mixed venous blood in the right ventricle, raising overall P_{O_2} in the right ventricle (Fig. 2–16). The composition of right atrial blood is unaffected by a ventricular shunt, and the P_{O_2} of its blood remains at the mixed venous value. In summary, Paola's right atrial blood had a P_{O_2} of 40 mm Hg because that was the value of her mixed venous P_{O_2}. Paola's right ventricular blood had a P_{O_2} of 70 mm Hg because arterialized blood from the left ventricle (P_{O_2}, 100 mm Hg) mixed with mixed venous blood (P_{O_2}, 40 mm Hg). The extent to which right ventricular P_{O_2} is greater than right atrial P_{O_2} depends on the size of the shunt—the larger the shunt, the higher the right ventricular P_{O_2}, and the greater the difference.

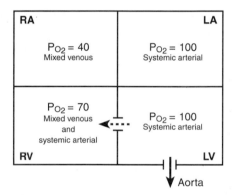

Figure 2–16 Values for P_{O_2} in the presence of a left-to-right ventricular shunt. (LA, left atrium; LV, left ventricle; RA, right atrium; RV, right ventricle.)

5. Paola had a normal value for systemic arterial P_{O_2} (100 mm Hg), as is characteristic of left-to-right shunts. The blood returning to her left heart was arterialized normally in the lungs. A portion of this blood, with its P_{O_2} of 100 mm Hg, was ejected into the systemic arteries; the presence of the shunt does not change the P_{O_2} of this blood.

6. Although Paola's ventricular septal defect was present before birth, it would not have produced a significant left-to-right shunt. What accounts for the difference between the prenatal and postnatal periods? The answer lies in the changes in pulmonary vascular resistance that occur following delivery. Before birth, there is no alveolar ventilation, and consequently there is alveolar hypoxia throughout the lungs. Global alveolar hypoxia causes vasoconstriction throughout the lungs (**hypoxic vasoconstriction**), which increases pulmonary vascular resistance. Increased pulmonary vascular resistance leads to increased pulmonary artery pressure and increased pressures on the right side of the heart; during systole, right ventricular pressure will be as high as left ventricular pressure. Thus, the ventricular septal defect does not cause a significant shunt prenatally because there is not a favorable pressure gradient between the left and right ventricles. At birth, alveolar ventilation begins, there is reversal of hypoxic vasoconstriction, and consequently there is a decrease in pulmonary artery pressure and pressures on the right side of the heart. When right ventricular pressure becomes less than left ventricular pressure during systole, flow through the shunt begins.

Key topics

Frank–Starling mechanism

Hypoxic vasoconstriction

Left-to-right shunt

Pansystolic murmur

S_1

S_2

Ventricular septal defect

Case 19

Aortic Stenosis

Joe Lombardy is an 82-year-old retired carpenter who still does "odd jobs" for friends and neighbors. His wife has pleaded with him to relax, but he ignores her. Despite having chest pains (angina) and periods of confusion, Joe doesn't trust doctors and has stubbornly refused to have a check-up. Recently, though, after several episodes of syncope (fainting) while he was hauling lumber, Joe grudgingly agreed to see a physician.

On physical examination, the physician noted a murmur during systole (described as systolic ejection murmur), a palpable S_4, and a significantly diminished aortic component of S_2. An electrocardiogram (ECG) was consistent with left ventricular hypertrophy. His carotid artery pulse was weak, and had a delayed upstroke. The physician ordered a cardiac catheterization, which showed a pressure gradient of 100 mm Hg between the left ventricle and the aorta during systole, consistent with aortic stenosis.

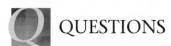 QUESTIONS

1. In aortic stenosis, there is significant narrowing of the aortic valve opening. Why does this narrowing cause a murmur?

2. In aortic stenosis, the murmur occurs during systole (i.e., a systolic ejection murmur). Why? What is the timing of the murmur with respect to S_1 and S_2?

3. What are the components of a normal S_2, and why did Joe have a diminished aortic (A_2) component of S_2?

4. What is the normal pressure gradient between the left ventricle and the aorta during systole? What is the significance of Joe's gradient being 100 mm Hg?

5. Why does left ventricle hypertrophy occur in aortic stenosis?

6. Why was Joe's cerebral arterial pulse weak, and why did it have a delayed upstroke?

7. What is the likely reason for Joe's fainting spells during physical exertion?

8. What is S_4, and why did Joe have a palpable S_4?

9. Congestive heart failure is one consequence of aortic stenosis. Which ventricle fails in aortic stenosis, and where is edema likely to occur?

ANSWERS AND EXPLANATIONS

1. A **murmur** is a sound produced by **turbulent blood flow.** Normally, blood flow is laminar and produces no sound. However, hemodynamic or structural abnormalities in the cardiovascular system can cause blood flow to become turbulent. In the case of aortic stenosis, when blood is ejected from the left ventricle through the partially obstructed aortic valve, it produces a sound (murmur) that is not present when the aortic valve is normal. The tendency of blood flow to be turbulent, rather than laminar, is predicted by the **Reynolds number,** as discussed in Case 14.

2. In **aortic stenosis**, the murmur occurs during ventricular systole (ventricular contraction), because it is during systole that blood flows from the ventricle, through the aortic valve, into the aorta. Ventricular systole consists of an isovolumetric phase and an ejection phase. During the isovolumetric phase, all valves are closed, and therefore no blood is ejected; the ejection phase begins when the aortic valve opens, and it ends when the aortic valve closes. Since the murmur of aortic stenosis occurs because blood is flowing through a stenosed aortic valve, it must occur during ventricular ejection (i.e., *systolic ejection murmur*).

   In aortic stenosis, the murmur begins after S_1 (mitral and tricuspid valve closure) and ends before S_2 (aortic and pulmonic valve closure); that is, it occurs **between S_1 and S_2.** In the left heart, the mitral valve closes at the beginning of isovolumetric contraction (S_1). Following S_1, there is a brief silence during isovolumetric contraction. After the silence, the aortic valve opens, and the murmur is heard as blood is ejected through the stenosed aortic valve. The murmur must end before the aortic valve closes (S_2), because no blood can be ejected through a closed aortic valve.

3. Normal S_2 results from aortic (A_2) and pulmonic (P_2) valve closure. The configuration of S_2 varies with the respiratory cycle. During **expiration,** A_2 occurs before P_2, but they are fused as a single sound. During **inspiration,** however, there is normal **"splitting"** in which A_2 still occurs first, but is separated from P_2, as is shown in Figure 2–17 and explained as follows. During inspiration, intrathoracic pressure becomes more negative, which increases venous return to the right heart; the resulting increase in right ventricular end-diastolic volume and right heart cardiac output delays closure of the pulmonic valve (there is more blood to eject). At the same time, since blood volume in the right heart is increased, venous return to left heart is decreased, which decreases left ventricular cardiac output and causes earlier closure of the aortic valve. Thus, S_2 is split during inspiration for two reasons: P_2 is later than during expiration, and A_2 is earlier than during expiration.

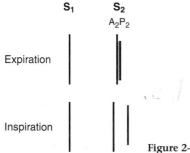

Figure 2–17   Components of normal S_1 and S_2 during inspiration and expiration.

   Joe had a **diminished A_2** because the stenotic aortic valve is relatively fixed; when it closes, it produces less sound than does normal valve closure.

4. During systole, the normal pressure gradient between the left ventricle and the aorta is close to zero. During left ventricular contraction, ventricular pressure increases, and as soon as it exceeds aortic pressure, the aortic valve opens and ejection of blood begins. Thus, during

ventricular ejection, ventricular pressure is normally only slightly higher than aortic pressure. Joe's pressure gradient of 100 mm Hg is very abnormal. During systole, his left ventricular pressure must increase to a value much greater than aortic pressure in order to open the stenosed aortic valve and to eject blood.

5. In aortic stenosis, the left ventricle undergoes **concentric hypertrophy** as a compensatory response. This type of hypertrophy (typical of the response to increased afterload) involves synthesis of new sarcomeres in parallel with old sarcomeres, such that **left ventricular wall thickness increases** but the radius of the left ventricular chamber is unchanged. The increase in wall thickness allows the left ventricle to generate the high pressures required to eject blood through the stenosed aortic valve. Once again, recall the description of these relationships by the **law of Laplace**:

$$P = \frac{HT}{r}$$

   where

   P = ventricular pressure
   H = ventricular wall thickness
   T = wall tension
   r = radius

6. Joe's cerebral arterial pulse was weak, with a delayed upstroke, because left ventricular cardiac output through the stenotic valve is impeded. In other words, blood is not ejected into the systemic arterial vasculature (as represented by the carotid arterial pulse) as swiftly or intensely as it is normally.

7. During exertion, Joe fainted **(syncope)** secondary to **decreased arterial pressure.** At rest, his left ventricle was able to maintain cardiac output (and arterial pressure): by increasing left ventricular pressure to very high levels, a normal cardiac output could be forced through the aortic valve. During exertion, however, he was *unable* to increase his cardiac output through the stenotic valve. Recall that during exercise, there is arteriolar vasodilation in skeletal muscle that results in decreased total peripheral resistance (TPR). **Decreased TPR**, combined with a lack of increase in cardiac output, results in a decrease in arterial pressure (P_a = cardiac output × TPR), a decrease in cerebral blood flow, and syncope.

8. S_4 (the fourth heart sound), when present, occurs late in diastole and coincides with **atrial contraction.** S_4 is not present in normal adults, but can be heard when the left (or right) atrium is filling a stiffened ventricle. In Joe's case, S_4 was present because when his left ventricle hypertrophied, it became stiff and noncompliant. Thus, as his left atrium filled his noncompliant left ventricle, it caused a palpable S_4.

   A related issue in aortic stenosis is that atrial contraction becomes more important when the atrium needs to fill a noncompliant left ventricle. (Normally, filling of the ventricle is primarily passive, and atrial contraction adds very little.) Over time, the left atrium also hypertrophies as a compensatory response to filling the noncompliant left ventricle.

9. Aortic stenosis can lead to **congestive heart failure.** As the stenosis worsens, eventually the left ventricle may not be able to raise its pressure enough to eject a normal cardiac output (i.e., *left* ventricular failure). When this happens, blood "backs up" behind the left ventricle, into the left atrium and pulmonary veins. The resulting increase in pulmonary venous pressure causes increased pulmonary capillary pressure, increased filtration from the pulmonary capillaries, and **pulmonary edema.**

Key topics

A_2

P_2

S_1

S_2

S_4

Aortic stenosis

Arterial pressure

Concentric hypertrophy

Congestive heart failure

Law of Laplace

Pulmonary edema

Reynolds number

Systolic ejection murmur

Turbulent blood flow

Case 20

Atrioventricular Conduction Block

Charles Doucette, who is 68 years old, retired from a middle management position in the automotive industry following an acute myocardial infarction. He was recovering in a local hospital, where the physicians closely monitored his ECG (Fig. 2–18).

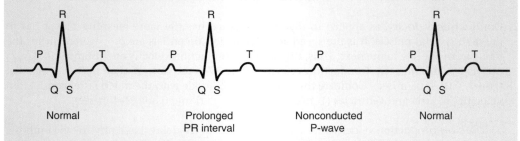

Normal   Prolonged   Nonconducted   Normal
PR interval   P-wave

Figure 2–18 Effect of atrioventricular conduction block on the electrocardiogram

    Mr. Doucette's PR intervals were longer than normal. Although his QRS complexes had a normal configuration, there were occasional P-waves that were not followed by QRS complexes (nonconducted P-waves). He fainted twice in the hospital. The physicians believed that the myocardial infarction caused a block in his atrioventricular (AV) conducting system. While they were discussing the possibility of treating him with atropine, his ECG returned to normal. Mr. Doucette had no more fainting episodes, and he was sent home without further treatment.

 QUESTIONS

1. What does the PR interval on the ECG represent? What units are used to express the PR interval? What is the normal value?

2. What does the term "conduction velocity" mean, as applied to myocardial tissue? What is the normal conduction velocity through the AV node? How does conduction velocity in the AV node compare with conduction velocity in other portions of the heart?

3. How does AV nodal conduction velocity correlate with PR interval? Why were Mr. Doucette's PR intervals longer than normal?

4. What does the QRS complex on the ECG represent? What is implied in the information that the QRS complexes on Mr. Doucette's ECG had a normal configuration?

5. How is it possible to have P-waves that are not followed by QRS complexes? Explain this phenomenon in light of a presumed decreased AV node conduction velocity.

6. Why did Mr. Doucette faint?

7. How might atropine have helped Mr. Doucette?

ANSWERS AND EXPLANATIONS

1. The **PR interval** on the ECG represents the time from initial depolarization of the atria to initial depolarization of the ventricles (i.e., beginning of the **P-wave** to beginning of the R-wave). Therefore, the PR interval includes the P-wave (atrial depolarization) and the **PR segment,** an isoelectric portion of the ECG that corresponds to conduction through the **AV node.** Because PR interval is a *time,* its units are given in seconds (sec) or milliseconds (msec). You may have needed to look up the normal value for PR interval, which is 120 to 200 msec (average, 160 msec).

2. **Conduction velocity,** as applied to myocardial tissue, has the same meaning that it has in nerve or skeletal muscle. It is the speed at which action potentials are propagated within the tissue from one site to the next. Thus, the units for conduction velocity are distance/time (e.g., meters/seconds [m/sec]). Conduction velocity in the AV is the slowest of all of the myocardial tissues (0.01–0.05 m/sec). Compare this value in the AV node with the much faster conduction velocities in atria and ventricles (1 m/sec) and in His–Purkinje tissue (2–4 m/sec).

   The slow conduction velocity through the AV node, or **AV delay,** has a physiologic purpose: it ensures that the ventricles will not be activated "too soon" after the atria are activated, thus allowing adequate time for ventricular filling prior to ventricular contraction.

3. The slower the conduction velocity through the AV node, the longer the PR interval (because the length of the PR segment is increased). Conversely, the faster the conduction velocity through the AV node, the shorter the PR interval. Mr. Doucette's PR intervals were longer than normal because the conduction velocity through the AV node was decreased, presumably because of tissue damage caused by the myocardial infarction.

4. The **QRS complex** on the ECG corresponds to electrical activation of the ventricles. The normal configuration of Mr. Doucette's QRS complexes implies that his ventricles were activated in the normal sequence (i.e., the spread of activation was from the AV node through the bundle of His to the ventricular muscle).

5. Mr. Doucette's ECG showed some P-waves that were not followed by QRS complexes. AV nodal conduction was slowed so much that some impulses were not conducted *at all* from atria to ventricles. This observation is consistent with increased AV delay and increased PR interval.

6. Mr. Doucette fainted because his arterial pressure was decreased, which caused a decrease in cerebral blood flow. The decrease in arterial pressure is likely related to the absent QRS complexes on the ECG. Each cardiac cycle without a QRS complex is a cardiac cycle in which electrical activation of the ventricles did not occur. If the ventricles were not activated electrically, they did not contract; if they did not contract, they did not eject blood, and mean arterial pressure decreased.

7. The rationale for treating Mr. Doucette with **atropine** is based on the effect of the **parasympathetic nervous system** on conduction velocity in the AV node. Parasympathetic nerves innervating the AV node release acetylcholine, which activates **muscarinic receptors** and decreases AV node conduction velocity. Therefore, atropine (a muscarinic receptor antagonist) opposes this parasympathetic effect and increases AV node conduction velocity.

Key topics

Atropine

Atrioventricular (AV) node

Atrioventricular (AV) delay

Conduction velocity

Electrocardiogram

Muscarinic receptors

P-wave

Parasympathetic nervous system

PR interval

PR segment

QRS complex

Respiratory Physiology

Case 21

Essential Respiratory Calculations: Lung Volumes, Dead Space, and Alveolar Ventilation

This case will guide you through some of the important, basic calculations involving the respiratory system. Use the information provided to answer the questions.

Figure 3–1 shows a record from a person breathing into and out of a spirometer. The volume displaced by the spirometer's bell is recorded on calibrated paper. The person took one normal breath followed by a maximal inhalation, a maximal exhalation, and another normal breath. (The volume remaining in the lungs after maximal expiration is not measurable by spirometry and was determined by other techniques.)

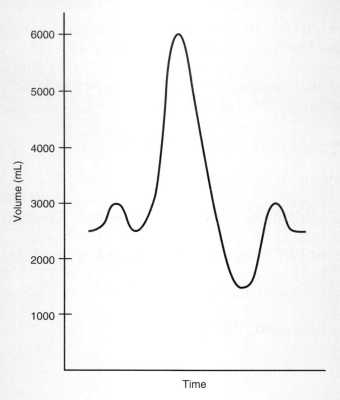

Figure 3–1 Spirometry diagram showing a tidal breath, followed by maximal inspiration and maximal expiration.

TABLE 3–1	*Respiratory Values for Case 21*
Breathing rate	12 breaths/min
Pa_{CO_2} (arterial P_{CO_2})	40 mm Hg
Pa_{O_2} (arterial P_{O_2})	100 mm Hg
Pe_{CO_2} (P_{CO_2} in expired air)	30 mm Hg
Pi_{O_2} (P_{O_2} in humidified inspired air)	150 mm Hg
Pi_{CO_2} (P_{CO_2} in inspired air)	0
$\dot{V}_{CO_2}$ (rate of CO_2 production)	200 mL/min
$\dot{V}_{O_2}$ (rate of O_2 consumption)	250 mL/min

P_{CO_2}, partial pressure of carbon dioxide; P_{O_2}, partial pressure of oxygen.

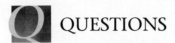 QUESTIONS

1. Using the information provided in Table 3–1 and Figure 3–1, what are the values for tidal volume, inspiratory capacity, expiratory reserve volume, functional residual capacity, vital capacity, and total lung capacity? (Hint: It may be helpful to label the spirometry diagram with the names of the lung volumes and capacities.)

2. What is the name of the volume remaining in the lungs after maximal expiration that is not measurable by spirometry? What other lung volumes or capacities are not measurable by spirometry?

3. What is the meaning of the term "physiologic dead space?" What assumptions are made in calculating the physiologic dead space? What is the volume of the physiologic dead space in this case?

4. What is the value for minute ventilation?

5. What is the value for alveolar ventilation?

6. What is the alveolar ventilation equation? What is the relationship between alveolar ventilation and alveolar P_{CO_2} ($P_{A_{CO_2}}$)?

7. What is the value for alveolar partial pressure of oxygen ($P_{A_{O_2}}$)?

ANSWERS AND EXPLANATIONS

1. Static **lung volumes** (except for residual volume) are measured by **spirometry**. They include the tidal volume, **inspiratory reserve volume**, expiratory reserve volume, and residual volume. **Lung capacities** include two or more lung volumes. If you began by labeling the lung volumes and capacities, as shown in Figure 3–2 and Table 3–2, then determining the numerical values should be a straightforward exercise.

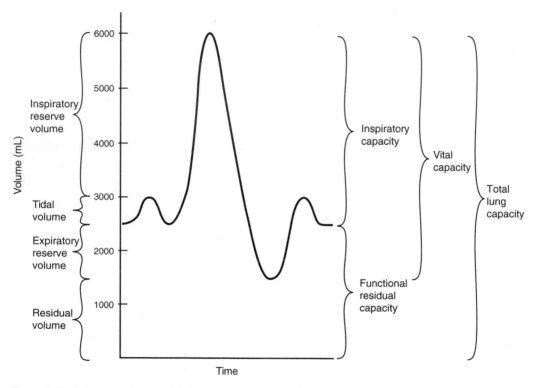

Figure 3–2 Spirometry diagram labeled with lung volumes and capacities.

TABLE 3–2	Lung Volumes and Capacities in Case 21
Tidal volume	500 mL
Inspiratory capacity	3,500 mL
Expiratory reserve volume	1,000 mL
Functional residual capacity	2,500 mL
Vital capacity	4,500 mL
Total lung capacity	6,000 mL

2. The volume remaining in the lungs after maximal expiration is called the **residual volume.** This volume is not measurable by spirometry. Therefore, any lung volume or capacity that includes the residual volume is also not measurable by spirometry (i.e., functional residual capacity, total lung capacity).

3. **Physiologic dead space** is the volume of air in the lungs that does not participate in gas exchange (i.e., it is "dead"). Physiologic dead space has two components: (i) **anatomic dead space**, which is the volume of conducting airways; and (ii) functional dead space, which is made up of alveoli that do not participate in gas exchange (i.e., alveoli that are ventilated, but are not perfused by pulmonary capillary blood). By comparing the physiologic dead space with the tidal volume, it is possible to estimate how much ventilation is "wasted."

The volume of the physiologic dead space is estimated with a method based on the P_{CO_2} of expired air ($P_{E_{CO_2}}$) that applies the following three assumptions. (i) There is no CO_2 in inspired air (i.e., $P_{I_{CO_2}} = 0$). (ii) The physiologic dead space does not participate in gas exchange; therefore, it does not contribute any CO_2 to expired air. (iii) All of the CO_2 in expired air comes from the exchange of CO_2 in functioning alveoli.

When discussing physiologic dead space, it is helpful to consider two examples, one in which there is *no* physiologic dead space and the other in which *some* degree of physiologic dead space is present. If there is *no* physiologic dead space, $P_{E_{CO_2}}$ should equal the P_{CO_2} in alveolar air ($P_{A_{CO_2}}$). If there *is* a physiologic dead space present, then $P_{E_{CO_2}}$ will be "diluted" by air expired from the dead space (air that contains no CO_2), and $P_{E_{CO_2}}$ will be less than $P_{A_{CO_2}}$.

One problem in comparing the P_{CO_2} of alveolar and expired air is that alveolar air cannot be sampled directly; in other words, we cannot measure $P_{A_{CO_2}}$. This problem can be solved, however, because alveolar gas normally equilibrates with pulmonary capillary blood (which becomes systemic arterial blood). Thus, by measuring arterial P_{CO_2} ($P_{a_{CO_2}}$), we can determine $P_{A_{CO_2}}$. Using the foregoing assumptions, **physiologic dead space** is calculated as follows:

$$V_D = V_T \times \frac{P_{a_{CO_2}} - P_{E_{CO_2}}}{P_{a_{CO_2}}}$$

where

$$V_D = \text{physiologic dead space (mL)}$$
$$V_T = \text{tidal volume (mL)}$$
$$P_{a_{CO_2}} = P_{CO_2} \text{ of arterial blood (mm Hg)}$$
$$P_{E_{CO_2}} = P_{CO_2} \text{ of expired air (mm Hg)}$$

In words, physiologic dead space is the tidal volume multiplied by a fraction that expresses the dilution of alveolar P_{CO_2} by dead-space air.

We have all of the values we need to calculate the physiologic dead space in this case. Tidal volume was determined from spirometry, and the values for $P_{a_{CO_2}}$ and $P_{E_{CO_2}}$ are given in the case data.

$$V_D = V_T \times \frac{P_{a_{CO_2}} - P_{E_{CO_2}}}{P_{a_{CO_2}}}$$

$$= 500 \text{ mL} \times \frac{40 \text{ mm Hg} - 30 \text{ mm Hg}}{40 \text{ mm Hg}}$$

$$= 500 \text{ mL} \times 0.25$$

$$= 125 \text{ mL}$$

Thus, in the tidal volume of 500 mL, 125 mL occupied the physiologic dead space (i.e., the conducting airways and nonfunctional alveoli). In other words, 125 mL was "wasted" in lung spaces that cannot participate in gas exchange.

4. **Minute ventilation** is the tidal volume multiplied by the number of breaths per minute. In this case:

$$\text{Minute ventilation} = V_T \times \text{breaths/min}$$
$$= 500 \text{ mL} \times 12/\text{min}$$
$$= 6{,}000 \text{ mL/min}$$

5. **Alveolar ventilation** ($\dot{V}_A$) is minute ventilation corrected for physiologic dead space, or:

$$\dot{V}_A = (V_T - V_D) \times \text{breaths/min}$$

where

$\dot{V}_A$ = alveolar ventilation (mL/min)
V_T = tidal volume (mL)
V_D = physiologic dead space (mL)

In this case, tidal volume was determined by spirometry (500 mL), and physiologic dead space was calculated in the previous question (125 mL). Thus, alveolar ventilation is:

$$\dot{V}_A = (500 \text{ mL} - 125 \text{ mL}) \times 12 \text{ breaths/min}$$
$$= 375 \text{ mL} \times 12 \text{ breaths/min}$$
$$= 4{,}500 \text{ mL/min}$$

6. In considering these questions about alveolar ventilation and alveolar P_{CO_2}, perhaps you wondered what alveolar ventilation has to do with alveolar P_{CO_2}. The answer is everything! The fundamental relationship in respiratory physiology is an inverse correlation between alveolar ventilation (the volume of air reaching functional alveoli per minute) and alveolar P_{CO_2}. If CO_2 production is constant, the higher the alveolar ventilation, the more CO_2 expired, and the lower the arterial P_{CO_2}. Since alveolar P_{CO_2} equilibrates with arterial P_{CO_2}, the higher the alveolar ventilation, the lower the alveolar P_{CO_2}. Conversely, the lower the alveolar ventilation, the less CO_2 expired, and the higher the arterial and alveolar P_{CO_2}. This relationship is expressed by the **alveolar ventilation equation:**

$$\dot{V}_A = \frac{\dot{V}_{CO_2} \times K}{P_{A_{CO_2}}}$$

where

$P_{A_{CO_2}}$ = alveolar P_{CO_2} (mm Hg)
$\dot{V}_A$ = alveolar ventilation (mL/min)
$\dot{V}_{CO_2}$ = rate of CO_2 production (mL/min)
K = constant (863 mm Hg at body temperature, ambient pressure, and gas saturated with water vapor)

7. Because we cannot sample alveolar gas, we cannot directly measure $P_{A_{O_2}}$. However, we can use the following approach to estimate its value. $P_{A_{O_2}}$ is determined by the balance between removal of O_2 from alveolar gas (to meet the body's demands for O_2) and replenishment of O_2 by alveolar ventilation. Therefore, if O_2 consumption is constant, alveolar P_{O_2} is determined by alveolar ventilation (just as alveolar P_{CO_2} is determined by alveolar ventilation).

This relationship is expressed by the **alveolar gas equation**, which incorporates the factors that determine $P_{A_{O_2}}$ (including partial pressure of O_2 in inspired air [$P_{I_{O_2}}$]), $P_{A_{CO_2}}$ (which reflects alveolar ventilation, as explained earlier), and **respiratory quotient** (R, the ratio of CO_2 production to O_2 consumption):

$$PA_{O_2} = PI_{O_2} - \frac{PA_{CO_2}}{R}$$

where

PA_{O2} = alveolar P_{O2} (mm Hg)
PI_{O2} = P_{O2} in inspired air (mm Hg)
PA_{CO2} = alveolar P_{CO2} (mm Hg)
R = respiratory quotient (ratio of CO_2 production to O_2 consumption)

In this case, the value for PI_{O2} (150 mm Hg) was given, the value for Pa_{CO2} and PA_{CO2} (40 mm Hg) was given, and the value for respiratory quotient can be calculated as the rate of CO_2 production (200 mL/min) divided by the rate of O_2 consumption (250 mL/min), or 0.8.

$$PA_{O_2} = 150 \text{ mm Hg} - \frac{40 \text{ mm Hg}}{0.8}$$
$$= 150 \text{ mm Hg} - 50 \text{ mm Hg}$$
$$= 100 \text{ mm Hg}$$

Key topics

Alveolar gas equation
Alveolar ventilation
Alveolar ventilation equation
Anatomic dead space
Expiratory reserve volume
Functional residual capacity
Inspiratory capacity
Inspiratory reserve volume
Minute ventilation
Physiologic dead space
Residual volume
Respiratory quotient
Spirometry
Tidal volume
Total lung capacity
Vital capacity

Case 22

Essential Respiratory Calculations: Gases and Gas Exchange

Using O_2 as an example, this case guides you through important, basic calculations involving partial pressures of gases and concentrations of gases in solutions such as blood. Use the information provided in Table 3–3 to answer the questions.

TABLE 3–3	Respiratory Values for Case 22	
P_B (barometric pressure)		760 mm Hg (at sea level)
P_{H_2O} (water vapor pressure)		47 mm Hg at 37°C
F_{IO_2} (fractional concentration of O_2 in inspired air)		0.21 (or 21%)
P_{AO_2} (alveolar P_{O_2})		100 mm Hg
Solubility of O_2 in blood		0.003 mL O_2/100 mL blood/mm Hg
Hemoglobin concentration of blood		15 g/dL
O_2-binding capacity of blood		20.1 mL O_2/100 mL blood
% Saturation		98%

P_{O_2} partial pressure of oxygen.

 QUESTIONS

1. What is the partial pressure of O_2 (P_{O_2}) in dry air at sea level?

2. When inspired air enters the trachea, it is saturated with water vapor (humidified). What is the P_{O_2} of humidified tracheal air at sea level?

3. The value for alveolar P_{O_2} (P_{AO_2}) is given as 100 mm Hg. Assuming complete equilibration of O_2 across the alveolar–pulmonary capillary barrier, what is the value for P_{O_2} in pulmonary capillary blood? How does this equilibration occur? What is the concentration of dissolved O_2 in that blood?

4. The total O_2 content of blood includes dissolved O_2 and O_2 bound to hemoglobin (O_2-hemoglobin). What is the total O_2 content of the blood in this case? What fraction of the total O_2 content is O_2-hemoglobin?

5. If the hemoglobin concentration is reduced from 15 g/dL to 9 g/dL, how would this reduction alter the amount of O_2-hemoglobin? How would it alter the amount of dissolved O_2? How would it alter the total O_2 content of blood?

6. If alveolar P_{O_2} is reduced from 100 mm Hg to 50 mm Hg, how would this reduction alter pulmonary capillary P_{O_2}? How would it alter the concentration of dissolved O_2 in pulmonary capillary blood? How would it alter the total O_2 content?

ANSWERS ON NEXT PAGE

ANSWERS AND EXPLANATIONS

1. **Dalton's law of partial pressures** states that the partial pressure of a gas in a mixture of gases (e.g., in atmospheric air) is the pressure that the gas would exert if it occupied the total volume of the mixture. Therefore, **partial pressure** is the total pressure (e.g., atmospheric pressure) multiplied by the fractional concentration of the gas:

   $$P_X = P_B \times F$$

   where

   P_X = partial pressure of the gas (mm Hg)
   P_B = barometric pressure (mm Hg)
   F = fractional concentration of the gas (no units)

   Thus, the P_{O_2} in dry air at a barometric pressure of 760 mm Hg is:

   $$
   \begin{aligned}
   P_{O_2} &= 760 \text{ mm Hg} \times 0.21 \\
   &= 159.6 \text{ mm Hg}
   \end{aligned}
   $$

2. When inspired air is humidified in the trachea, water vapor becomes an obligatory component of the gas mixture. To calculate the P_{O_2} of humidified air, barometric pressure must be corrected for water vapor pressure:

   $$P_X = (P_B - P_{H_2O}) \times F$$

   where

   P_X = partial pressure of the gas in humidified air (mm Hg)
   P_B = barometric pressure (mm Hg)
   F = fractional concentration of the gas (no units)
   P_{H_2O} = water vapor pressure (47 mm Hg at 37°C)

   Thus, the P_{O_2} of humidified tracheal air is:

   $$
   \begin{aligned}
   P_{O_2} &= (760 \text{ mm Hg} - 47 \text{ mm Hg}) \times 0.21 \\
   &= 149.7 \text{ mm Hg}
   \end{aligned}
   $$

3. Normally, pulmonary capillary blood equilibrates almost completely with alveolar gas. Therefore, if alveolar gas has a P_{O_2} of 100 mm Hg, pulmonary capillary blood will also have a P_{O_2} of 100 mm Hg, which occurs as follows. O_2 is transferred from alveolar gas into pulmonary capillary blood by **simple diffusion**. The driving force for this diffusion is the partial pressure difference for O_2 between alveolar gas and pulmonary capillary blood (Fig. 3–3).

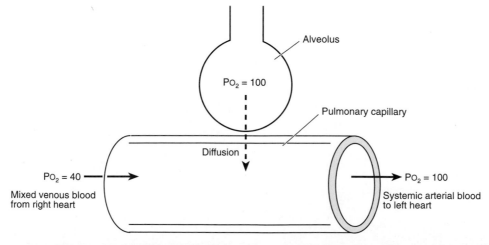

Figure 3–3 Diffusion of O_2 from alveolar gas into pulmonary capillary blood. (P_{O_2}, partial pressure of oxygen.)

Mixed venous blood from the right side of the heart enters the pulmonary capillaries with a relatively low P_{O_2} (approximately 40 mm Hg). Alveolar gas has a much higher P_{O_2} (approximately 100 mm Hg). Thus, initially, there is a large partial pressure gradient (driving force) for diffusion of O_2 from alveolar gas into the pulmonary capillary. O_2 diffuses into the blood until the P_{O_2} of pulmonary capillary blood is equal to the P_{CO_2} of alveolar gas (100 mm Hg). Once equilibration has occurred, there is no longer a driving force for further diffusion of O_2. This equilibrated blood leaves the pulmonary capillaries, enters the left side of the heart, and becomes systemic arterial blood.

According to **Henry's law,** the *concentration* of dissolved O_2 depends on the partial pressure of O_2 in the liquid phase (e.g., blood) and the solubility of O_2 in that liquid:

Cx = Px × solubility

where

$\quad\quad\quad$ Cx = concentration of dissolved gas (mL gas/100 mL blood)
$\quad\quad\quad$ Px = partial pressure of the gas (mm Hg)
$\quad$ Solubility = solubility of gas in blood (mL gas/100 mL blood/mm Hg)

As discussed earlier, the P_{O_2} of pulmonary capillary blood is 100 mm Hg. The solubility of O_2 is given in the case as 0.003 mL O_2/100 mL blood/mm Hg. Thus:

$\quad$ Dissolved $[O_2]$ = 100 mm Hg × 0.003 mL O_2/100 mL blood/mm Hg
$\quad\quad\quad\quad\quad\quad$ = 0.3 mL O_2/100 mL blood

4. The **O_2 content of blood** includes dissolved O_2 and O_2 bound to hemoglobin. In the previous question, we discussed the dissolved form of O_2 (which depends on P_{O_2} and the solubility of O_2 in blood) and calculated its value.

Now, what determines the amount of O_2 present as **O_2-hemoglobin** (the bound form)? The amount of O_2-hemoglobin depends on the **hemoglobin concentration** of the blood, the **O_2-binding capacity** of the hemoglobin (i.e., the maximum amount of O_2 that can be bound), and the **percent saturation** of hemoglobin by O_2. This last point is very important! The hemoglobin molecule has four subunits, each of which can bind one molecule of O_2, for a total of four O_2 molecules per hemoglobin. Thus, 100% saturation means four O_2 molecules per hemoglobin, 75% saturation means three O_2 molecules per hemoglobin, and so forth. The percent saturation of hemoglobin depends on the P_{O_2} of the blood, as described by the **O_2–hemoglobin dissociation curve** (Fig. 3–4). When P_{O_2} is 100 mm Hg, hemoglobin is 100% saturated; when P_{O_2} is 50 mm Hg, hemoglobin is approximately 85% saturated; and when P_{O_2} is 25 mm Hg, hemoglobin is 50% saturated. (The P_{O_2} at which hemoglobin is 50% saturated is called the **P_{50}**.)

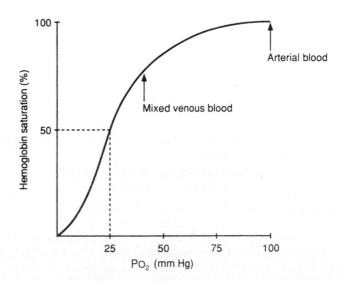

Figure 3–4 O_2–hemoglobin dissociation curve. (P_{O_2}, partial pressure of oxygen.)

Thus, the amount of O_2 bound to hemoglobin is calculated by multiplying the O_2-binding capacity of hemoglobin times the percent saturation, both of which are given in the case.

$$O_2\text{-hemoglobin} = O_2\text{-binding capacity} \times \%\text{ saturation}$$
$$= 20.1 \text{ mL } O_2/100 \text{ mL blood} \times 98\%$$
$$= 19.7 \text{ mL } O_2/100 \text{ mL blood}$$

Finally, the total O_2 content is the sum of dissolved O_2 and O_2-hemoglobin:

$$\text{Total } O_2 \text{ content} = \text{dissolved } O_2 + O_2\text{-hemoglobin}$$
$$= 0.3 \text{ mL } O_2/100 \text{ blood} + 19.7 \text{ mL } O_2/100 \text{ mL blood}$$
$$= 20.0 \text{ mL } O_2/100 \text{ mL blood}$$

O_2-hemoglobin is 98% of the total O_2 content (i.e., 19.7/20.0).

5. If the hemoglobin concentration is 9 g/dL instead of 15 g/dL, the O_2 content of blood is reduced because the O_2-hemoglobin component is reduced. What is the new value for the total O_2 content? In the previous calculation of O_2-hemoglobin content, we didn't use the hemoglobin concentration because the O_2-binding capacity of the blood was given (20.1 mL O_2/100 mL). To determine the effect of a reduction in hemoglobin concentration on the O_2-hemoglobin content, we simply need to calculate how such a change will alter the O_2-binding capacity of blood (i.e., in this case, it will be reduced to 9/15 of the original O_2-binding capacity).

$$O_2\text{-binding capacity} = 9/15 \times 20.1 \text{ mL } O_2/100 \text{ mL blood}$$
$$= 12.1 \text{ mL } O_2/100 \text{ mL blood}$$

Now we can calculate the amount of O_2 bound to hemoglobin, assuming that percent saturation is not affected by a reduction in hemoglobin concentration:

$$O_2\text{-hemoglobin} = O_2\text{-binding capacity} \times \%\text{ saturation}$$
$$= 12.1 \text{ mL } O_2/100 \text{ mL blood} \times 98\%$$
$$= 11.9 \text{ mL } O_2/100 \text{ mL blood}$$

We know that the total O_2 content is the sum of O_2-hemoglobin and dissolved O_2. We also know that O_2-hemoglobin is quantitatively much more important than dissolved O_2 and that O_2-hemoglobin is decreased by a decrease in hemoglobin concentration (discussed earlier). However, might dissolved O_2 also be altered by such a change in hemoglobin concentration, perhaps because of a change in P_{O_2}? The answer is that, if anything, P_{O_2} will be slightly increased. (If less O_2 is bound to hemoglobin, because less hemoglobin is available, more O_2 will be free in solution.) However, normally, the contribution of dissolved O_2 to total O_2 content is so small that it is insignificant. For this reason, we can safely use the original value for dissolved O_2 (0.3 mL O_2/100 mL blood) that we calculated in Question 3. Therefore, total O_2 content at a reduced hemoglobin concentration of 9 g/dL is:

$$\text{Total } O_2 \text{ content} = O_2\text{-hemoglobin} + \text{dissolved } O_2$$
$$= 11.9 \text{ mL } O_2/100 \text{ mL blood} + 0.3 \text{ mL } O_2/100 \text{ mL blood}$$
$$= 12.2 \text{ mL } O_2/100 \text{ mL blood}$$

Such a reduction in hemoglobin concentration (e.g., as occurs in **anemia**) has a profound effect on the O_2 content of the blood; the total O_2 content is reduced to 60% of normal (i.e., 12.2/20.0)!

6. If alveolar P_{O_2} is 50 mm Hg and O_2 equilibration is assumed to be normal, then pulmonary capillary P_{O_2} is also 50 mm Hg. The dissolved O_2 concentration is the P_{O_2} multiplied by the solubility of O_2 in blood, or:

$$\text{Dissolved } [O_2] = 50 \text{ mm Hg} \times 0.003 \text{ mL } O_2/100 \text{ mL blood/mm Hg}$$
$$= 0.15 \text{ mL } O_2/100 \text{ mL blood}$$

What about the amount of O_2 that is bound to hemoglobin? Will it be altered if P_{O_2} is reduced to 50 mm Hg? Recall that the amount of O_2 bound to hemoglobin depends on the O_2-binding capacity, hemoglobin concentration, the number of available binding sites, and the percent saturation of hemoglobin by O_2. When the P_{O_2} is 50 mm Hg, the percent saturation is reduced, which reduces the amount of O_2 bound to hemoglobin. Using the O_2–hemoglobin dissociation curve (see Fig. 3–4), the percent saturation at a P_{O_2} of 50 mm Hg can be estimated to be approximately 85%.

$$
\begin{aligned}
O_2\text{-hemoglobin} &= O_2\text{-binding capacity of blood} \times \%\text{ saturation} \\
&= 20.1 \text{ mL } O_2/100 \text{ mL blood} \times 85\% \\
&= 17.1 \text{ mL } O_2/100 \text{ mL blood}
\end{aligned}
$$

Using these calculated values of dissolved O_2 and O_2-hemoglobin, the total O_2 content at a P_{O_2} of 50 mm Hg is:

$$
\begin{aligned}
\text{Total } O_2 \text{ content} &= \text{dissolved } O_2 + O_2\text{-hemoglobin} \\
&= 0.15 \text{ mL } O_2/100 \text{ mL blood} + 17.1 \text{ mL } O_2/100 \text{ mL blood} \\
&= 17.3 \text{ mL } O_2/100 \text{ mL blood}
\end{aligned}
$$

Thus, at a P_{O_2} of 50 mm Hg (assuming a normal hemoglobin concentration and normal O_2-binding capacity), the total amount of O_2 in blood is severely reduced compared with normal, *primarily* because the amount of O_2 bound to hemoglobin is reduced. (The change in dissolved O_2 makes little difference.)

Key topics

Dalton's law of partial pressures

Diffusion

Henry's law

O_2-binding capacity

O_2 content of blood

O_2-hemoglobin

O_2-hemoglobin dissociation curve

Partial pressure

P_{50}

Percent saturation

Case 23

Ascent to High Altitude

Dan Hsieh celebrated his graduation from college by joining a mountain climbing expedition in the French Alps. Dan is in excellent physical condition: he runs 3 to 5 miles daily, and he played intramural soccer, volleyball, and rugby throughout college. At the insistence of his parents, Dan underwent a complete medical examination before the climb, which he passed with flying colors. He was off to the Alps!

 QUESTIONS

1. Mont Blanc, the highest elevation in the French Alps, is 15,771 feet above sea level. The barometric pressure on Mont Blanc is approximately 420 mm Hg. (The barometric pressure at sea level is 760 mm Hg.) What is the fractional concentration of O_2 (F_{IO_2}) in atmospheric air on Mont Blanc? What is the partial pressure of oxygen (P_{O_2}) of humidified air on Mont Blanc? How does this value of P_{O_2} compare with the P_{O_2} of humidified air at sea level?

2. At his physical examination (performed at sea level), Dan's arterial P_{O_2} (Pa_{O_2}) was 100 mm Hg. If Dan's Pa_{O_2} had been measured when he arrived on Mont Blanc, it would have been approximately 50 mm Hg. Why would his Pa_{O_2} be decreased at the higher elevation? What was Dan's alveolar P_{O_2} (PA_{O_2}) on Mont Blanc?

3. Predict whether each of the following parameters would be increased, decreased, or unchanged on Mont Blanc. Explain why each of the predicted changes would occur.

   - Breathing rate.
   - Percent saturation of hemoglobin.
   - P_{O_2} at which hemoglobin is 50% saturated (P_{50}).
   - Pulmonary artery pressure.

4. If Dan's arterial P_{CO_2} (Pa_{CO_2}) had been measured on Mont Blanc, would it have been increased, decreased, or unchanged compared with normal? Why? If you predicted a change in Pa_{CO_2}, what effect would this change have had on arterial pH? What acid–base disorder would it have caused?

5. The climbers were encouraged to breathe from tanks of 100% O_2. What is the P_{O_2} of 100% humidified O_2 on Mont Blanc? What effect would breathing 100% O_2 have had on Dan's Pa_{O_2}? What effect would it have had on his breathing rate?

6. The physician suggested that Dan take acetazolamide, a carbonic anhydrase inhibitor, prophylactically. Which of the responses and changes that you predicted in Questions 3 and 4 would have been eliminated or offset if Dan took acetazolamide?

ANSWERS ON NEXT PAGE

ANSWERS AND EXPLANATIONS

1. Although the barometric pressure on Mont Blanc is much lower than that at sea level, the F_{IO_2} is the same (0.21, or 21%). We calculate the P_{O_2} in humidified air by correcting the barometric pressure (P_B) for water vapor pressure (P_{H_2O}), and then multiplying this figure by F_{IO_2} (as described in Case 22).

$$\begin{aligned} P_{O_2} \text{ (Mont Blanc)} &= (P_B - P_{H_2O}) \times F_{IO_2} \\ &= (420 \text{ mm Hg} - 47 \text{ mm Hg}) \times 0.21 \\ &= 78.3 \text{ mm Hg} \\ P_{O_2} \text{ (sea level)} &= (P_B - P_{H_2O}) \times F_{IO_2} \\ &= (760 \text{ mm Hg} - 47 \text{ mm Hg}) \times 0.21 \\ &= 149.7 \text{ mm Hg} \end{aligned}$$

Thus, the P_{O_2} of humidified air on Mont Blanc is much lower than the P_{O_2} of humidified air at sea level because of the lower barometric pressure at the higher altitude.

2. Dan's P_{aO_2} would be greatly reduced (**hypoxemia**) on Mont Blanc because, as demonstrated in the previous question, the air he breathed on Mont Blanc had a much lower P_{O_2} (78.3 mm Hg) than the air he breathed at sea level (149.7 mm Hg).

Such a decrease in inspired P_{O_2} would be reflected in a decreased alveolar P_{O_2} (P_{AO_2}). How can we estimate what his P_{AO_2} might have been? One approach is to assume that O_2 equilibrates between alveolar gas and pulmonary capillary blood (systemic arterial blood). If Dan's measured P_{aO_2} was 50 mm Hg, then his P_{AO_2} can be assumed to be 50 mm Hg.

3. On Mont Blanc, the following changes are predicted:

- Dan's breathing rate would be *increased* (**hyperventilation**) because decreased P_{aO_2} stimulates **peripheral chemoreceptors** in the carotid bodies located near the bifurcation of the common carotid arteries. When **P_{aO_2} is less than 60 mm Hg**, these chemoreceptors are strongly stimulated. This information is then relayed to medullary respiratory centers that direct an increase in breathing rate. In other words, the body is calling for more O_2!

- **Percent saturation of hemoglobin** would be *decreased* because P_{aO_2} is decreased. Figure 3–5 shows the effect of P_{O_2} on percent saturation of hemoglobin.

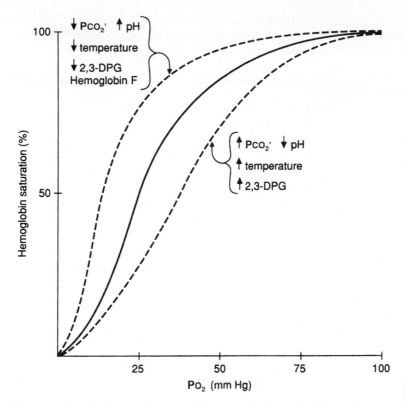

Figure 3–5 Changes in the O_2–hemoglobin dissociation curve showing the effects of partial pressure of carbon dioxide (P_{CO2}), pH, temperature, 2,3-diphosphoglycerate (DPG), and fetal hemoglobin (hemoglobin F). (P_{O2}, partial pressure of oxygen.) (Reprinted, with permission, from Costanzo LS. *BRS Physiology.* 4th ed. Baltimore: Lippincott Williams & Wilkins; 2007:132.)

In Figure 3–5, the solid line shows the normal O_2 hemoglobin relationship that was discussed in Case 21. At a Pa_{O2} of 50 mm Hg, hemoglobin would be approximately 85% saturated, which would significantly decrease the total O_2 content of Dan's blood and compromise O_2 delivery to his tissues.

- P_{50} would be *increased* because there is a **right shift of the O_2–hemoglobin dissociation curve** on ascent to high altitude. This right shift occurs because hypoxemia stimulates the synthesis of **2,3-diphosphoglycerate (DPG)**. 2,3-DPG binds to hemoglobin and decreases its affinity for O_2. This **decreased affinity** is a helpful adaptation at high altitude that facilitates unloading of O_2 in the tissues.

  Notice also the effect of the right shift on percent saturation; at a P_{O2} of 50 mm Hg, hemoglobin is approximately 75% saturated on the right-shifted curve, which is less than the 85% saturation we estimated from the normal curve.

- Pulmonary artery pressure would be *increased* because alveolar hypoxia causes vasoconstriction of pulmonary arterioles **(hypoxic vasoconstriction)**. Vasoconstriction leads to increased pulmonary vascular resistance, which increases pulmonary arterial pressure. (Recall from cardiovascular physiology that arterial pressure = blood flow × resistance.) Hypoxic vasoconstriction is a unique phenomenon in the lungs that shunts blood flow away from hypoxic regions; in contrast, in other tissues, hypoxia is vasodilatory.

4. Dan's Pa_{CO2} would have been *decreased* secondary to hyperventilation. As discussed earlier, hypoxemia (Pa_{O2}, 50 mm Hg) stimulated Dan's peripheral chemoreceptors and increased his

breathing rate (hyperventilation). Hyperventilation drives off extra CO_2 from the lungs and causes a decrease in arterial P_{CO_2}. (Recall from Case 21 that if CO_2 production is constant, arterial P_{CO_2} is determined by alveolar ventilation.)

Decreased Pa_{CO_2} causes an increase in arterial pH, according to the **Henderson–Hasselbalch equation**, which states that:

$$pH = 6.1 + \log \frac{HCO_3^-}{P_{CO_2}}$$

where

$$pH = -\log_{10} [H^+]$$
$$6.1 = pK \text{ of } HCO_3^-/CO_2 \text{ buffer}$$
$$HCO_3^- = HCO_3^- \text{ concentration of arterial blood}$$
$$P_{CO_2} = P_{CO_2} \text{ of arterial blood}$$

The acid–base disorder that is caused by hyperventilation is **respiratory alkalosis.** As the name implies, the alkaline blood pH results from a respiratory problem (in this case, hyperventilation that produced a decreased P_{CO_2}).

5. To calculate the P_{O_2} of 100% O_2 saturated with water vapor, we use the same approach that was described in Question 1. Note that $F_{I_{O_2}}$ is now 1.0 (or 100%). Thus:

$$P_{O_2} = (P_B - P_{H_2O}) \times 1.0$$
$$= (420 \text{ mm Hg} - 47 \text{ mm Hg}) \times 1.0$$
$$= 373 \text{ mm Hg}$$

Thus, breathing 100% O_2 would be expected to increase the P_{O_2} of Dan's inspired air to 373 mm Hg, which would be expected to increase his alveolar and arterial P_{O_2}. According to the O_2–hemoglobin curve, such an increase in arterial P_{O_2} would increase the percent saturation of hemoglobin and thereby increase O_2 delivery to Dan's tissues. Dan would no longer be hypoxemic, there would no longer be a hypoxemic stimulation of peripheral chemoreceptors, and his breathing rate would return to normal.

6. **Acetazolamide,** a carbonic anhydrase inhibitor, inhibits renal HCO_3^- reabsorption and increases HCO_3^- excretion in the urine. Increased urinary HCO_3^- excretion leads to decreased HCO_3^- concentration in the blood (**metabolic acidosis).**

Dan's physician suggested that he take acetazolamide to produce a mild metabolic acidosis that would offset or negate the respiratory alkalosis caused by hyperventilation. The Henderson–Hasselbalch equation shows how this offset occurs:

$$pH = 6.1 + \log \frac{HCO_3^-}{P_{CO_2}}$$

Hypoxemia causes hyperventilation by stimulating peripheral chemoreceptors. Hyperventilation causes a decrease in P_{CO_2} that, by decreasing the denominator of the Henderson–Hasselbalch equation, causes an increase in blood pH. Acetazolamide causes a decrease in blood HCO_3^- concentration, which decreases the numerator in the Henderson–Hasselbalch equation. If the numerator (HCO_3^-) and the denominator (P_{CO_2}) decrease to the same extent, then the pH is normalized.

Of all of the responses predicted to occur at high altitude, the only one that would be offset by acetazolamide is the increased blood pH. Dan would still be breathing air with a low P_{O_2}. Thus, he would still have a low Pa_{O_2} and a low percent saturation, and he would still be hyperventilating secondary to hypoxemia.

Key topics

Acetazolamide

2,3-diphosphoglycerate (DPG)

Henderson–Hasselbalch equation

High altitude

Hyperventilation

Hypoxemia

Hypoxic vasoconstriction

Metabolic acidosis

O_2–hemoglobin

O_2–hemoglobin dissociation curve

P_{50}

Peripheral chemoreceptors

Respiratory alkalosis

Right shift of the O_2–hemoglobin curve

Case 24

Asthma: Obstructive Lung Disease

Ralph Grundy was a 43-year-old lineman for a Midwestern power company. He was married and the father of four children who were 24, 22, 21, and 18 years of age. Ralph had a history of asthma since childhood. His asthma attacks, which were characterized by wheezing and shortness of breath, were often precipitated by high pollen levels and cold weather. He used an inhaled bronchodilator (albuterol, a β_2-adrenergic agonist) to treat the attacks. At the time of his death, Ralph had been trying desperately to get "inside" work. His asthma attacks were becoming more frequent and more severe, and he had been taken to the emergency room five times in the past year.

Three days before his death, Ralph had an upper respiratory infection, with nasal and chest congestion and a fever of 101.8°F. He was exhausted from "just trying to breathe," and the bronchodilator inhaler wasn't working. On the third day of the illness, Ralph's oldest son took him to the emergency room of the local community hospital. He had inspiratory and expiratory wheezes and was in severe respiratory distress. Table 3–4 shows the information obtained when he arrived at the emergency room at 4 PM.

TABLE 3–4	*Ralph's Respiratory Values at 4 PM.*
Respiratory rate	30 breaths/min (normal, 12–15)
F_{IO_2} (fractional concentration of O_2)	0.21 (room air)
pH	7.48 (normal, 7.4)
Pa_{O_2} (arterial P_{O_2})	55 mm Hg (normal, 100 mm Hg)
Pa_{CO_2} (arterial P_{CO_2})	32 mm Hg (normal, 40 mm Hg)

The emergency room staff treated Ralph with an inhaled bronchodilator and had him breathe 50% O_2 (F_{IO_2}, 0.5). At 6 PM, his condition had not improved; in fact, it had worsened, and Ralph was obtunded (sleepy and inattentive). Before proceeding with more aggressive treatment (e.g., anti-inflammatory drugs and intubation), the emergency room staff obtained a second set of measurements (Table 3–5).

TABLE 3–5	*Ralph's Respiratory Values at 6 PM.*
Respiratory rate	8 breaths/min
F_{IO_2} (fractional concentration of O_2)	0.5
pH	7.02 (normal, 7.4)
Pa_{O_2} (arterial P_{O_2})	45 mm Hg (normal, 100 mm Hg)
Pa_{CO_2} (arterial P_{CO_2})	80 mm Hg (normal, 40 mm Hg)

Ralph died before aggressive treatment could be initiated. At autopsy, his airways were almost totally occluded by mucus plugs.

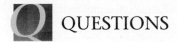

QUESTIONS

1. Asthma is an obstructive disease in which the airways narrow, increasing the resistance to airflow into and out of the lungs. What are the relationships between airflow, resistance, and airway diameter? Use equations to support your answers.

2. Figure 3–6 shows the results of pulmonary function tests performed on Ralph during an asthma attack the previous year. For the test, Ralph first took a normal tidal breath, then a maximal inspiration, followed by maximal expiration. The test was repeated after he inhaled a bronchodilator, a β_2-adrenergic agonist.

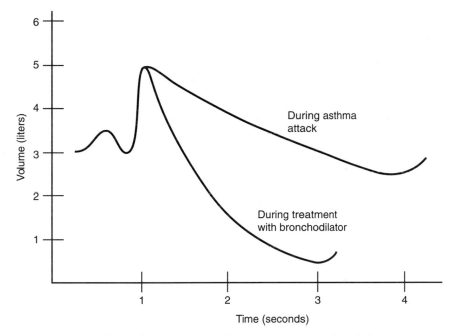

Figure 3–6 Lung volumes during forced expiration during an asthma attack and during treatment with an inhaled bronchodilator.

What was Ralph's tidal volume? What was his forced vital capacity (FVC) during the asthma attack and after treatment with the bronchodilator? What was his FEV_1 (volume expired in the first second of forced expiration) during the attack and after bronchodilator treatment? What was Ralph's FEV_1/FVC during the attack and after treatment? What is the significance of the changes in FVC, FEV_1, and FEV_1/FVC that were produced by the bronchodilator?

3. What effect did Ralph's asthma have on residual volume and functional residual capacity (FRC)?

4. Why was Ralph exhausted from "just trying to breathe?" How does obstructive lung disease increase the work of breathing?

5. Why was Ralph's arterial P_{O_2} (Pa_{O_2}) decreased at 4 PM? (Hint: Consider how changes in the ventilation–perfusion [$\dot{V}/\dot{Q}$] ratio might alter Pa_{O_2}.)

6. What is an A–a gradient, and what is its significance? What was Ralph's A–a gradient at 4 PM? (Assume that his respiratory quotient was 0.8.)

7. Why was Ralph hyperventilating at 4 PM? Why was his arterial P_{CO_2} (Pa_{CO_2}) decreased (compared with normal)? What acid–base abnormality did he have at 4 PM?

8. What was Ralph's A–a gradient at 6 PM? (Assume that his respiratory quotient remained at 0.8.) What is the significance of the change in A–a gradient that occurred between 4 PM and 6 PM?

9. Why was Ralph's Pa_{CO_2} increased at 6 PM? What acid–base abnormality did he have at that time? Why was he obtunded?

ANSWERS ON NEXT PAGE

ANSWERS AND EXPLANATIONS

1. **Asthma** is characterized by inflammation of the airways. The inflammatory process leads to swelling of airway linings, increased mucus production, and release of mediators that cause contraction of airway smooth muscle, or **bronchospasm.** As a consequence, there is a decrease in airway diameter. **Airway resistance** is inversely correlated with airway diameter or **radius.** As the radius of an airway decreases, resistance to airflow increases, according to **Poiseuille's law:**

$$R = \frac{8 \eta l}{\pi r^4}$$

where

R = resistance of the airway
η = viscosity of inspired air
l = length of the airway
r = radius of the airway

This relationship, which is especially powerful because of the fourth-power dependence on radius, should be familiar from cardiovascular physiology.

   Airflow is inversely proportional to airway resistance, according to the now-familiar relationship between **flow, pressure, and resistance:**

$$Q = \frac{\Delta P}{R}$$

where

Q = airflow (L/min)
ΔP = pressure difference (mm Hg or cm H_2O)
R = airway resistance (cm H_2O/L per sec)

Thus, airflow (Q) is directly proportional to the pressure difference (ΔP) between the inlet and the outlet of the airway (e.g., between the mouth and the alveoli), and inversely proportional to the resistance of the airway (R). The pressure difference is the *driving force* for airflow; resistance is the *impediment* to airflow.

   By combining the relationships for airway radius, resistance, and airflow, we conclude that the larger the radius of the airway, the smaller the resistance and the higher the airflow. Conversely, the smaller the radius, the larger the resistance and the lower the airflow.

   Note that although the resistance of a single airway is inversely correlated with its radius, the **medium-sized bronchi** are actually the site of highest airway resistance in the intact respiratory system (even though it seems that the smallest airways should have the highest resistance). This apparent discrepancy is explained by the parallel arrangement of the small airways. When resistances are arranged in parallel, the total resistance is lower than the individual resistances.

2. **Tidal volume** is the volume inspired and expired during normal breathing. **Forced vital capacity (FVC)** is the volume that can be forcibly expired after a maximal inspiration. **FEV_1** is the volume expired in the first second of the forced expiration. **FEV_1/FVC** is the fraction of FVC expired in the first second. In healthy people, FEV_1/FVC is approximately 0.8 (or 80%); in other words, normally, most of the vital capacity is expired in the first second of forced expiration (Table 3–6).

TABLE 3-6	*Ralph's Lung Volumes and Capacities During an Asthma Attack and During Treatment with a Bronchodilator*	
	During Asthma Attack	**During Bronchodilator Treatment**
Tidal volume	0.5 L	0.5 L
FVC	2.5 L	4.5 L
FEV_1	1.2 L	3.5 L
FEV_1/FVC	0.48	0.78

FVC, forced vital capacity; FEV_1, volume expired in the first second of forced expiration.

Ralph had asthma, an **obstructive pulmonary disease** that is characterized by inflammation and narrowing of the airways. This narrowing (i.e., decreased airway radius) led to **increased resistance** and decreased airflow, as discussed in the previous question. Ralph's **wheezes** were the sounds produced when he expired forcibly through these narrowed airways.

In asthma, the airways are narrowed for three major reasons: (i) hyperresponsiveness of bronchial smooth muscle to a variety of stimuli, which causes bronchospasm and **bronchoconstriction** during an attack; (ii) thickening and edema of the bronchial walls secondary to **inflammation;** and (iii) increased production of bronchial **mucus** that obstructs the airways. The first mechanism (bronchoconstriction) can be reversed by administering bronchodilator drugs, such as β_2-**adrenergic agonists** (e.g., **albuterol**).

Increases in airway resistance, such as those seen in asthma, lead to *decreases in all expiratory parameters,* including FVC, FEV_1, and FEV_1/FVC. The higher the airway resistance, the more difficult it is to expire air from the lungs. Airway resistance is especially increased during *forced* expiration, when intrapleural pressure becomes positive and tends to compress, or even close, the airways (Fig. 3–7). Therefore, FVC decreases during an asthma attack because the airways close prematurely during expiration. One result of this **premature closure of the airways** is that air that should have been expired remains in the lungs (**air trapping**).

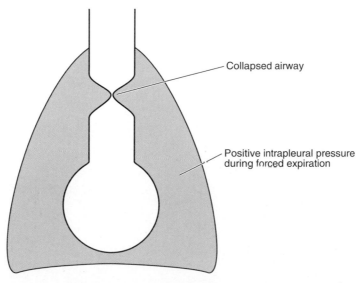

Figure 3–7   Airway collapse during forced expiration as a result of positive intrapleural pressure.

The inhaled **bronchodilator** relaxed Ralph's airways, increasing their radii and decreasing their resistance to airflow. The decrease in airway resistance improved Ralph's expiratory functions, as evidenced by the increased FEV_1 and FEV_1/FVC. Also, because his airways did not close prematurely, his FVC was increased.

3. Ralph's asthma was associated with increased airway resistance, which compromised his expiratory functions. As a result, air that should have been expired remained in the lungs, increasing his residual volume and his **functional residual capacity (FRC).** Recall that FRC is the resting, or equilibrium, position of the lungs (i.e., the volume in the lungs between breaths). Because Ralph's FRC was increased, his normal "tidal" breathing had to occur at higher lung volumes.

4. The work of breathing is determined by how much pressure change is required to move air into and out of the lungs. In obstructive lung diseases, such as asthma, the **work of breathing** is increased for two reasons. (i) A person with asthma breathes at higher lung volumes (because of the higher FRC), as discussed earlier. During *inspiration,* a person with asthma must lower intrathoracic pressure more than a healthy person to bring air into the lungs; thus, more work is required during inspiration. (ii) During *expiration,* because airway resistance is increased, higher pressures must be created to force air out of the lungs; this greater expiratory effort requires the use of accessory muscles. (In healthy people, expiration is passive and does not require the assistance of accessory muscles.) Increased work of breathing is reflected in higher rates of O_2 consumption and CO_2 production.

5. Recall the **ventilation–perfusion ($\dot{V}/\dot{Q}$) relationship** in the lungs. Ventilation ($\dot{V}$) and perfusion ($\dot{Q}$) are normally matched such that ventilated alveoli lie in close proximity to perfused capillaries. This $\dot{V}/\dot{Q}$ matching (i.e., $\dot{V}/\dot{Q} \cong 1.0$) allows O_2 exchange to proceed normally (as shown in the upper portion of Figure 3–8). O_2 diffuses from alveolar gas into pulmonary capillary blood until alveolar P_{O_2} and pulmonary capillary P_{O_2} are equal (normally 100 mm Hg).

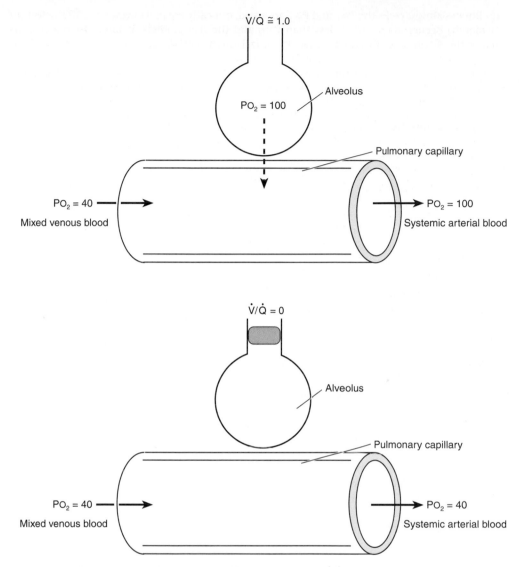

Figure 3–8 Effect of airway obstruction on ventilation–perfusion ($\dot{V}/\dot{Q}$) ratio and O_2 exchange. (P_{O_2}, partial pressure of oxygen.)

Ralph's arterial P_{O_2} (Pa_{O_2}) was decreased **(hypoxemia)** because he had a $\dot{V}/\dot{Q}$ **defect** (or mismatch). Bronchoconstriction and obstruction of some airways prevented adequate ventilation of some regions of his lungs. In these unventilated regions, fresh air, with its supply of O_2, did not reach the alveoli for gas exchange. Therefore, the pulmonary capillary blood that perfused these unventilated alveoli was not oxygenated. As shown in the lower portion of Figure 3–8, the P_{O_2} of the blood in these capillaries remained the same as that of mixed venous blood. This portion of the pulmonary blood flow is called a **shunt** because the blood flow bypasses ventilated alveoli and is not oxygenated. Ralph's pulmonary venous blood (which becomes systemic arterial blood) was a mixture of blood from well-ventilated and poorly ventilated regions of the lungs; therefore, his systemic arterial blood had a P_{O_2} of less than 100 mm Hg.

6. **The A–a gradient** is the difference between alveolar P_{O_2} (PA_{O_2}, or "A") and arterial P_{O_2} (Pa_{O_2}, or "a"). The A–a gradient tells us whether O_2 is equilibrating normally between alveolar gas and pulmonary capillary blood. For example, the normal A–a gradient is close to zero because O_2

equilibrates almost perfectly: $P_{A_{O_2}}$ and $P_{a_{O_2}}$ are equal, or nearly equal. However, if a $\dot{V}/\dot{Q}$ defect (or mismatch) occurs, then $P_{a_{O_2}}$ is less than $P_{A_{O_2}}$ and the A–a gradient is larger than zero. The greater the disturbance in O_2 exchange, the larger the A–a gradient.

The A–a gradient is determined by measuring "a" (the P_{O_2} of arterial blood, or $P_{a_{O_2}}$) and calculating "A" (the P_{O_2} of alveolar gas, or $P_{A_{O_2}}$) with the **alveolar gas equation** (described in Case 21). Therefore, at 4 PM:

"a" = 55 mm Hg

$$\text{"A"} = P_{I_{O_2}} - \frac{P_{A_{CO_2}}}{R}$$

$$= (P_B - P_{H_2O}) \times F_{I_{O_2}} - \frac{P_{A_{CO_2}}}{R}$$

$$= (760 \text{ mm Hg} - 47 \text{ mm Hg}) \times 0.21 - \frac{32 \text{ mm Hg}}{0.8}$$

$$= 150 \text{ mm Hg} - \frac{32 \text{ mm Hg}}{0.8}$$

$$= 110 \text{ mm Hg}$$

$$\text{A–a} = 110 \text{ mm Hg} - 55 \text{ mm Hg}$$

$$= 55 \text{ mm Hg}$$

Compared with a healthy person, whose A–a gradient is close to zero, Ralph's A–a gradient was greatly increased. In other words, O_2 could not equilibrate between alveolar gas and pulmonary capillary blood because of Ralph's $\dot{V}/\dot{Q}$ **defect** (specifically, a *decreased* $\dot{V}/\dot{Q}$ **ratio**).

7. Ralph was hyperventilating at 4 PM because **hypoxemia** stimulated **peripheral chemoreceptors** located in the carotid bodies. This stimulation led to an increased breathing rate **(hyperventilation)**. At 4 PM, Ralph's arterial P_{CO_2} ($P_{a_{CO_2}}$) was decreased *secondary* to the hyperventilation. (Recall that $P_{a_{CO_2}}$ is inversely correlated with alveolar ventilation.) This decrease in $P_{a_{CO_2}}$ caused an acid–base disorder called **respiratory alkalosis**. The pH of arterial blood is determined by the ratio of HCO_3^- to CO_2, as described by the **Henderson–Hasselbalch equation:**

$$\textbf{pH} = \textbf{6.1} + \textbf{log} \frac{\textbf{HCO}_3^-}{\textbf{P}_{\textbf{CO}_2}}$$

where

$$\text{pH} = -\log_{10} [H^+]$$
$$6.1 = \text{pK of the } HCO_3^-/CO_2 \text{ buffer}$$
$$HCO_3^- = HCO_3^- \text{ concentration of arterial blood}$$
$$P_{CO_2} = P_{CO_2} \text{ of arterial blood}$$

The decrease in P_{CO_2} (secondary to hyperventilation) decreased the denominator of the Henderson–Hasselbalch equation and, consequently, increased the pH of Ralph's arterial blood (i.e., respiratory alkalosis).

8. At 6 PM, Ralph's A–a gradient was as follows (note that F_{IO_2} was increased from 0.21 to 0.5, or 50%):

"a" = 45 mm Hg

$$"A" = P_{IO_2} - \frac{PA_{CO_2}}{R}$$

$$= (760 \text{ mm Hg} - 47 \text{ mm Hg}) \times 0.5 - \frac{80 \text{ mm Hg}}{0.8}$$

$$= 357 \text{ mm Hg} - 100 \text{ mm Hg}$$

$$= 257 \text{ mm Hg}$$

$$A-a = 257 \text{ mm Hg} - 45 \text{ mm Hg}$$

$$= 212 \text{ mm Hg}$$

Ralph's A–a gradient had increased further at 6 PM! Increasing F_{IO_2} to 0.5 caused Ralph's alveolar P_{O_2} ("A") to increase from 110 to 257 mm Hg. However, this change did not improve Ralph's blood oxygenation. In fact, at 6 PM, his arterial P_{O_2} ("a") had decreased further, to 45 mm Hg. The fact that Ralph's A–a gradient widened (or increased) suggests that even more regions of his lungs were receiving inadequate ventilation; as a result, the $\dot{V}/\dot{Q}$ defect was even greater.

9. At 6 PM, Ralph's Pa_{CO_2} was 80 mm Hg. This value was significantly elevated compared with both the normal value of 40 mm Hg and Ralph's value at 4 PM (which was lower than normal). We have already discussed why Ralph's Pa_{CO_2} was reduced at 4 PM (i.e., he was hyperventilating secondary to hypoxemia). The dramatic increase in Ralph's arterial P_{CO_2} between 4 PM and 6 PM reflects significant worsening of his condition. Undoubtedly, Ralph's airways had become more obstructed (a suspicion that was confirmed at autopsy), his work of breathing was further increased, he was **hypoventilating**, and he could not eliminate the CO_2 that his body produced. Retention of CO_2 elevated his Pa_{CO_2} and caused **respiratory acidosis**, as predicted by the Henderson–Hasselbalch equation:

$$pH = 6.1 + \log \frac{HCO_3^-}{P_{CO_2}}$$

The increase in P_{CO_2} (in the denominator) caused his arterial pH to decrease to 7.01 (respiratory acidosis). Ralph was obtunded as a result of the narcotic effect of high P_{CO_2}

Key topics

A–a gradient

β_2-adrenergic agonists

Airflow, pressure, resistance relationship

Air trapping

Airway resistance

Albuterol

Alveolar gas equation

Asthma

Bronchoconstriction

Bronchodilator drugs

FEV_1

FEV_1/FVC

Forced vital capacity (FVC)

Functional residual capacity (FRC)

Hyperventilation

Hypoventilation

Hypoxemia

Obstructive pulmonary disease

Peripheral chemoreceptors

Poiseuille's law

Respiratory acidosis

Respiratory alkalosis

Tidal volume

Ventilation–perfusion ($\dot{V}/\dot{Q}$) defect, or mismatch

$\dot{V}/\dot{Q}$ ratio

Work of breathing

Case 25

Chronic Obstructive Pulmonary Disease

Bernice Betweiler is a 73-year-old retired seamstress who has never been married. She worked in the alterations department of a men's clothier for 48 years. Bernice is a chain smoker. On the job, she was never found without a cigarette hanging from her lips. When her employer announced that smoking would no longer be allowed in the store, Bernice retired. Since her retirement 3 years ago, Bernice has not been feeling well. She fatigues easily, even with light exertion. She has shortness of breath and recently has begun to sleep on two pillows. However, despite these problems, she has refused to stop smoking.

Bernice made an appointment with her physician, who noted a prolonged expiratory phase in her breathing, expiratory wheezes, and increased anteroposterior chest diameter. Her nail beds were cyanotic, and she had moderate pitting edema of her ankles. Based on these observations and the results of laboratory and pulmonary tests, the physician concluded that Bernice has a combination of emphysema and bronchitis, called chronic obstructive pulmonary disease (COPD), which resulted from her long history of smoking.

The results of pulmonary function and laboratory tests are shown in Tables 3–7 and 3–8, respectively.

TABLE 3–7	*Bernice's Pulmonary Function Tests*
Vital capacity	Decreased
Residual volume	Increased
Functional residual capacity	Increased
Expiratory flow rate	Decreased

TABLE 3–8	*Bernice's Laboratory Values*
Hemoglobin	14.5 g/dL (normal for women, 12–15 g/dL)
Pa_{O_2} (arterial P_{O_2})	48 mm Hg (normal, 100 mm Hg)
O_2 saturation	78% (normal, 98–100%)
Pa_{CO_2} (arterial P_{CO_2})	69 mm Hg (normal, 40 mm Hg)
HCO_3^-	34 mEq/L (normal, 24 mEq/L)

 QUESTIONS

1. Bernice's chronic bronchitis is associated with inflammation of the airways and hypersecretion of mucus, which led to obstruction of her airways and increased airway resistance. Her emphysema is associated with loss of alveolar–capillary units and decreased lung elasticity. How do these changes in airway resistance and lung elasticity explain the results of Bernice's pulmonary function tests?

2. The curves in Figure 3–9 show expiratory airflow during *forced expiration* in a healthy person and in a person with COPD. Each subject first inspired maximally (not shown) and then expired forcibly. The curves show the expiratory flow rates and lung volumes during forced expiration.

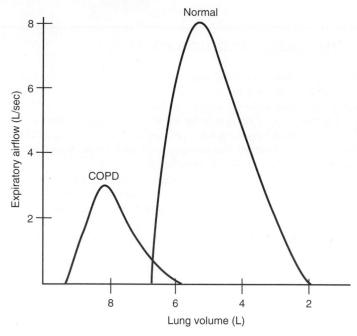

Figure 3–9 Expiratory flow rate during forced expiration in healthy people and in patients with chronic obstructive pulmonary disease (COPD).

What is the value for forced vital capacity (FVC) in the healthy person and the person with COPD? What is the value for peak expiratory flow rate in each person? What is the value for residual volume in each person?

3. How is Bernice's increased anteroposterior (AP) chest diameter explained by the results of her pulmonary function tests and by your answers to Question 1?

4. Why does Bernice have a decrease in arterial P_{O_2} (Pa_{CO_2})?

5. Why is her percent O_2 saturation decreased, and what are the implications for O_2 delivery to the tissues?

6. Why are Bernice's nail beds cyanotic (blue)?

7. Bernice's hemoglobin concentration is normal. If her hemoglobin concentration had been decreased, would that have altered her Pa_{O_2}? If so, in what direction?

8. Why does Bernice have an increase in arterial P_{CO_2} (Pa_{CO_2})?

9. What is Bernice's arterial pH? (Assume that the CO_2 concentration of arterial blood is $P_{CO_2} \times 0.03$.) What acid–base disorder does she have, and what is the cause? Why is her HCO_3^- concentration increased?

10. How does respiratory acidosis alter the delivery of O_2 to the tissues? (Think about the effect of CO_2 on the O_2–hemoglobin dissociation curve.) Is this effect helpful or harmful?

11. Why does Bernice have ankle edema? (Hint: Think sequentially, starting with her lungs.)

ANSWERS ON NEXT PAGE

ANSWERS AND EXPLANATIONS

1. The pulmonary function tests showed that Bernice had increased residual volume, increased functional residual capacity (FRC), decreased vital capacity, and decreased expiratory flow rate. Recall that **residual volume** is the volume that remains in the lungs after forced maximal expiration; **functional residual capacity (FRC)** is the volume that remains in the lungs after expiration of a normal tidal volume. Two components of Bernice's disease led to these pulmonary changes: increased resistance of her airways and decreased elasticity of her lung tissues.

   The bronchitic component of Bernice's **COPD (chronic bronchitis)** caused narrowing and obstruction of her airways. The resulting **increased resistance** of the airways caused a decrease in airflow, especially during expiration. Because the expiratory phase was compromised, air was trapped in the lungs, and residual volume was increased. Because FRC includes residual volume, FRC was also increased.

   The emphysematous component of Bernice's disease **(emphysema)** caused **decreased elasticity** of her lung tissues, which also compromised expiration. To understand how lung elasticity is related to expiratory function, it is necessary to recall that **elastance** is inversely correlated with **compliance** (where compliance = volume/pressure). To illustrate the relationship between elastance and compliance, consider two rubber bands, one thick and one thin. The thick rubber band has a large amount of elastic "tissue"; thus, it has high elastance and high elastic recoil strength, but low compliance. The thin rubber band has a smaller amount of elastic "tissue"; thus, it has lower elastance and lower elastic recoil strength, but high compliance. In emphysema, there is loss of elastic tissue in the lung structures; as a result, elastance is decreased and **compliance is increased.** These changes in elastance and compliance have two important implications for the expiratory functions of the lungs: (i) Normal expiration is driven by elastic recoil forces that compress the air in the lungs, increase alveolar pressure, and drive the air out of the lungs. When elastic tissue is lost, elastic recoil force is decreased and expiration is impaired. (ii) Normally, the airways are kept open during expiration by radial traction. This traction is created by elastic recoil forces acting on the airway walls. When elastic recoil strength decreases, the airways are deprived of this radial traction. As a result, they may collapse and close during expiration. When the airways collapse, airway resistance increases, expiration ends "early," and air that should have been expired is trapped in the lungs.

   One consequence of air being trapped in the lungs, which increases the residual volume, is that the **vital capacity is decreased.** (Recall from Case 21 that vital capacity is the maximal volume of air that can be inspired above the residual volume.) Because the residual volume occupies a greater fraction of total lung capacity, it encroaches on and decreases the vital capacity.

2. To answer these numerical questions, first note that the curves show expiratory airflow as a function of lung volume. Each person has just inspired maximally. The curves show the lung volume and airflow during the forced expiration that follows.

   The *healthy person* inspired maximally to a lung volume of 6.8 L, and then started the forced expiration. During expiration, the **peak (maximal) expiratory flow rate** was 8 L/sec. At the completion of the forced expiration, 2 L remained in the lungs. Thus, the healthy person's residual volume was 2 L, and his FVC (the total volume expired) was 4.8 L (6.8 L − 2 L).

   The *person with COPD* inspired maximally to a lung volume of 9.3 L, and then started the forced expiration. The peak expiratory flow rate was much less than in the healthy person (3 L/sec). At the completion of the forced expiration, 5.8 L remained in the lungs. Thus, the person with COPD had a higher residual volume (5.8 L) and a lower FVC (3.5 L [9.3 L − 5.8 L]) than the healthy person.

3. Bernice's **anteroposterior (AP) chest diameter** was increased because her expiratory functions were compromised. As a result, Bernice had **air trapping**, increased residual volume, and increased FRC. Because of air trapping and increased FRC, people with COPD have **barrel-shaped chests** and are said to "breathe at higher lung volumes."

4. Bernice's arterial P_{O_2} (Pa_{O_2}) was 48 mm Hg, much lower than the normal value of 100 mm Hg. In other words, she was **hypoxemic**. Recall that a normal value of Pa_{O_2} indicates normal oxygenation of blood in the lungs. Normal oxygenation requires ventilation–perfusion ($\dot{V}/\dot{Q}$) matching, whereby ventilated alveoli lie in close proximity to perfused capillaries. Bernice had a $\dot{V}/\dot{Q}$ **defect** as a result of impaired ventilation. A portion of her pulmonary blood flow perfused lung regions that were not ventilated **(intrapulmonary shunt)**. Those regions had a **decreased $\dot{V}/\dot{Q}$ ratio.** In other words, the denominator ($\dot{Q}$) became relatively higher than the numerator ($\dot{V}$). The blood serving these lung regions could not be oxygenated. This poorly oxygenated blood from shunt regions mixed with blood from regions of the lung that were well oxygenated. As a result, the overall P_{O_2} of blood leaving the lungs (and becoming systemic arterial blood) was decreased.

5. The **percent saturation** of hemoglobin was reduced because Bernice's P_{O_2} was reduced. Recall the important relationship between P_{O_2} and percent saturation from the discussion of the O_2–hemoglobin dissociation curve in Case 23 (see Fig. 3–5).

   According to the curve, percent saturation is approximately 80% at an arterial P_{O_2} of 48 mm Hg. This number is in good agreement with Bernice's measured value of 78%. This percent saturation is clearly *reduced* from the normal value of 100%, and it corresponds to about three O_2 molecules per hemoglobin molecule (rather than the normal four O_2 molecules per hemoglobin molecule). Such a change would impair O_2 delivery to the tissues because the O_2 content of the blood is largely dependent on the amount of O_2 bound to hemoglobin. Thus, at 78% saturation, the delivery and content of O_2 are approximately 78% of normal. (Recall that dissolved O_2, the other form of O_2 in blood, contributes little to the total O_2 content.)

6. Bernice's nail beds were **cyanotic** (they had a dusky blue appearance) because there was an increased concentration of **deoxygenated hemoglobin** in her blood. This deoxygenated hemoglobin was visible in capillary beds near the skin surface. Oxygenated hemoglobin is red; deoxygenated hemoglobin is blue. Because Bernice's P_{O_2} was decreased, she had a decreased percent saturation of hemoglobin. With less hemoglobin present in the oxygenated form, more hemoglobin was present in the deoxygenated form. As a result, the blood appeared blue rather than red.

7. You may have thought that a decrease in hemoglobin concentration automatically means there is a decrease in Pa_{O_2}; however, this is not the case. Although decreased hemoglobin causes decreased O_2 *content* of blood (because the total amount of O_2 bound to hemoglobin is decreased), Pa_{O_2} is determined by the *free*, unbound O_2 (see Case 22), which is not directly affected by the hemoglobin concentration.

8. Bernice's Pa_{CO_2} was increased **(hypercapnia)** because she could not eliminate all of the CO_2 that her tissues produced. As her disease progressed, she was unable to maintain alveolar ventilation (due to increased work of breathing), and thus retained CO_2.

9. Bernice had **respiratory acidosis** secondary to CO_2 retention. Her arterial pH can be calculated with the **Henderson–Hasselbalch equation** as follows:

$$pH = 6.1 + \log \frac{HCO_3^-}{P_{CO_2} \times 0.03}$$

$$= 6.1 + \log \frac{34 \text{ mM}}{69 \text{ mm Hg} \times 0.03}$$

$$= 6.1 + \log \frac{34 \text{ mM}}{2.07 \text{ mM}}$$

$$= 6.1 + 1.22$$

$$= 7.32$$

An arterial pH of 7.32 is considered acidemia because it is lower than the normal pH of 7.4. Bernice had acidemia secondary to an elevated P_{CO_2}, which increased the denominator of the Henderson–Hasselbalch equation.

Bernice's HCO_3^- concentration was increased because she has *chronic* respiratory acidosis, in which **renal compensation** occurs. The renal compensation for respiratory acidosis is increased reabsorption of HCO_3^- (a process that is aided by the high level of P_{CO_2}). When HCO_3^- reabsorption increases, the blood HCO_3^- concentration increases. This increase in HCO_3^- concentration is "compensatory" in the sense that it helps to restore normal arterial pH. Amazingly, although Bernice had a severely elevated Pa_{CO_2}, her pH was only *slightly* acidic. This is explained by the fact that her HCO_3^- concentration was also elevated, almost to the same extent as her P_{CO_2}. As a result, the ratio of HCO_3^- to CO_2 was nearly normal, and her pH was nearly normal.

10. The only "good news" for Bernice is that her increased P_{CO_2} caused a **right shift of the O_2–hemoglobin dissociation curve** (see Fig. 3–5). Increases in P_{CO_2} (and acidosis) cause a decrease in the affinity of hemoglobin for O_2 (**Bohr effect**), which appears as a right shift of the curve. For a given value of P_{O_2}, the percent saturation of hemoglobin is decreased. In Bernice's case, the right shift was helpful; although the O_2 content of her blood was significantly decreased (secondary to hypoxemia), the **decreased affinity** made it easier for hemoglobin to unload O_2 in the tissues. The "bad news" is that the right shift with its decreased affinity also made it more difficult to load O_2 in the lungs.

11. The "hint" in the question suggests that Bernice had edema on the systemic side of the circulation (in the ankles) because of problems in her lungs. In patients with COPD, pulmonary artery pressure is often elevated secondary to **increased pulmonary vascular resistance.** Pulmonary vascular resistance is increased for two reasons: (i) COPD is associated with loss of alveolar–capillary units. The loss of capillary beds increases pulmonary resistance. (ii) Alveolar hypoxia (secondary to hypoventilation) causes **hypoxic vasoconstriction.** The increased pulmonary vascular resistance leads to increased pulmonary artery pressure, which is the afterload of the right ventricle. Increased afterload on the right ventricle causes **decreased cardiac output,** or **cor pulmonale (right ventricular failure** secondary to **pulmonary hypertension).** Blood that is not ejected from the right ventricle "backs up" into the right atrium and the systemic veins. Increased systemic venous pressure increases capillary hydrostatic pressure, leading to increased filtration of fluid into the interstitium **(edema).**

Although hypoxic vasoconstriction (discussed earlier) is "bad" in the sense that it causes pulmonary hypertension and subsequent right ventricular failure, it is "good" in the sense that it is attempting to improve $\dot{V}/\dot{Q}$ matching. Poorly ventilated regions of the lung are hypoxic; this hypoxia causes vasoconstriction of nearby arterioles and directs blood flow away from regions where gas exchange cannot possibly occur. Therefore, this process attempts to redirect (or shunt) blood flow to regions that are ventilated.

A final note on this case: patients with COPD are classified as "pink puffers" (type A) or "blue bloaters" (type B), depending on whether their disease is primarily emphysema (pink puffers) or bronchitis (blue bloaters). Bernice is a **blue bloater:** she has severe hypoxemia with cyanosis, hypercapnia, right ventricular failure, and systemic edema. **Pink puffers** are tachypneic (have an increased breathing rate), have mild hypoxemia, and are hypocapnic or normocapnic.

Key topics

Air trapping

Anteroposterior (AP) chest diameter

Blue bloater

Bohr effect

Bronchitis

Chronic obstructive pulmonary disease (COPD)

Compliance

Cor pulmonale

Cyanosis

Elastance

Emphysema

Functional residual capacity (FRC)

Right-ventricular heart failure

Henderson–Hasselbalch equation

Hypercapnia

Hypoxemia

Hypoxic vasoconstriction

Intrapulmonary shunt

Peak expiratory flow rate

Percent saturation

Pink puffer

Pulmonary hypertension

Pulmonary vascular resistance

Renal compensation

Residual volume

Respiratory acidosis

Right ventricular failure

Right shift of the O_2–hemoglobin dissociation curve

Ventilation–perfusion ($\dot{V}/\dot{Q}$) defect

$\dot{V}/\dot{Q}$ ratio

Case 26

Interstitial Fibrosis: Restrictive Lung Disease

Simone Paciocco, a 42-year-old wife and mother of two teenagers, was diagnosed 3 years ago with diffuse interstitial pulmonary fibrosis. As much as possible, Simone has tried to continue her normal activities, which include working as an assistant manager at a bank. However, keeping up with the demands of day-to-day life has become increasingly difficult. Simone tires easily and can no longer climb a flight of stairs without becoming extremely short of breath. She is being closely followed by her physician, a pulmonologist.

Tables 3–9 and 3–10 show the information obtained at a recent physical examination. After these results were obtained at rest, Simone was asked to exercise on a stair climber. After only 2 minutes, she became extremely fatigued and had to discontinue the test. The arterial blood gas measurements were repeated, with the results shown in Table 3–11.

think about 10 rubber bands around hand instead of 1

TABLE 3–9	Simone's Arterial Blood Gases at Rest
Pa_{O_2} (arterial P_{O_2})	76 mm Hg (normal, 100 mm Hg)
Pa_{CO_2} (arterial P_{CO_2})	37 mm Hg (normal, 40 mm Hg)
% Saturation	97% (normal, 95–100%)

TABLE 3–10	Results of Simone's Pulmonary Function Tests at Rest
Total lung capacity	Decreased
Functional residual capacity	Decreased
Residual volume	Decreased
$D_{L_{CO}}$	Decreased
FEV_1/FVC	Increased

$D_{L_{CO}}$, lung diffusing capacity; FEV_1, volume expired in the first second of forced expiration; FVC, forced vital capacity.

→ more of a diagnostic indicator in obstructive lung disease where it would be decreased

TABLE 3–11	Simone's Arterial Blood Gases During Exercise
Pa_{O_2} (arterial P_{O_2})	62 mm Hg (normal, 100 mm Hg)
Pa_{CO_2} (arterial P_{CO_2})	36 mm Hg (normal, 40 mm Hg)
% Saturation	90%

 QUESTIONS

1. Diffuse interstitial fibrosis is a restrictive pulmonary disease characterized by decreased compliance of lung tissues. Use this information to explain Simone's decreased total lung capacity, decreased functional residual capacity (FRC), and decreased residual volume at rest. Why was there an increase in her FEV_1/FVC (fraction of the forced vital capacity [FVC] expired in the first second of expiration)?

2. Lung diffusing capacity (D_L) is measured with carbon monoxide. Why carbon monoxide? What is the meaning of Simone's decreased $D_{L_{CO}}$?

3. In addition to changes in lung compliance, diffuse interstitial fibrosis is also characterized by thickening of alveolar membranes. Use this information to explain Simone's decreased arterial P_{O_2} (Pa_{O_2}) at rest.

4. Use Figure 3–10 to explain why O_2 exchange between alveolar gas and pulmonary capillary blood in healthy people is considered a "perfusion-limited" process. In fibrosis, why does O_2 exchange convert to a "diffusion-limited" process? How does this conversion affect Pa_{O_2}?

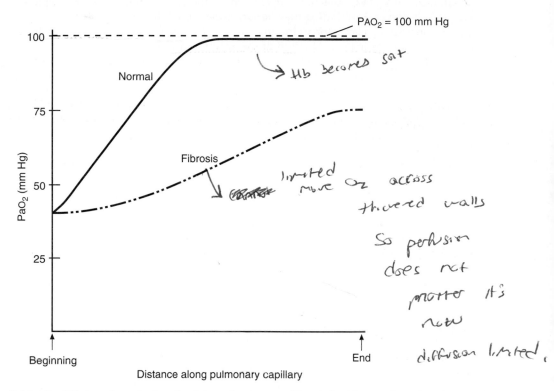

Figure 3–10 O_2 diffusion along the length of the pulmonary capillary in healthy people and patients with fibrosis. ($P_{A_{O_2}}$, partial pressure of oxygen in alveolar gas; Pa_{O_2}, partial pressure of oxygen in arterial blood.)

5. What was the total O_2 content of Simone's blood while she was at rest? Assume that the O_2-binding capacity of her blood was 1.34 mL O_2/g hemoglobin, her hemoglobin concentration was 15 g/dL, and the solubility of O_2 in blood is 0.003 mL O_2/100 mL blood/mm Hg.

6. While exercising on the stair climber, Simone's Pa_{O_2} decreased even further, to 62 mm Hg. Propose a mechanism for this further decrease in Pa_{O_2}.

7. Why did the percent saturation of hemoglobin in Simone's blood decrease (from 97% to 90%) when she exercised? How did the decrease in percent saturation affect Simone's exercise tolerance?

8. Simone was hypoxemic (i.e., she had a decreased Pa_{O_2}). However, she was not hypercapnic (i.e., she did not have CO_2 retention or an increased Pa_{CO_2}). In fact, at 37 mm Hg, her Pa_{CO_2} was slightly lower than normal. Simone clearly has a problem with O_2 exchange, but she doesn't seem to have a problem with CO_2 exchange. How can hypoxemia occur in the absence of hypercapnia?

[handwritten: q in elasun. have an inverse relationship btw compliance + elasticity]

[handwritten: elastance holds the lung open]

A ANSWERS AND EXPLANATIONS

1. Simone had decreased total lung capacity, decreased FRC, and decreased residual volume. In explaining these findings, it is important to understand that **restrictive pulmonary diseases** (e.g., interstitial fibrosis) are associated with **decreased compliance** of lung tissues. Because the lungs are stiff and noncompliant, greater changes in pulmonary pressures and greater effort are needed to expand the lungs during inspiration. As a result, all lung volumes and capacities are compromised (or decreased).

[handwritten: alveoli get scarred which dec. SA for diffusion]

   Simone's **FEV$_1$/FVC** (the fraction expired in the first second of forced expiration) was *increased,* however. This finding may be surprising. Recall, however, that the airways are normally held open by elastic forces in lung tissues. The greater the elastance of the lung tissues, the greater the elastic forces that tether the airways open. Thus, in fibrosis and other restrictive diseases in which compliance is decreased and **elastance is increased,** the airways are more dilated than normal. (In fibrotic lungs, the dilated airways, surrounded by scar tissue, have a characteristic **honeycomb** appearance.) The increased airway diameter results in decreased resistance to airflow, which is evidenced by an increased FEV$_1$/FVC. Although FVC (like the other lung volumes and capacities) is decreased, the *fraction* expired in the first second actually can be increased.

2. **Lung diffusing capacity (D$_L$),** estimates the permeability of the alveolar-pulmonary capillary barrier. D$_L$ includes the diffusion coefficient of the gas, the surface area available for diffusion, and the thickness of the barrier. D$_L$ is measured with **carbon monoxide (CO)** as follows. In the single-breath method, a subject maximally inspires air containing CO, holds his or her breath for 10 seconds, and then expires. The amount of CO that is transferred from alveolar gas into pulmonary capillary blood is measured to assess the diffusion characteristics of the alveolar–pulmonary capillary barrier.

   Why use CO? Why not use some other gas? CO is used because it is **diffusion-limited** (i.e., its transfer from alveolar gas into pulmonary capillary blood depends *solely* on the diffusion process). To understand this point, recall two important principles concerning the diffusion of gases: (i) The partial pressure of a gas in solution depends on the concentration of free, unbound gas. (ii) The diffusion of gas is driven by a difference in partial pressure. In the **single-breath method,** the partial pressure of CO in alveolar gas is very high and the partial pressure of CO in pulmonary capillary blood is initially zero. (Normally, we have no CO in our blood.) Thus, the partial pressure gradient across the alveolar–pulmonary capillary barrier is initially very high. The gradient remains high, even after CO begins to diffuse from alveolar gas into the blood, because CO binds avidly to hemoglobin in the blood, forming **carboxyhemoglobin.** Binding of CO to hemoglobin keeps both the free, unbound CO concentration and the partial pressure of CO in the blood low. Thus, the **driving force for CO diffusion is maintained** along the length of the pulmonary capillary. Consequently (because the driving force for CO diffusion never dissipates), the amount of CO that is transferred from alveolar gas into pulmonary capillary blood depends solely on the diffusion characteristics of the alveolar–pulmonary barrier (e.g., its thickness).

   Simone's D$_{LCO}$ was decreased because interstitial fibrosis is associated with **thickening of the alveolar walls**. This thickening increases the diffusion distance for gases such as CO and O$_2$ and decreases the total amount of gas that can be transferred across the alveolar wall.

3. At rest, Simone's Pa$_{O_2}$ was 76 mm Hg, which is lower than the normal value (100 mm Hg). Before we discuss why Simone's Pa$_{O_2}$ was decreased, let's consider how the value of 100 mm Hg is achieved in healthy people. Equilibration of O$_2$ occurs across the alveolar–pulmonary capillary barrier as follows. O$_2$ diffuses readily from alveolar gas into pulmonary capillary blood, driven by its partial pressure gradient, until the P$_{O_2}$ of the blood equals that of alveolar gas (approximately 100 mm Hg). Thus, the normal equilibration process results in a Pa$_{O_2}$ of 100 mm Hg.

In Simone's case, however, perfect equilibration of O_2 was impossible: thickening of the alveolar walls impaired O_2 diffusion (as detected in a decreased DL_{CO}), and Pa_{O2} could not become equal to alveolar P_{O2} (PA_{O2}).

4. Figure 3–10 shows the relationship between arterial P_{O2} (Pa_{O2}) and distance, or length, along the pulmonary capillary. For reference, alveolar P_{O2} (PA_{O2}) is represented by the dashed horizontal line at 100 mm Hg.

   The curve for healthy people **(normal)** shows how O_2 equilibrates across the alveolar–pulmonary capillary barrier, as described in Question 3. Mixed venous blood enters the pulmonary capillary with a P_{O2} of 40 mm Hg. At the beginning of the capillary, there is a large partial pressure gradient for O_2 diffusion because the P_{O2} of alveolar gas is much higher than that of mixed venous blood. O_2 readily diffuses down this partial pressure gradient, from alveolar gas into the pulmonary capillary blood. Initially, as O_2 enters the capillary, it binds to hemoglobin, which keeps the capillary P_{O2} low and maintains the partial pressure gradient for O_2 diffusion. However, after all of the binding sites on hemoglobin are occupied, the P_{O2} of the blood rapidly increases and becomes equal to the PA_{O2}. This equilibration point occurs approximately one-third of the distance along the capillary. From that point on, no further net diffusion of O_2 can occur because there is no longer a partial pressure gradient, or driving force. Blood leaves the capillary and becomes systemic arterial blood with a Pa_{O2} equal to PA_{O2} (100 mm Hg). In healthy people, this process is described as **perfusion-limited** because equilibration of O_2 occurs *early* along the length of the pulmonary capillary. The only way to increase the amount of O_2 transferred into the blood is to provide more blood flow, or *perfusion.*

   In patients with **fibrosis,** let's presume (for the sake of discussion) that mixed venous blood enters the pulmonary capillary at the same P_{O2} as in healthy people (40 mm Hg). Thus, the driving force for O_2 diffusion is initially identical to that of healthy people. However, in fibrotic lungs, O_2 diffusion is severely impaired because of thickening of the alveolar walls. As a result, the rate of O_2 diffusion is much lower than in normal lungs. Although P_{O2} gradually increases along the length of the capillary, O_2 never equilibrates. The blood that leaves the pulmonary capillary (to become systemic arterial blood) has a much lower P_{O2} than alveolar gas (in Simone's case, 76 mm Hg). Thus, in fibrosis, O_2 exchange becomes **diffusion-limited.** The partial pressure gradient for O_2 is maintained along the entire length of the pulmonary capillary, and equilibration never occurs. (For purposes of discussion, mixed venous blood was shown entering the pulmonary capillary with a normal P_{O2} of 40 mm Hg. However, because the disease process decreases Pa_{O2}, it is expected that venous P_{O2} would eventually be decreased as well. This simplification does not detract from the major point of the question.)

5. The **total O_2 content of blood** has two components: (i) free, dissolved O_2 and (ii) O_2-hemoglobin. By now, you know that **O_2-hemoglobin** is by far the greater contributor to total O_2 content. However, to be thorough, let's calculate both dissolved and bound O_2 for Simone at rest, as described in Case 22.

$$\begin{aligned} \text{Dissolved } O_2 &= P_{O2} \times \text{solubility} \\ &= 76 \text{ mm Hg} \times 0.003 \text{ mL } O_2/100 \text{ blood/mm Hg} \\ &= 0.23 \text{ mL } O_2/100 \text{ mL blood} \\ \\ O_2\text{-hemoglobin} &= O_2\text{-binding capacity} \times \% \text{ saturation} \\ &= (\text{hemoglobin concentration} \times O_2\text{-binding capacity}) \times \% \text{ saturation} \\ &= (15 \text{ g/dL} \times 1.34 \text{ mL } O_2/\text{g hemoglobin}) \times \% \text{ saturation} \\ &= 20.1 \text{ mL } O_2/100 \text{ mL blood} \times 97\% \\ &= 19.5 \text{ mL } O_2/100 \text{ mL blood} \\ \\ \text{Total } O_2 \text{ content} &= \text{dissolved } O_2 + O_2\text{-hemoglobin} \\ &= 0.23 \text{ mL } O_2/100 \text{ mL blood} + 19.5 \text{ mL } O_2/100 \text{ mL blood} \\ &= 19.7 \text{ mL } O_2/100 \text{ mL blood} \end{aligned}$$

6. You were asked to suggest possible reasons why Simone's Pa_{O_2} decreased further when she exercised. Worsening of **hypoxemia** during exercise is typical in pulmonary fibrosis. We know that thickening of the alveolar walls compromises O_2 diffusion and lowered Simone's Pa_{O_2} at rest. But why should O_2 exchange *worsen* during exercise? Perhaps, based on the discussions of the importance of ventilation–perfusion ($\dot{V}/\dot{Q}$) matching in this chapter, you wondered whether exercise might induce a $\dot{V}/\dot{Q}$ defect in fibrosis. Good thinking!

During exercise, we expect both ventilation and perfusion (cardiac output) to increase to meet the body's greater demand for O_2. However, in fibrosis, these increases in ventilation and cardiac output are limited, and because of the limitations, hypoxemia worsens with exercise. Because of the restrictive nature of fibrosis, it is difficult for patients to increase their tidal volume as a mechanism for increasing ventilation; instead, they tend to increase breathing rate. This rapid, shallow breathing **increases dead space ventilation.** Increasing dead space causes a $\dot{V}/\dot{Q}$ **defect** and worsens hypoxemia. Also in fibrosis, there are associated increases in pulmonary vascular resistance, which increase afterload on the heart and limit the increase in cardiac output. The limited increase in cardiac output and tissue blood flow results in *increased tissue extraction of O_2,* which decreases venous P_{O_2}. Thus, when patients with fibrosis exercise, the mixed venous blood entering the lungs has a P_{O_2} that is lower than at rest. This lower "starting point," coupled with the diffusion defect already discussed, causes arterial blood to have an *even lower P_{O_2} during exercise* than at rest.

7. Simone's percent saturation was further decreased during exercise because her Pa_{O_2} was further decreased. The **O_2-hemoglobin dissociation curve** (discussed in Case 22) describes the relationship between percent O_2 saturation of hemoglobin and P_{O_2} (see Fig. 3–4). At a P_{O_2} of 100 mm Hg, hemoglobin is 100% saturated (four O_2 molecules per hemoglobin molecule). At a P_{O_2} of 76 mm Hg (Simone at rest), hemoglobin is approximately 97% saturated. At a P_{O_2} of 62 mm Hg (Simone during exercise), hemoglobin is approximately 90% saturated.

Because her percent saturation was decreased, the total O_2 content of Simone's blood was lower during exercise than at rest. How did this change affect **O_2 delivery to the tissues?** O_2 delivery is the product of blood flow (cardiac output) and O_2 content of the blood. Although Simone's cardiac output was undoubtedly increased during exercise (but less than in a healthy person), her O_2 content was decreased because the amount of O_2 bound to hemoglobin was decreased. Given the increased O_2 requirement of the body during exercise, it is not surprising that O_2 delivery to the tissues was insufficient to meet the demand (i.e., Simone's exercise tolerance was very poor).

8. Although Simone has a problem with O_2 exchange and is hypoxemic (she has a decreased Pa_{O_2}), she does not seem to have a problem with CO_2 exchange. That is, she is not hypercapnic (she does not have CO_2 retention or an increased Pa_{CO_2}). In fact, both at rest and during exercise, Simone's Pa_{CO_2} was slightly lower than the normal value of 40 mm Hg. This pattern is common in patients with respiratory diseases: *hypoxemia can occur without hypercapnia.* But why?

Consider the sequence of events in Simone's lungs that created this pattern of arterial blood gases. The fibrotic disease affected some, but not all, regions of her lungs. The diseased regions had thickening of the alveolar walls and the diffusion barrier for O_2 and CO_2. The diffusion problem caused hypoxemia (decreased Pa_{O_2}) and may have briefly caused hypercapnia (increased Pa_{CO_2}). However, because the **central chemoreceptors** are exquisitely sensitive to small changes in P_{CO_2}, they responded to hypercapnia by increasing the ventilation rate. The increase in alveolar ventilation in healthy regions of the lungs eliminated excess CO_2 that was retained in unhealthy regions. In other words, by increasing alveolar ventilation, healthy regions of the lungs could compensate for unhealthy regions with respect to CO_2 exchange. As a result, Simone's P_{CO_2} returned to normal. Later in the course of her disease, **hypercapnia** *may* develop if she does not have enough healthy lung tissue to compensate for the unhealthy tissue, or if the **work of breathing** becomes so great that she cannot increase her alveolar ventilation sufficiently.

At this point, you may legitimately ask: If increased alveolar ventilation can rid the body of excess CO_2 that is retained by unhealthy regions of the lungs, why can't increased alveolar ventilation also correct the **hypoxia?** The answer lies in the characteristics of the O_2–hemoglobin curve. Increased alveolar ventilation does little to increase the total O_2 content of blood in healthy regions of the lung because of the saturation properties of hemoglobin. Once hemoglobin is 100% saturated (i.e., four O_2 molecules per hemoglobin molecule), further O_2 diffusion increases the P_{O_2} of the pulmonary capillary blood until it equals the P_{O_2} of alveolar gas. Once equilibration occurs, there is no further diffusion of O_2. The O_2 added to this blood is mostly in the dissolved form, which adds little to total O_2 content. Furthermore, well-oxygenated blood from healthy regions of the lung is always mixing with, and being diluted by, poorly oxygenated blood from unhealthy regions. As a result, the P_{aO_2} of the mixture (systemic arterial blood) will always be lower than normal.

Another question may arise from this discussion: Can the degree of hyperventilation be so great that the patient actually becomes hypocapnic (has decreased P_{aCO_2})? Absolutely! In fact, Simone's P_{aCO_2} is slightly lower than normal. If P_{aO_2} is low enough to stimulate the **peripheral chemoreceptors** (i.e., < 60 mm Hg), hyperventilation occurs, even greater amounts of CO_2 are expired by healthy regions of the lung, and P_{aCO_2} falls below the normal value of 40 mm Hg.

In summary, it is not uncommon for a patient with lung disease to pass through three stages of abnormal arterial blood gases: (i) mild hypoxemia with normocapnia; (ii) more severe hypoxemia (P_{aO_2} < 60 mm Hg) with **hypocapnia**, which results in **respiratory alkalosis;** and (iii) severe hypoxemia with hypercapnia, which results in **respiratory acidosis.** At this point in her disease, Simone is somewhere between the first and the second stage.

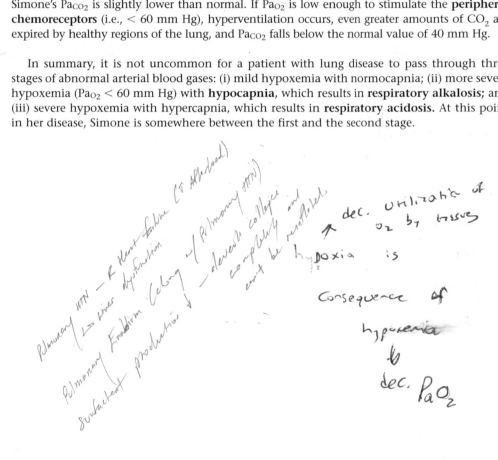

Key topics

Carbon monoxide

Carboxyhemoglobin

Central chemoreceptors

Compliance

Diffusion-limited gas exchange

D_L

$D_{L_{CO}}$

Elastance

FEV_1

FEV_1/FVC

Hypercapnia

Hypocapnia

Hypoxemia

Hypoxia

Lung diffusing capacity (D_L)

O_2 content of blood

O_2 delivery to tissues

O_2–hemoglobin dissociation curve

Perfusion-limited gas exchange

Peripheral chemoreceptors

Pulmonary fibrosis

Respiratory acidosis

Respiratory alkalosis

Restrictive lung disease

Single-breath method

Ventilation–perfusion ($\dot{V}/\dot{Q}$) defect

$\dot{V}/\dot{Q}$ ratio

Work of breathing

Case 27

Carbon Monoxide Poisoning

Herman Neiswander is a 65-year-old retired landscape architect in northern Wisconsin. One cold January morning, he decided to warm his car in the garage. Forty minutes later, Mr. Neiswander's wife found him slumped in the front seat of the car, confused and breathing rapidly. He was taken to a nearby emergency department, where he was diagnosed with acute carbon monoxide poisoning and given 100% O_2 to breathe. An arterial blood sample had an unusual cherry-red color. The values obtained in the blood sample are shown in Table 3–12.

TABLE 3–12	Mr. Neiswander's Arterial Blood Gases	
Pa_{O_2} (arterial P_{O_2})	660 mm Hg (normal, 100 mm Hg, room air)	
Pa_{CO_2} (arterial P_{CO_2})	36 mm Hg (normal, 40 mm Hg)	
% Saturation	50% (normal, 95–100%)	

 QUESTIONS

1. In healthy people, the percent O_2 saturation of hemoglobin in arterial blood is 95% to 100%. Why was Mr. Neiswander's O_2 saturation reduced to 50%?

2. What percentage of the heme groups on his hemoglobin were bound to carbon monoxide (CO)?

3. Draw a normal O_2–hemoglobin dissociation curve, and superimpose the O_2–hemoglobin dissociation curve that would have been obtained on Mr. Neiswander in the emergency department. What effect did CO poisoning have on his O_2-binding capacity? What effect did CO poisoning have on the affinity of hemoglobin for O_2?

4. How did CO poisoning alter O_2 delivery to Mr. Neiswander's tissues?

5. What was the rationale for giving Mr. Neiswander 100% O_2 to breathe?

6. In healthy people breathing room air, arterial P_{O_2} (Pa_{O_2}) is approximately 100 mm Hg. Mr. Neiswander had a Pa_{O_2} of 660 mm Hg while breathing 100% O_2. How is a value of 660 mm Hg possible? (Hint: There is a calculation that will help you to determine whether this value makes sense. For that calculation, assume that Mr. Neiswander's respiratory quotient [CO_2 production/O_2 consumption] was 0.8.)

7. What is an A–a gradient? What physiologic process does the presence or absence of an A–a gradient reflect? What was the value of Mr. Neiswander's A–a gradient while he was breathing 100% O_2? What interpretation can you offer for this value?

ANSWERS AND EXPLANATIONS

1. Mr. Neiswander's **percent O_2 saturation** was only 50% (normal, 95–100%) because CO occupied O_2-binding sites on hemoglobin. In fact, CO binds avidly to hemoglobin, with an affinity that is more than 200 times that of O_2. Thus, heme groups that should be bound to O_2 were instead bound to CO. Hemoglobin that is bound to CO is called **carboxyhemoglobin** and has a characteristic **cherry-red color.**

2. Because the percent saturation of O_2 was 50%, we can conclude that the remaining 50% of the heme sites were occupied by CO.

3. In the presence of CO, the **O_2–hemoglobin dissociation curve** is altered (Fig. 3–11). The maximum percent saturation of hemoglobin by O_2 was decreased (in Mr. Neiswander's case, to 50%), resulting in **decreased O_2-binding capacity.** A **left shift** of the curve also occurred because of a conformational change in the hemoglobin molecule caused by binding of CO. This conformational change increased the affinity of hemoglobin for the *remaining* bound O_2.

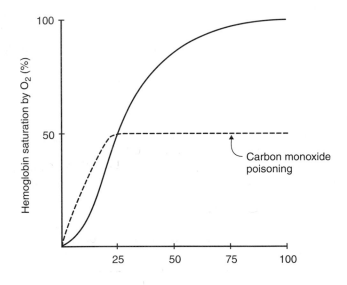

Figure 3–11   Effect of carbon monoxide on the O_2–hemoglobin dissociation curve.

4. **O_2 delivery** to the tissues is the product of blood flow (cardiac output) and O_2 content of the blood, as follows:

O_2 delivery = cardiac output × O_2 content of blood

The O_2 content of blood is the sum of dissolved O_2 and O_2 bound to hemoglobin. Of these two components, O_2-hemoglobin is by far the most important. In Mr. Neiswander's case, O_2 delivery to the tissues was significantly reduced for two reasons: (i) CO occupied O_2-binding sites on hemoglobin, decreasing the total amount of O_2 carried on hemoglobin in the blood. (ii) The remaining heme sites (those not occupied by CO) bound O_2 with a higher affinity (consistent with a left shift of the O_2–hemoglobin curve). This increase in affinity made it more difficult to unload O_2 in the tissues. These two effects of CO combined to cause severe O_2 deprivation in the tissues (**hypoxia**).

5. Mr. Neiswander was given **100% O_2** to breathe for two reasons: (i) to competitively displace as much CO from hemoglobin as possible and (ii) to increase the dissolved O_2 content in his blood. As you have learned, dissolved O_2 normally contributes little to the total O_2 content of

blood. However, in CO poisoning, the O_2-carrying capacity of hemoglobin is severely reduced (in this case, by 50%), and dissolved O_2 becomes, by default, relatively more significant. By increasing the fraction of O_2 in inspired air to 100% (room air is 21% O_2), the P_{O_2} in Mr. Neiswander's alveolar gas and arterial blood will be increased, which will increase the dissolved O_2 content (dissolved O_2 = P_{O_2} × solubility of O_2 in blood).

6. While Mr. Neiswander was breathing 100% O_2, the measured value for Pa_{O2} was strikingly high (660 mm Hg). Because pulmonary capillary blood normally equilibrates with alveolar gas, arterial P_{O2} (Pa_{O2}) should be equal to alveolar P_{O2} (PA_{O2}). Therefore, the question that we really need to answer is: *Why was the PA_{O2} 660 mm Hg?*

The **alveolar gas equation** is used to calculate the expected value for PA_{O2} (as described in Case 21). For the alveolar gas equation, we need to know the values for P_{O2} of inspired air (PI_{O2}), PA_{CO2}, and respiratory quotient. PI_{O2} is calculated from the barometric pressure (corrected for water vapor pressure) and the fraction of O_2 in inspired air (FI_{O2}). In Mr. Neiswander's case, FI_{O2} is 1.0, or 100%. PA_{CO2} is equal to Pa_{CO2}, which is given. The respiratory quotient is 0.8. Thus:

$$PI_{O_2} = (P_B - P_{H_2O}) \times FI_{O_2}$$

$$= (760 \text{ mm Hg} - 47 \text{ mm Hg}) \times 1.0$$

$$= 713 \text{ mm Hg}$$

$$PA_{O_2} = PI_{O_2} - \frac{PA_{CO_2}}{R}$$

$$= 713 \text{ mm Hg} - \frac{36 \text{ mm Hg}}{0.8}$$

$$= 668 \text{ mm Hg}$$

From this calculation, we know that when Mr. Neiswander breathed 100% O_2, his alveolar P_{O2} (PA_{O2}) was expected to be 668 mm Hg. Assuming that his systemic arterial blood was equilibrated with alveolar gas, the measured Pa_{O2} of 660 mm Hg makes perfect sense.

7. The **A–a gradient** is the difference in P_{O2} between alveolar gas ("A") and arterial blood ("a"). In other words, the A–a gradient tells us whether equilibration of O_2 between alveolar gas and pulmonary capillary blood has occurred. If the A–a gradient is zero or close to zero, then perfect (or nearly perfect) equilibration of O_2 occurred, as is normally the case. Increases in the A–a gradient indicate a lack of equilibration, as with a **ventilation–perfusion ($\dot{V}/\dot{Q}$) defect** (e.g., obstructive lung disease), when a diffusion defect is present (e.g., fibrosis), or with a **right-to-left cardiac shunt** (i.e., a portion of the cardiac output bypasses the lungs and is not oxygenated).

Mr. Neiswander's PA_{O2} was calculated from the alveolar gas equation (see Question 6), and his Pa_{O2} was measured in arterial blood. His A–a gradient is the difference between the two values:

$$\text{A–a gradient} = PA_{O2} - Pa_{O2}$$
$$= 668 \text{ mm Hg} - 660 \text{ mm Hg}$$
$$= 8 \text{ mm Hg}$$

This small difference between the P_{O2} of alveolar gas and the P_{O2} of arterial blood implies that pulmonary capillary blood equilibrated almost perfectly with alveolar gas. In other words, CO poisoning caused *no problems* with $\dot{V}/\dot{Q}$ matching or O_2 diffusion.

Key topics

A–a gradient

Alveolar gas equation

Carbon monoxide (CO) poisoning

Carboxyhemoglobin

Hypoxia

Left shift of the O_2–hemoglobin dissociation curve

O_2 delivery

O_2–hemoglobin dissociation curve

Right-to-left cardiac shunt

Ventilation–perfusion ($\dot{V}/\dot{Q}$) ratio

Case 28

Pneumothorax

Serena Cervantes and her boyfriend left their senior prom and were on the way to the post-prom party when a limousine carrying other students slammed broadside into their sport utility vehicle. Serena was not wearing a seatbelt, and she was thrown from the vehicle and landed on a fence. When the emergency medical crew arrived, it was clear that she had multiple injuries, including penetrating chest trauma that caused a pneumothorax. She was having difficulty breathing, and pulse oximetry showed an O_2 saturation of 85%. In the emergency department, a chest x-ray confirmed that her left lung had collapsed, and a large-bore chest tube was placed in her thoracic cavity.

 QUESTIONS

1. Following a traumatic pneumothorax, the pressure in the intrapleural space becomes zero. What is the normal intrapleural pressure, and what does this pressure of zero mean?

2. Why did the pneumothorax cause her left lung to collapse?

3. Pneumothorax also causes the chest wall to "spring out." Why?

4. The chest tube was connected to a vacuum pump. What is the purpose of creating a vacuum in the thoracic cavity?

5. Serena's O_2 saturation of 85% was much lower than normal. What is the significance of this number, and what caused it to be low?

ANSWERS AND EXPLANATIONS

1. Normal intrapleural pressure is negative, or less than atmospheric pressure. **Negative intrapleural pressure** is created by the elastic forces of the lungs and chest wall pulling in opposite direction on the intrapleural space. (Note that the intrapleural space is not a literal space, but a virtual space between the visceral and parietal pleura.) When the system is at equilibrium (i.e., at functional residual capacity, FRC), the lungs, with their elastic properties, are naturally inclined to collapse, and the chest wall, with its elastic properties, is inclined to spring out. These two equal and opposite forces pulling on the intrapleural space create a vacuum, or negative pressure, in the space.

    When Serena sustained a penetrating chest wound in the accident, her chest wall was punctured and her intrapleural space was opened to the atmosphere. Her intrapleural pressure was "zero," meaning that intrapleural pressure was equal to atmospheric pressure. (By convention, lung pressures are always expressed relative to atmospheric pressure.)

2. **Pneumothorax** caused her lung to collapse because the injury eliminated the normal, negative intrapleural pressure. Normally, the lungs are held open by the negative intrapleural pressure outside of them. Without this negative outside pressure, the lungs follow their natural tendency to collapse (owing to their elastic properties), as shown in Figure 3–12.

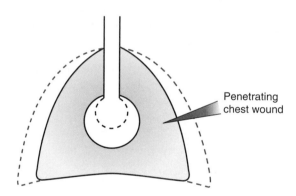

Penetrating
chest wound

Figure 3–12 Pneumothorax. The solid lines show the original position of the lungs and chest wall. The *dashed lines* show that the lungs collapse and the chest wall springs out following a pneumothorax.

3. The elastic properties of the chest wall are such that it is naturally inclined to "spring out" (like a compressed coil). This tendency of the chest wall is normally opposed by the negative intrapleural pressure. (Just as the negative intrapleural pressure keeps the lungs from collapsing, it also keeps the chest wall from springing out.) When the negative intrapleural pressure is eliminated by a traumatic pneumothorax, the chest wall springs out because there is no longer a force opposing its natural tendency (also shown in Figure 3–12).

4. A large-bore tube connected to vacuum was inserted in Serena's chest. The vacuum restored the negative pressure that is normally present in the intrapleural space, which would have the effect of reinflating her collapsed lung.

5. While Serena's left lung was collapsed, pulse oximetry estimated her **O_2 saturation** at 85%. This measurement refers to **percent saturation of hemoglobin by O_2;** a value of 85% means that 85% of heme groups are bound to O_2, and 15% are not bound. Percent saturation of hemoglobin is a way of **approximating arterial P_{O_2}** according to the **O_2-hemoglobin dissociation curve** shown in Figure 3–13. Eighty-five percent saturation corresponds to an arterial P_{O_2} of approximately 50 mm Hg.

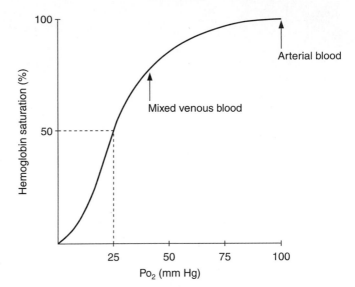

Figure 3–13 O_2–hemoglobin dissociation curve.

Serena's estimated arterial P_{O_2} of 50 mm Hg is significantly lower than the normal value of 100 mm Hg—she had severe **hypoxemia**, which is caused by a **ventilation–perfusion ($\dot{V}/\dot{Q}$) defect.** Secondary to the pneumothorax, her left lung collapsed and was not being ventilated; consequently, the blood flow to her left lung became a **shunt**, in which there is perfusion of lung regions with no ventilation. The blood perfusing her left lung, the shunt, had the same P_{O_2} as mixed venous blood, typically 40 mm Hg. This shunted blood from the left lung mixes with blood flow to the ventilated right lung, and dilutes the overall P_{O_2} of systemic arterial blood **(venous admixture).**

Key topics
Hypoxemia
Intrapleural pressure
O_2–hemoglobin dissociation curve
O_2 saturation
Pneumothorax
Venous admixture
Ventilation–perfusion ($\dot{V}/\dot{Q}$) defect

Renal and Acid–Base Physiology

Case 29

Essential Calculations in Renal Physiology

This case will guide you through some of the basic equations and calculations in renal physiology. Use the data provided in Table 4–1 to answer the questions.

TABLE 4–1	*Renal Physiology Values for Case 29*
$\dot{V}$ (urine flow rate)	1 mL/min
P_{inulin} (plasma concentration of inulin)	100 mg/mL
U_{inulin} (urine concentration of inulin)	12 g/mL
RA_{PAH} (renal artery concentration of PAH)	1.2 mg/mL
RV_{PAH} (renal vein concentration of PAH)	0.1 mg/mL
U_{PAH} (urine concentration of PAH)	650 mg/mL
P_A (plasma concentration of A)	10 mg/mL
U_A (urine concentration of A)	2 g/mL
P_B (plasma concentration of B)	10 mg/mL
U_B (urine concentration of B)	10 mg/mL
Hematocrit	0.45

PAH, para-aminohippuric acid; A, Substance A; B, Substance B.

Q QUESTIONS

1. What is the value for the glomerular filtration rate (GFR)?

2. What is the value for the "true" renal *plasma* flow? What is the value for the "true" renal *blood* flow? What is the value for the "effective" renal plasma flow? Why is effective renal plasma flow different from true renal plasma flow?

3. What is the value for the filtration fraction, and what is the meaning of this value?

4. Assuming that Substance A is freely filtered (i.e., not bound to plasma proteins), what is the filtered load of Substance A? Is Substance A reabsorbed or secreted? What is the rate of reabsorption or secretion?

5. What is the fractional excretion of Substance A?

6. What is the clearance of Substance A? Is this value for clearance consistent with the conclusion you reached in Question 4 about whether Substance A is reabsorbed or secreted?

7. Substance B is 30% bound to plasma proteins. Is Substance B reabsorbed or secreted? What is the rate of reabsorption or secretion?

ANSWERS ON NEXT PAGE

ANSWERS AND EXPLANATIONS

1. The **glomerular filtration rate** (GFR) is measured by the clearance of a glomerular marker. A **glomerular marker** is a substance that is freely filtered across the glomerular capillaries and is neither reabsorbed nor secreted by the renal tubules. The ideal glomerular marker is **inulin**. Thus, the clearance of inulin is the GFR.

The generic equation for **clearance** of any substance, X, is:

$$C_x = \frac{U_x \times \dot{V}}{P_x}$$

where

C_x = clearance (mL/min)
U_x = urine concentration of substance X (e.g., mg/mL)
P_x = plasma concentration of substance X (e.g., mg/mL)
$\dot{V}$ = urine flow rate (mL/min)

The **GFR**, or the clearance of inulin, is expressed as:

$$GFR = \frac{U_{inulin} \times \dot{V}}{P_{inulin}}$$

where

GFR = glomerular filtration rate (mL/min)
U_{inulin} = urine concentration of inulin (e.g., mg/mL)
P_{inulin} = plasma concentration of inulin (e.g., mg/mL)
$\dot{V}$ = urine flow rate (mL/min)

In this case, the value for GFR (clearance of inulin) is:

$$GFR = \frac{U_{inulin} \times \dot{V}}{P_{inulin}}$$

$$= \frac{12 \text{ g/mL} \times 1 \text{ mL/min}}{100 \text{ mg/mL}}$$

$$= \frac{12,000 \text{ mg/mL} \times 1 \text{ mL/min}}{100 \text{ mg/mL}}$$

$$= 120 \text{ mg/mL}$$

2. Renal plasma flow is measured with an organic acid called ***para*-aminohippuric acid (PAH)**. The properties of PAH are very different from those of inulin. PAH is both filtered across the glomerular capillaries *and* secreted by the renal tubules, whereas inulin is only filtered. The equation for measuring "true" renal plasma flow with PAH is based on the Fick principle of conservation of mass. The Fick principle states that the amount of PAH entering the kidney through the renal artery equals the amount of PAH leaving the kidney through the renal vein and the ureter. Therefore, the equation for **"true" renal plasma flow** is as follows:

$$RPF = \frac{U_{PAH} \times \dot{V}}{RA_{PAH} - RV_{PAH}}$$

where

RPF = renal plasma flow (mL/min)
U_{PAH} = urine concentration of PAH (e.g., mg/mL)

RA_{PAH} = renal artery concentration of PAH (e.g., mg/mL)
RV_{PAH} = renal vein concentration of PAH (e.g., mg/mL)
$\dot{V}$ = urine flow rate (mL/min)

Thus, in this case, the "true" renal plasma flow is:

$$RPF = \frac{650 \text{ mg/mL} \times 1 \text{ mL/min}}{1.2 \text{ mg/mL} - 0.1 \text{ mg/mL}}$$

$$RPF = \frac{650 \text{ mg/min}}{1.1 \text{ mg/mL}}$$

$$= 591 \text{ mL/min}$$

Renal blood flow is calculated from the measured renal plasma flow and the hematocrit, as follows:

$$\textbf{RBF} = \frac{\textbf{RPF}}{\textbf{1 - Hct}}$$

where

RBF = renal blood flow (mL/min)
RPF = renal plasma flow (mL/min)
Hct = hematocrit (no units)

In words, RBF is RPF divided by 1 minus the hematocrit. **Hematocrit** is the fractional blood volume occupied by red blood cells. Thus, 1 minus the hematocrit is the fractional blood volume occupied by plasma. In this case, RBF is:

$$RBF = \frac{591 \text{ mL/min}}{1 - 0.45}$$

$$= 1,075 \text{ mL/min}$$

Looking at the equation for "true" renal plasma flow, you can appreciate that this measurement would be difficult to make in human beings—blood from the renal artery and renal vein would have to be sampled directly! The measurement can be simplified, however, by applying two reasonable assumptions. (i) The concentration of PAH in the renal vein is zero, or nearly zero, because all of the PAH that enters the kidney is excreted in the urine through a combination of filtration and secretion processes. (ii) The concentration of PAH in the renal artery equals the concentration of PAH in any systemic vein (other than the renal vein). This second assumption is based on the fact that no organ, other than the kidney, extracts PAH. With these two assumptions (i.e., renal vein PAH is zero and renal artery PAH is the same as systemic venous plasma PAH), we have a much simplified version of the equation, which is now called "effective" renal plasma flow. Note that **effective renal plasma flow** is also the **clearance of PAH**, as follows:

$$\textbf{Effective RPF} = \frac{\textbf{U}_{PAH} \times \dot{\textbf{V}}}{\textbf{P}_{PAH}} = \textbf{C}_{PAH}$$

For this case, effective RPF is:

$$\text{Effective RPF} = \frac{650 \text{ mg/mL} \times 1 \text{ mL/min}}{1.2 \text{ mg/mL}} = 542 \text{ mL/min}$$

Effective RPF (542 mL/min) is less than true RPF (591 mL/min). Thus, the effective RPF underestimates the true RPF by approximately 10% [(591 − 542)/591 = 0.11, or 11%]. This underestimation occurs because the renal vein concentration of PAH is *not exactly* zero (as we had assumed), it is *nearly* zero. Approximately 10% of the RPF serves renal tissue that is not involved in the filtration and secretion of PAH (e.g., renal adipose tissue). The PAH in that portion of the RPF appears in renal venous blood, not in the urine.

Naturally, you are wondering, "When should I calculate true RPF and when should I calculate effective RPF?" Although there are no hard and fast rules among examiners, it is safe to assume that if you are given values for renal artery and renal vein PAH, you will use them to calculate true RPF. If you are given only the systemic venous plasma concentration of PAH, then you will calculate effective RPF.

3. Filtration fraction is the fraction of the renal plasma flow that is filtered across the glomerular capillaries. In other words, **filtration fraction** is GFR divided by RPF:

$$\textbf{Filtration fraction} = \frac{\textbf{GFR}}{\textbf{RPF}}$$

In this case:

$$\text{Filtration fraction} = \frac{120 \, \text{mL/min}}{591 \, \text{mL/min}}$$

$$= 0.20$$

This value for filtration fraction (0.20, or 20%) is typical for normal kidneys. It means that approximately 20% of the renal plasma flow entering the kidneys through the renal arteries is filtered across the glomerular capillaries. The remaining 80% of the renal plasma flow leaves the glomerular capillaries through the efferent arterioles and becomes the peritubular capillary blood flow.

4. These questions concern the calculation of filtered load, excretion rate, and reabsorption or secretion rate of Substance A (Fig. 4–1).

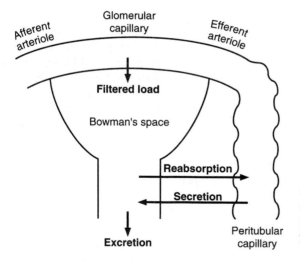

Figure 4–1 Processes of filtration, reabsorption, secretion, and excretion in the nephron. (Reprinted, with permission, from Costanzo LS: *BRS Physiology.* 4th ed. Baltimore: Lippincott Williams & Wilkins; 2007:160.)

An interstitial-type fluid is filtered from glomerular capillary blood into the Bowman space (the first part of the proximal convoluted tubule). The amount of a substance filtered per unit time is called the **filtered load**. This glomerular filtrate is subsequently modified by reabsorption and secretion processes in the epithelial cells that line the nephron. With **reabsorption**, a substance that was previously filtered is transported *from* the lumen of the nephron into the peritubular capillary blood. Many substances are reabsorbed, including Na^+, Cl^-, HCO_3^-, amino acids, and water. With **secretion**, a substance is transported from peritubular capillary blood *into* the lumen of the nephron. A few substances are secreted, including K^+, H^+, and organic acids and bases. **Excretion rate** is the amount of a substance that is excreted per unit time; it is the sum, or net result, of the three processes of filtration, reabsorption, and secretion.

We can determine whether net reabsorption or net secretion of a substance has occurred by comparing its excretion rate with its filtered load. If the excretion rate is *less than* the filtered load, the substance was reabsorbed. If the excretion rate is *greater than* the filtered load, the substance was secreted. Thus, it is necessary to know how to calculate filtered load and excretion rate. With this information, we can then calculate reabsorption or secretion rate intuitively.

The filtered load of any substance, X, is the product of GFR and the plasma concentration of X, as follows:

Filtered load $= GFR \times P_x$

where

Filtered load = amount of X filtered per minute (e.g., mg/min)
$\quad$ GFR = glomerular filtration rate (mL/min)
$\quad\quad P_x$ = plasma concentration of X (e.g., mg/mL)

The excretion rate of any substance, X, is the product of urine flow rate and the urine concentration of X:

Excretion rate $= \dot{V} \times U_x$

where

Excretion rate = amount of X excreted per minute (e.g., mg/min)
$\quad\quad \dot{V}$ = urine flow rate (mL/min)
$\quad\quad U_x$ = urine concentration of X (e.g., mg/mL)

Now we are ready to calculate the values for filtered load and excretion rate of Substance A, and to determine whether Substance A is reabsorbed or secreted. The GFR was previously calculated from the clearance of inulin as 120 mL/min.

$$\text{Filtered load of A} = GFR \times P_A$$
$$= 120 \text{ mL/min} \times 10 \text{ mg/mL}$$
$$= 1{,}200 \text{ mg/min}$$
$$\text{Excretion rate of A} = \dot{V} \times U_A$$
$$= 1 \text{ mL/min} \times 2 \text{ g/mL}$$
$$= 1 \text{ mL/min} \times 2{,}000 \text{ mg/mL}$$
$$= 2{,}000 \text{ mg/min}$$

The filtered load of Substance A is 1,200 mg/min, and the excretion rate of Substance A is 2,000 mg/min. How can there be more of Substance A excreted in the urine than was originally filtered? Substance A must have been *secreted* from the peritubular capillary blood into the tubular fluid (urine). Intuitively, we can determine that the net rate of secretion of Substance A is 800 mg/min (the difference between the excretion rate and the filtered load).

5. The **fractional excretion** of a substance is the fraction (or percent) of the filtered load that is excreted in the urine. Therefore, fractional excretion is excretion rate ($U_x \times \dot{V}$) divided by filtered load ($GFR \times P_x$), as follows:

$$\text{Fractional excretion} = \frac{U_x \times \dot{V}}{GFR \times P_x}$$

where

Fractional excretion = fraction of the filtered load excreted in the urine
U_x = urine concentration of X (e.g., mg/mL)
P_x = plasma concentration of X (e.g., mg/mL)
$\dot{V}$ = urine flow rate (mL/min)
GFR = glomerular filtration rate (mL/min)

For Substance A, fractional excretion is:

$$\text{Filtration fraction} = \frac{\text{Excretion rate}}{\text{Filtered load}}$$

$$= \frac{U_A \times \dot{V}}{GFR \times P_A}$$

$$= \frac{2 \text{ g/mL} \times 1 \text{ mL/min}}{120 \text{ mL/min} \times 10 \text{ mg/mL}}$$

$$= \frac{2000 \text{ mg/min}}{1200 \text{ mg/min}}$$

$$= 1.67, \text{ or } 167\%$$

You may question how this number is possible. Can we actually excrete 167% of the amount that was originally filtered? Yes, we can if secretion adds a large amount of Substance A to the urine, over and above the amount that was originally filtered.

6. The concept of clearance and the clearance equation were discussed in Question 1. The renal clearance of Substance A is calculated with the clearance equation:

$$C_A = \frac{U_A \times \dot{V}}{P_A}$$

$$= \frac{2 \text{ g/mL} \times 1 \text{ mL/min}}{10 \text{ mg/mL}}$$

$$= \frac{2000 \text{ mg/mL} \times 1 \text{ mL/min}}{10 \text{ mg/mL}}$$

$$= 200 \text{ mL/min}$$

The question asked whether this calculated value of clearance is consistent with the conclusion reached in Questions 4 and 5. (The conclusion from Questions 4 and 5 was that Substance A is secreted by the renal tubule.) To answer this question, compare the clearance of Substance A (200 mL/min) with the clearance of inulin (120 mL/min). Inulin is a pure glomerular marker that is filtered, but neither reabsorbed nor secreted. The clearance of Substance A is higher than the clearance of inulin because Substance A is both filtered and secreted, whereas inulin is only filtered. Thus, comparing the clearance of Substance A with the clearance of inulin gives the same qualitative answer as the calculations in Questions 4 and 5—Substance A is secreted.

7. The approach to this question is the same as that used in Question 4, except that Substance B is 30% bound to plasma proteins. Because plasma proteins are not filtered, 30% of Substance B in plasma cannot be filtered across the glomerular capillaries; only 70% of Substance B in plasma is filterable. This correction is applied in the calculation of filtered load.

Filtered load of B = GFR × P_B × % filterable
= 120 mL/min × 10 mg/mL × 0.7
= 840 mg/min

Excretion rate of B = $\dot{V} \times U_B$
$$= 1 \text{ mL/min} \times 10 \text{ mg/mL}$$
$$= 10 \text{ mg/min}$$

Because the excretion rate of Substance B (10 mg/min) is much less than the filtered load (840 mg/min), Substance B must have been reabsorbed. The rate of net reabsorption, calculated intuitively from the difference between filtered load and excretion rate, is 830 mg/min.

Key topics

Clearance

Effective renal plasma flow

Excretion rate

Filtered load

Filtration fraction

Fractional excretion

Glomerular filtration rate (GFR)

Hematocrit

Reabsorption

Renal blood flow

Renal plasma flow

Secretion

Case 30

Essential Calculations in Acid–Base Physiology

This case will guide you through essential calculations in acid–base physiology. Use the values provided in Table 4–2 to answer the questions.

TABLE 4–2	Constants for Case 30	
pK of HCO_3^-/CO_2		6.1
$[CO_2]$		$P_{CO_2} \times 0.03$

 QUESTIONS

1. If the H^+ concentration of a blood sample is 40×10^{-9} Eq/L, what is the pH of the blood?

2. A weak acid, HA, dissociates in solution into H^+ and the conjugate base, A^-. If the pK of this weak acid is 4.5, will the concentration of HA or A^- be higher at a pH of 7.4? How much higher will it be?

3. For the three sets of information shown in Table 4–3, calculate the missing values.

TABLE 4–3	Acid–Base Values for Case 30		
	pH	HCO_3^-	P_{CO_2}
A		14 mEq/L	36 mm Hg
B	7.6		48 mm Hg
C	7.2	26 mEq/L	

4. A man with chronic obstructive pulmonary disease is hypoventilating. The hypoventilation caused him to retain CO_2 and to increase his arterial P_{CO_2} to 70 mm Hg (much higher than the normal value of 40 mm Hg). If his arterial HCO_3^- concentration is normal (24 mEq/L), what is his arterial pH? Is this value compatible with life? What value of arterial HCO_3^- would make his arterial pH 7.4?

5. Figure 4–2 shows a titration curve for a hypothetical buffer, a weak acid.

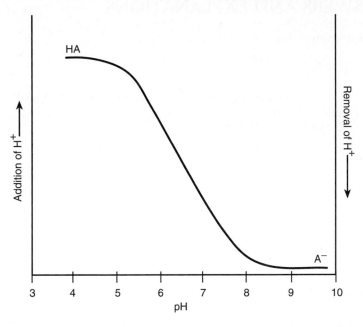

Figure 4–2 Titration curve for a weak acid. (HA, weak acid; A⁻, conjugate base.)

What is the approximate pK of this buffer? At a pH of 7.4, which is the predominant form of the buffer, HA or A⁻? If H⁺ was added to a solution containing this buffer, would the greatest change in pH occur between pH 8 and 9, between pH 6 and 7, or between pH 5 and 6?

A ANSWERS AND EXPLANATIONS

1. The **pH** of a solution is $-\log_{10}$ of the H^+ concentration:

$$pH = -\log_{10} [H^+]$$

Thus, the pH of a blood sample with an H^+ concentration of 40×10^{-9} Eq/L is:

$$
\begin{aligned}
pH &= -\log_{10} 40 \times 10^{-9} \text{ Eq/L} \\
&= -\log_{10} 4 \times 10^{-8} \text{ Eq/L} \\
&= -\log_{10} (4) + -\log_{10} (10^{-8}) \\
&= -0.6 + (-)(-8) \\
&= -0.6 + 8 \\
&= 7.4
\end{aligned}
$$

In performing this basic calculation, you were reminded that: (i) a logarithmic term is more than a "button on my calculator"; (ii) a blood pH of 7.4 (the normal value) corresponds to an H^+ concentration of 40×10^{-9} Eq/L; and (iii) the H^+ concentration of blood is *very low!*

2. The **Henderson–Hasselbalch equation** is used to calculate the pH of a buffered solution when the concentrations of the **weak acid** (HA) and the **conjugate base** (A^-) are known. Or, it can be used to calculate the relative concentrations of HA and A^- if the pH is known.

$$\mathbf{pH = pK + \log \dfrac{A^-}{HA}}$$

where

$pH = -\log_{10} [H^+]$
$pK = -\log_{10}$ of the equilibrium constant
$A^- =$ concentration of the conjugate base, the proton acceptor
$HA =$ concentration of the weak acid, the proton donor

For this question, you were given the pK of a **buffer** (4.5) and the pH of a solution containing this buffer (7.4), and you were asked to calculate the relative concentrations of A^- and HA.

$$pH = pK + \log \dfrac{A^-}{HA}$$

$$7.4 = 4.5 + \log \dfrac{A^-}{HA}$$

$$2.9 = \log \dfrac{A^-}{HA}$$

Taking the antilog of both sides of the equation:

$$794 = A^-/HA$$

Thus, at pH 7.4, for a weak acid with a pK of 4.5, much more of the A^- form than the HA form is present (794 times more).

3. These questions concern calculations with the HCO_3^-/CO_2 **buffer** pair, which has a pK of 6.1. For this buffer, HCO_3^- is the conjugate base (A^-) and CO_2 is the weak acid (HA). The Henderson–Hasselbalch equation, as applied to the HCO_3^-/CO_2 buffer, is written as follows:

$$pH = 6.1 + \log \dfrac{HCO_3^-}{CO_2}$$

Although values for CO_2 are usually reported as P_{CO_2}, for this calculation we need to know the CO_2 *concentration*. The CO_2 concentration is calculated as $P_{CO_2} \times 0.03$. (The conversion factor, 0.03, converts P_{CO_2} in mm Hg to CO_2 concentration in mmol/L.)

$$pH = 6.1 + \log \frac{HCO_3^-}{P_{CO_2} \times 0.03}$$

where

$$pH = -\log_{10} \text{ of } [H^+]$$
$$6.1 = pK \text{ of the } HCO_3^-/CO_2 \text{ buffer}$$
$$HCO_3^- = HCO_3^- \text{ concentration (mmol/L or mEq/L)}$$
$$P_{CO_2} = \text{partial pressure of } CO_2 \text{ (mm Hg)}$$
$$0.03 = \text{factor that converts } P_{CO_2} \text{ to } CO_2 \text{ concentration in blood (mmol/L per mm Hg)}$$

A. $pH = 6.1 + \log \dfrac{14}{36 \times 0.03}$

   $= 6.1 + \log 12.96$

   $= 6.1 + 1.11$

   $= 7.21$

B. $7.6 = 6.1 + \log \dfrac{HCO_3^-}{48 \times 0.03}$

   $7.6 = 6.1 + \log \dfrac{HCO_3^-}{1.44}$

   $1.5 = \log \dfrac{HCO_3^-}{1.44}$

   Taking the antilog of both sides:

   $31.62 = \dfrac{HCO_3^-}{1.44}$

   $HCO_3^- = 45.5 \text{ mEq/L}$

C. $7.2 = 6.1 + \log \dfrac{26}{P_{CO_2} \times 0.03}$

   $1.10 = \log \dfrac{26}{P_{CO_2} \times 0.03}$

   Taking the antilog of both sides:

   $12.6 = \dfrac{26}{P_{CO_2} \times 0.03}$

   $P_{CO_2} \times 0.03 = \dfrac{26}{12.6}$

   $P_{CO_2} \times 0.03 = 2.06$

   $P_{CO_2} = 69 \text{ mm Hg}$

4. For this question, we were given a P_{CO_2} of 70 mm Hg and an HCO_3^- concentration of 24 mEq/L. We apply the Henderson–Hasselbalch equation to calculate the pH.

$$pH = 6.1 + \log \frac{HCO_3^-}{P_{CO_2} \times 0.03}$$

$$= 6.1 + \log \frac{24}{70 \times 0.03}$$

$$= 6.1 + \log 11.4$$

$$= 6.1 + 1.06$$

$$= 7.16$$

The lowest arterial pH that is compatible with life is 6.8. Technically, this calculated pH of 7.16 is compatible with life, but it represents severe acidemia (acidic pH of the blood). To make the person's pH normal (7.4), his or her blood HCO_3^- concentration would have to be:

$$7.4 = 6.1 + \log \frac{HCO_3^-}{70 \times 0.03}$$

$$= 6.1 + \log \frac{HCO_3^-}{2.1}$$

$$1.3 = \log \frac{HCO_3^-}{2.1}$$

Taking the antilog of both sides:

$$19.95 = \frac{HCO_3^-}{2.1}$$

$$HCO_3^- = 41.9 \, mEq/L$$

This calculation is not just an algebraic exercise; it also illustrates the concept of **"compensation,"** which is applied in several cases in this chapter. In acid–base balance, compensation refers to processes that help correct the pH toward normal. This exercise with the Henderson–Hasselbalch equation shows how a normal pH can be achieved in a person with an abnormally high P_{CO_2}. (A normal pH can be achieved if the HCO_3^- concentration is increased proportionately as much as the P_{CO_2} is increased.) Note, however, that in real-life situations, compensatory mechanisms may restore the pH nearly (but never perfectly) to 7.4.

5. **Titration curves** are useful visual aids for understanding buffering and the Henderson–Hasselbalch equation. The **pK of the buffer** shown in Figure 4–2 is the pH at which the concentrations of the HA and the A$^-$ forms are equal (i.e., pH = 6.5). This pH coincides with the midpoint of the linear range of the titration curve, where addition or removal of H$^+$ causes the smallest change in pH of the solution. To determine which form of the buffer predominates at pH 7.4, locate pH 7.4 on the x-axis; visually, you can see that the predominant form at this pH is A$^-$. If H$^+$ were added to a solution containing this buffer, the greatest change in pH (of the stated choices) would occur between pH 8 and 9.

Key topics

Buffers

Conjugate base

HCO_3^-/CO_2 buffer

Henderson–Hasselbalch equation

pH

pK

Titration curves

Weak acid

Case 31

Glucosuria: Diabetes Mellitus

David Mandel was diagnosed with type I (insulin-dependent) diabetes mellitus when he was 12 years old, right after he started middle school. David was an excellent student, particularly in math and science, and had many friends, most of whom he had known since nursery school. Then, at a sleepover party, the unimaginable happened: David wet his sleeping bag! He might not have told his parents if he had not been worried about other symptoms he was experiencing. He was constantly thirsty (drinking a total of 3 to 4 quarts of liquids daily) and was urinating every 30 to 40 minutes. (The night of the accident, he had already been to the bathroom four times.) Furthermore, despite a voracious appetite, he seemed to be losing weight. David's parents panicked: they had heard that these were classic symptoms of diabetes mellitus. A urine dipstick test was positive for glucose, and David was immediately seen by his pediatrician. Table 4–4 shows the findings on physical examination and the results of laboratory tests.

TABLE 4–4	*David's Physical Examination Findings and Laboratory Values*
Height	5 feet, 3 inches
Weight	100 lb (115 lb at his annual checkup 2 months earlier)
Blood pressure	90/55 (lying)
	75/45 (standing)
Fasting plasma glucose	320 mg/dL (normal, 70–110 mg/dL)
Plasma Na^+	143 mEq/L (normal, 140 mEq/L)
Urine glucose	4+ (normal, none)
Urine ketones	2+ (normal, none)
Urine Na^+	Increased

In addition, David had decreased skin turgor, sunken eyes, and a dry mouth.

All of the physical findings and laboratory results were consistent with type I diabetes mellitus. David's pancreatic beta cells had stopped secreting insulin (perhaps secondary to autoimmune destruction after a viral infection). His insulin deficiency caused hyperglycemia (an increase in blood glucose concentration) through two effects: (i) increased hepatic gluconeogenesis and (ii) inhibition of glucose uptake and utilization by his cells. Insulin deficiency also increased lipolysis and hepatic ketogenesis. The resulting ketoacids (acetoacetic acid and β-OH butyric acid) were excreted in David's urine (urinary ketones).

David immediately started taking injectable insulin and learned how to monitor his blood glucose level. In high school, he excelled academically and served as captain of the wrestling team and as class president. Based on his extraordinary record, he won a full scholarship to the state university, where he is currently a premedical student and is planning a career in pediatric endocrinology.

Q QUESTIONS

1. How is glucose normally handled in the nephron? (Discuss filtration, reabsorption, and excretion of glucose.) What transporters are involved in the reabsorption process?

2. At the time of the diagnosis, David's blood sugar level was significantly elevated (320 mg/dL). Use Figure 4–3, which shows a glucose titration curve, to explain why David was excreting glucose in his urine (glucosuria).

Does the fact that David was excreting glucose in his urine indicate a defect in his renal threshold for glucose, in his transport maximum (T_m) for glucose, or in neither?

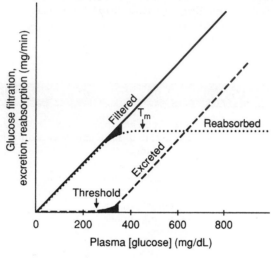

Figure 4–3 Glucose titration curve. Glucose filtration, excretion, and reabsorption are shown as a function of plasma glucose concentration. *Shaded areas* indicate the "splay." (T_m, transport maximum.) (Reprinted, with permission, from Costanzo LS: *BRS Physiology.* 4th ed. Baltimore: Lippincott Williams & Wilkins; 2007:161.)

3. David's glucosuria abated after he started receiving insulin injections. Why?

4. Why was David polyuric (increased urine production)? Why was his urinary Na^+ excretion elevated?

5. Plasma osmolarity (mOsm/L) can be estimated from the plasma Na^+ concentration (in mEq/L), the plasma glucose (in mg/dL), and the blood urea nitrogen (BUN, in mg/dL), as follows:

$$\text{Plasma omolarity} \cong 2 \times \text{plasma} \left[Na^+\right] + \frac{\text{glucose}}{18} + \frac{\text{BUN}}{2.8}$$

Why does this formula give a reasonable estimate of plasma osmolarity? Use the formula to estimate David's plasma osmolarity (assuming that his BUN is normal at 10 mg/dL). Is David's plasma osmolarity normal, increased, or decreased compared with normal?

6. Why was David constantly thirsty?

7. Why was David's blood pressure lower than normal? Why did his blood pressure decrease further when he stood up?

ANSWERS ON NEXT PAGE

ANSWERS AND EXPLANATIONS

1. The nephron handles glucose by a combination of **filtration** and **reabsorption,** as follows. Glucose is freely filtered across the glomerular capillaries. The filtered glucose is subsequently reabsorbed by epithelial cells that line the early renal proximal tubule (Fig. 4–4). The luminal membrane of these early proximal tubule cells contains an **Na^+-glucose cotransporter** that brings both Na^+ and glucose from the lumen of the nephron into the cell. The cotransporter is energized by the Na^+ gradient across the cell membrane **(secondary active transport).** Once glucose is inside the cell, it is transported across the basolateral membranes into the blood by **facilitated diffusion.** At a normal blood glucose concentration (and normal filtered load of glucose), all of the filtered glucose is reabsorbed, and none is excreted in the urine.

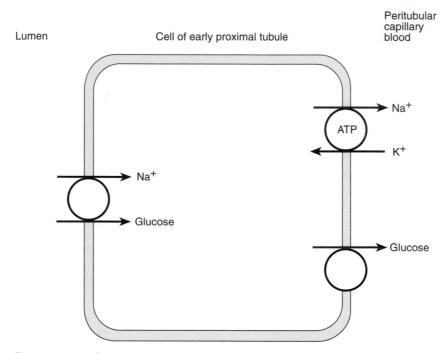

Figure 4–4 Mechanism of glucose reabsorption in the early proximal tubule.

2. The **glucose titration curve** (see Fig. 4–3) shows the relationship between plasma glucose concentration and rate of glucose reabsorption. Filtered load and excretion rate of glucose are shown on the same graph for comparison. By interpreting these three curves simultaneously, we can understand why David was "spilling" (excreting) glucose in his urine. The filtered load of glucose is the product of GFR and plasma glucose concentration. Therefore, as the plasma glucose concentration increases, the filtered load increases in a linear fashion. In contrast, the curves for reabsorption and excretion are not linear. (i) When the plasma glucose concentration is less than 200 mg/dL, all of the filtered glucose is reabsorbed because the Na^+-glucose cotransporters are not yet saturated. In this range, reabsorption equals filtered load, and no glucose is "left over" to be excreted in the urine. (ii) When the plasma glucose concentration is between 200 and 250 mg/dL, the reabsorption curve starts to "bend." At this point, the cotransporters are nearing saturation, and some of the filtered glucose escapes reabsorption and is excreted. The plasma glucose concentration at which glucose is first excreted in the urine (approximately 200 mg/dL) is called the **threshold,** or renal threshold. (iii) At a plasma glucose concentration of 350 mg/dL, the cotransporters are fully saturated and the reabsorption rate levels off at its maximal value **(transport maximum,** or T_m). Now the curve for excretion increases steeply, paralleling that for filtered load.

You may be puzzled as to why *any* glucose is excreted in the urine before the transporters are completely saturated. Stated differently: Why does threshold occur at a lower plasma glucose concentration than does T_m (called **splay**)? Splay has two explanations. (i) All nephrons don't have the same T_m (i.e., there is nephron heterogeneity). Nephrons that have a lower T_m excrete glucose in the urine before nephrons that have a higher T_m. (Of course, the final urine is a mixture from all nephrons.) Therefore, glucose is excreted in the urine before the average T_m of all of the nephrons is reached. (ii) The affinity of the Na^+-glucose cotransporter is low. Thus, approaching T_m, if a glucose molecule becomes detached from the carrier, it will likely be excreted in the urine, even though a few binding sites are available on the transporters.

In healthy persons, the fasting plasma glucose concentration of 70 to 110 mg/dL is below the threshold for glucose excretion. In other words, healthy fasting persons excrete *no* glucose in their urine because the plasma glucose concentration is low enough for all of the filtered glucose to be reabsorbed.

Because of his insulin deficiency, David's fasting plasma glucose value was elevated (320 mg/dL); this value is well above the threshold for glucose excretion. His Na^+-glucose cotransporters were nearing saturation, and any filtered glucose that escaped reabsorption was excreted in the urine (**glucosuria**).

Now we can answer the question of whether David was "spilling" glucose in his urine because of a defect in his renal threshold (increased splay) *or* a defect in his T_m. The answer is: neither! David was spilling glucose in his urine simply because he was hyperglycemic. His elevated plasma glucose level resulted in an increased filtered load that exceeded the reabsorptive capacity of his Na^+-glucose cotransporters.

3. After treatment, David was no longer glucosuric because insulin decreased his plasma glucose concentration, and he was no longer hyperglycemic. With his plasma glucose level in the normal range, he could reabsorb all of the filtered glucose, and no glucose was left behind to be excreted in his urine.

4. David was **polyuric** (had increased urine production) because unreabsorbed glucose acts as an **osmotic diuretic.** The presence of unreabsorbed glucose in the tubular fluid draws Na^+ and water osmotically from peritubular blood into the lumen. This back-flux of Na^+ and water (primarily in the proximal tubule) leads to increased excretion of Na^+ and water (diuresis and polyuria).

5. **Osmolarity** is the total concentration of solute particles in a solution (i.e., mOsm/L). The expression shown in the question can be used to estimate plasma osmolarity from plasma Na^+, glucose, and BUN because these are the major solutes (osmoles) of extracellular fluid and plasma. Multiplying the Na^+ concentration by two reflects the fact that Na^+ is balanced by an equal concentration of anions. (In plasma, these anions are Cl^- and HCO_3^-.) The glucose concentration (in mg/dL) is converted to mOsm/L when it is divided by 18. BUN (in mg/dL) is converted to mOsm/L when it is divided by 2.8.

David's estimated **plasma osmolarity (P_{osm})** is:

$$P_{osm} = 2 \times [Na^+] + \frac{glucose}{18} + \frac{BUN}{2.8}$$

$$= 2 \times 143 + \frac{320}{18} + \frac{10}{2.8}$$

$$= 286 + 17.8 + 3.6$$

$$= 307 \text{ mOsm/L}$$

The normal value for plasma osmolarity is 290 mOsm/L. At 307 mOsm/L, David's osmolarity was significantly elevated.

6. There are two likely reasons why David was constantly thirsty **(polydipsic)**. (i) His plasma osmolarity, as calculated in the previous question, was elevated at 307 mOsm/L (normal, 290 mOsm/L). The reason for this elevation was **hyperglycemia**; the increased concentration of glucose in plasma caused an increase in the total solute concentration. The increased plasma osmolarity stimulated thirst and drinking behavior through **osmoreceptors** in the hypothalamus. (ii) As discussed for Question 4, the presence of unreabsorbed glucose in the urine produced an osmotic diuresis, with increased Na$^+$ and water excretion. Increased Na$^+$ excretion led to decreased Na$^+$ content in the extracellular fluid (ECF) and decreased ECF volume **(volume contraction)**. ECF volume contraction activates the renin–angiotensin II–aldosterone system. The increased levels of **angiotensin II** stimulate thirst.

7. David's **arterial blood pressure** was lower than that of a normal 12-year-old boy because osmotic diuresis caused ECF **volume contraction.** Decreases in ECF volume are associated with decreases in blood volume and blood pressure. Recall from cardiovascular physiology that decreases in blood volume lead to decreased venous return and decreased cardiac output, which decreases arterial pressure. Other signs of ECF volume contraction were his decreased tissue turgor and his dry mouth, which signify decreased interstitial fluid volume (a component of ECF).

David's blood pressure decreased further when he stood up **(orthostatic hypotension)** because blood pooled in his lower extremities; venous return and cardiac output were further compromised, resulting in further lowering of arterial pressure.

Key topics

Diabetes mellitus type I

ECF volume contraction

Glucose titration curve

Glucosuria

Hyperglycemia

Hypotension

Na$^+$ glucose contransporter

Orthostatic hypotension

Osmoreceptors

Osmotic diuretic

Plasma osmolarity

Polydipsia

Polyuria

Reabsorption

Splay

Threshold

Transport maximum (T$_m$)

Volume contraction (extracellular fluid volume contraction)

Case 32

Hyperaldosteronism: Conn's Syndrome

Seymour Simon is a 54-year-old college physics professor who maintains a healthy lifestyle. He exercises regularly, doesn't smoke or drink alcohol, and keeps his weight in the normal range. Recently, however, he experienced generalized muscle weakness and headaches that "just won't quit." He attributed the headaches to the stress of preparing his grant renewal. Over-the-counter pain medication did not help. Professor Simon's wife was very concerned and made an appointment for him to see his primary care physician.

On physical examination, he appeared healthy. However, his blood pressure was significantly elevated at 180/100, both in the lying (supine) and the standing positions. His physician ordered laboratory tests on his blood and urine that yielded the information shown in Table 4–5.

TABLE 4–5	Professor Simon's Laboratory Values
Arterial Blood	
pH	7.50 (normal, 7.4)
P_{CO_2}	48 mm Hg (normal, 40 mm Hg)
Venous Blood	
Na^+	142 mEq/L (normal, 140 mEq/L)
K^+	2.0 mEq/L (normal, 4.5 mEq/L)
Total CO_2 (HCO_3^-)	36 mEq/L (normal, 24 mEq/L)
Cl^-	98 mEq/L (normal, 105 mEq/L)
Creatinine	1.1 mg/dL (normal, 1.2 mg/dL)
Urine	
Na^+ excretion	200 mEq/24 hr (normal)
K^+ excretion	1,350 mEq/24 hr (elevated)
Creatinine excretion	1,980 mg/24 hr
24-hr urinary catecholamines	Normal

 QUESTIONS

1. Professor Simon's arterial blood pressure was elevated in both the supine and the standing positions. Consider the factors that regulate arterial pressure, and suggest several potential causes for his hypertension. What specific etiology is ruled out by the normal value for 24-hour urinary catecholamine excretion?

2. The physician suspected that Professor Simon's hypertension was caused by an abnormality in the renin–angiotensin II–aldosterone system. He ordered additional tests, including a plasma renin activity, a serum aldosterone, and a serum cortisol, which yielded the information shown in Table 4–6. Using your knowledge of the renin-angiotensin II-aldosterone system, suggest a pathophysiologic explanation for Professor Simon's hypertension that is consistent with these findings.

TABLE 4–6	Professor Simon's Additional Laboratory Values
Plasma renin activity	Decreased
Serum aldosterone	Increased
Serum cortisol	Normal

3. The physician suspected that Professor Simon had primary hyperaldosteronism (Conn's syndrome), which means that the *primary* problem was that his adrenal gland was secreting too much aldosterone. How does an increased aldosterone level cause increased arterial pressure?

4. What effect would you expect primary hyperaldosteronism to have on urinary Na^+ excretion? In light of your prediction, explain the observation that Professor Simon's urinary Na^+ excretion was normal.

5. What explanation can you give for Professor Simon's hypokalemia? If the physician had given him an injection of KCl, would the injection have corrected his hypokalemia?

6. Explain Professor Simon's muscle weakness based on his severe hypokalemia. (Hint: Think about the resting membrane potential of skeletal muscle.)

7. What acid–base abnormality did Professor Simon have? What was its etiology? What is the appropriate compensation for this disorder? Did appropriate compensation occur?

8. What was Professor Simon's glomerular filtration rate?

9. What was his fractional Na^+ excretion?

10. A computed tomographic scan confirmed the presence of a single adenoma on the left adrenal gland. Professor Simon was referred to a surgeon, who wanted to schedule surgery immediately to remove the adenoma. Professor Simon requested a 2-week delay so that he could meet his grant deadline. The surgeon reluctantly agreed on the condition that Professor Simon take a specific diuretic in the meantime. What diuretic did the physician prescribe, and what are its actions? Which abnormalities would be improved by the diuretic?

ANSWERS ON NEXT PAGE

ANSWERS AND EXPLANATIONS

1. To answer this question about the etiology of hypertension, recall from cardiovascular physiology the determinants of **arterial pressure (P_a).** The equation for P_a is a variation on the pressure, flow, resistance relationship, as follows:

$$P_a = \text{cardiac output} \times \text{TPR}$$

In words, arterial pressure depends on the volume ejected from the ventricle per unit time (cardiac output) and the resistance of the arterioles **(total peripheral resistance, or TPR).** Thus, arterial pressure will increase if there is an increase in cardiac output, an increase in TPR, or an increase in both.

Cardiac output is the product of stroke volume and heart rate. Thus, cardiac output increases if there is an increase in either stroke volume or heart rate. An increase in stroke volume is produced by an increase in contractility (e.g., by catecholamines) or by an increase in preload or end-diastolic volume (e.g., by increases in extracellular fluid volume). An increase in heart rate is produced by catecholamines. An increase in **TPR** is produced by substances that cause vasoconstriction of arterioles (e.g., norepinephrine, angiotensin II, thromboxane, antidiuretic hormone) and by atherosclerotic disease. Thus, hypertension can be caused by an increase in cardiac output (secondary to increased contractility, heart rate, or preload) or an increase in TPR.

One of the potential causes of Professor Simon's hypertension (i.e., increased circulating catecholamines from an adrenal medullary tumor, or **pheochromocytoma**) was ruled out by the normal value for 24-hour urinary catecholamine excretion.

2. This question asked you to explain how the findings of an increased aldosterone level, a decreased renin level, and a normal level of **cortisol** could explain Professor Simon's hypertension.

Figure 2–10 (see Case 14) shows the **renin–angiotensin II–aldosterone system.** This figure shows how **aldosterone** secretion is increased secondary to a decrease in arterial pressure (e.g., caused by hemorrhage, diarrhea, or vomiting). Decreased arterial pressure leads to decreased renal perfusion pressure, which increases renin secretion. **Renin,** an enzyme, catalyzes the conversion of angiotensinogen to angiotensin I. Angiotensin-converting enzyme then catalyzes the conversion of angiotensin I to angiotensin II. **Angiotensin II** stimulates the secretion of aldosterone by the adrenal cortex. Clearly, Professor Simon's elevated aldosterone level *could not* have been caused by decreased blood pressure as shown in Figure 2–10; his blood pressure was *increased.*

Another possibility, also based on the renin–angiotensin II–aldosterone system, is **renal artery stenosis** (narrowing of the renal artery). Renal artery stenosis leads to decreased renal perfusion pressure, which increases renin secretion, increases aldosterone secretion, and causes hypertension (so-called **renovascular hypertension).** In that scenario, both renin levels and aldosterone levels are increased, a picture that is also inconsistent with Professor Simon's results: his renin levels were decreased, not increased.

Finally, Professor Simon's aldosterone levels could be increased if his adrenal cortex autonomously secreted too much aldosterone **(primary hyperaldosteronism).** In that case, high levels of aldosterone would lead to increases in Na^+ reabsorption, extracellular fluid (ECF) and blood volume, and blood pressure. The increased blood pressure would then cause *increased* renal perfusion pressure, which would inhibit renin secretion. This picture is entirely consistent with Professor Simon's increased aldosterone level and decreased **plasma renin activity.**

The normal level of cortisol suggests that an adrenal cortical tumor was selectively secreting aldosterone. If the entire adrenal cortex was oversecreting hormones (e.g., Cushing's disease), then cortisol levels would be elevated as well (see Fig. 6–6 in Case 52).

3. **Primary hyperaldosteronism (Conn's syndrome)** is associated with increased circulating levels of aldosterone, which increases Na^+ reabsorption in the **principal cells** of the late distal tubule and collecting ducts. Since the amount of Na^+ in the ECF determines the ECF volume, increased Na^+ reabsorption produces an increase in ECF volume and blood volume. Increased blood volume produces an increase in venous return and, through the **Frank–Starling mechanism,** an increase in cardiac output. As discussed in Question 1, increased cardiac output leads to an increase in arterial pressure (see Fig. 4–6).

4. In the initial phase of primary hyperaldosteronism, because aldosterone increases renal Na^+ reabsorption, we expect urinary **Na^+ excretion** to be decreased. However, as a consequence of the Na^+-retaining action of aldosterone, both the Na^+ content and the volume of ECF are increased (ECF volume expansion). **ECF volume expansion** then *inhibits* Na^+ reabsorption in the proximal tubule. In this later phase (when Professor Simon's urinary Na^+ excretion was measured), urinary Na^+ excretion increases toward normal, although ECF volume remains high.

This so-called "escape" from aldosterone (or **mineralocorticoid escape**) is a safety mechanism that limits the extent to which hyperaldosteronism can cause ECF volume expansion. Three physiologic mechanisms underlie mineralocorticoid escape, and all of them lead to an increase in Na^+ excretion. (i) ECF volume expansion inhibits renal sympathetic nerve activity. This **decreased sympathetic nerve activity** inhibits Na^+ reabsorption in the proximal tubule. (ii) ECF volume expansion causes dilution of the peritubular capillary protein concentration. The resulting decrease in peritubular capillary oncotic pressure causes a decrease in Na^+ reabsorption in the proximal tubule (by decreasing the **Starling forces** that drive reabsorption). (iii) ECF volume expansion stimulates the secretion of **atrial natriuretic peptide (ANP, or atrialpeptin).** ANP simultaneously causes dilation of renal afferent arterioles and constriction of renal efferent arterioles. The combined effect on the two sets of arterioles is to increase the **glomerular filtration rate (GFR).** As the GFR increases, more Na^+ is filtered; the more Na^+ that is filtered, the more Na^+ that is excreted. ANP may also directly inhibit Na^+ reabsorption in the collecting ducts.

5. Professor Simon's **hypokalemia** was another consequence of his primary hyperaldosteronism. In addition to increasing Na^+ reabsorption, aldosterone stimulates K^+ secretion by the **principal cells** of the late distal tubule and collecting ducts. Increased K^+ secretion leads to excessive urinary K^+ loss, **negative K^+ balance**, and hypokalemia. If Professor Simon's physician had given him an injection of KCl, it would *not* have effectively corrected his hypokalemia. Because of his high aldosterone level, the injected K^+ would simply have been excreted in the urine (Fig. 4–5, and see Figure 4–6).

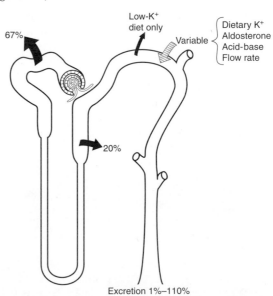

Figure 4–5 K^+ handling along the nephron. *Arrows* indicate reabsorption or secretion of K^+. *Numbers* indicate the percentage of the filtered load of K^+ that is reabsorbed, secreted, or excreted. (Reprinted, with permission, from Costanzo LS: *BRS Physiology.* 4th ed. Baltimore: Lippincott Williams & Wilkins; 2007:168.)

6. Hypokalemia was responsible for Professor Simon's generalized **skeletal muscle weakness.** Remember that, at rest, excitable cells (e.g., nerve, skeletal muscle) are very permeable to K^+. In fact, the **resting membrane potential** is close to the K^+ **equilibrium potential,** as described by the **Nernst equation.** (Intracellular K^+ concentration is high, and extracellular K^+ concentration is low; K^+ diffuses down this concentration gradient, creating an inside-negative membrane potential.) When the extracellular K^+ concentration is lower than normal (i.e., hypokalemia), as in Professor Simon's case, the resting membrane potential becomes even more negative (**hyperpolarization**). When the resting potential is hyperpolarized, it is further from threshold, and it is more difficult to fire action potentials in the muscle (see Case 4).

7. The alkaline arterial pH of 7.50 and the elevated HCO_3^- concentration of 36 mEq/L are consistent with **metabolic alkalosis.** The elevated P_{CO_2} of 48 mm Hg is the result of hypoventilation, which is the respiratory compensation for metabolic alkalosis. Decreased ventilation caused CO_2 retention, which decreased (compensated) the pH toward normal.

   We can apply the **Henderson–Hasselbalch equation** to the HCO_3^-/CO_2 buffer pair to demonstrate why hypoventilation is a compensation for metabolic alkalosis:

   $$pH = pK + \log \frac{HCO_3^-}{P_{CO_2}}$$

   In metabolic alkalosis, the primary disturbance is an increase in HCO_3^- concentration. By itself, this change would profoundly increase blood pH. However, the **respiratory compensation** (hypoventilation) elevates P_{CO_2}, which tends to normalize the ratio of HCO_3^- to CO_2 and decrease the pH toward normal. Respiratory compensation never corrects the pH perfectly and, as you can see, Professor Simon's pH was still alkaline (7.5).

   The "renal rules" shown in the Appendix provide a method for determining whether the degree of respiratory compensation for metabolic alkalosis is appropriate. According to the rules, in simple metabolic alkalosis, P_{CO_2} should increase by 0.7 mm Hg for every 1 mEq/L increase in HCO_3^-. Therefore, in Professor Simon's case:

   Increase in HCO_3^- (above normal value of 24 mEq/L) = +12 mEq/L
   $$Predicted\ increase\ in\ P_{CO_2} = 0.7 \times 12\ mEq/L$$
   $$= +8.4\ mm\ Hg$$
   $$Predicted\ P_{CO_2} = 40\ mm\ Hg + 8.4\ mm\ Hg$$
   $$= 48.4\ mm\ Hg$$

   Based on this renal rules calculation, the *predicted* P_{CO_2} is 48.4 mm Hg, which is virtually identical to Professor Simon's *actual* P_{CO_2} of 48 mm Hg. Thus, he had simple metabolic alkalosis with appropriate respiratory compensation.

The etiology of Professor Simon's metabolic alkalosis was hyperaldosteronism. Recall that, in addition to its actions to increase Na^+ reabsorption and K^+ secretion, aldosterone stimulates H^+ secretion by the **α-intercalated cells** of the late distal tubule and collecting ducts. This H^+ secretion is linked to the synthesis and reabsorption of new HCO_3^-, which elevates the blood HCO_3^- concentration and produces metabolic alkalosis (Figure 4–6).

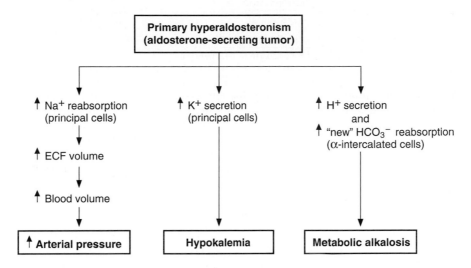

Figure 4–6   Consequences of primary hyperaldosteronism (aldosterone-secreting tumor). (ECF, extracellular fluid volume.)

8. **GFR** is calculated from the inulin clearance or the **creatinine clearance.** Because creatinine is an endogenous substance and inulin is not, the creatinine clearance is often preferred.

$$GFR = C_{creatinine}$$

$$= \frac{U_{creatinine} \times \dot{V}}{P_{creatinine}}$$

The plasma creatinine concentration is provided in the laboratory data, although the urine creatinine concentration and urine flow rate are not provided. Are we stuck? Not at all. To perform the calculation, you must realize that the numerator of the clearance equation, $U \times \dot{V}$, is equal to excretion rate. The 24-hour excretion rate of creatinine is provided in the laboratory data. Thus, the calculation is as follows:

$$GFR = C_{creatinine}$$

$$= \frac{U_{creatinine} \times \dot{V}}{P_{creatinine}}$$

$$= \frac{Creatine\ excretion\ rate}{P_{creatinine}}$$

$$= \frac{1980\ mg/24\ hr}{1.1\ mg/dL}$$

$$= \frac{1980\ mg/24\ hr}{11\ mg/L}$$

$$= 180\ L/24\ hr,\ or\ 180\ L/day$$

9. In words, **fractional Na$^+$ excretion** is the fraction of the filtered load of Na$^+$ that is excreted in urine. It is calculated as follows:

$$\text{Fractional Na}^+\text{excretion} = \frac{\text{Na}^+\text{excretion}}{\text{Filtered load of Na}^+}$$

$$= \frac{\text{Na}^+\text{excretion}}{\text{GFR} \times \text{P}_{\text{Na}}}$$

$$= \frac{200 \text{ mEq/24 hr}}{180 \text{ L/24 hr} \times 142 \text{ mEq/L}}$$

10. While Professor Simon awaited surgery for removal of the aldosterone-secreting tumor, he was treated with **spironolactone,** an aldosterone antagonist. Spironolactone blocks the actions of aldosterone by preventing aldosterone from entering the nucleus of its target cells in the late distal tubule and collecting ducts. (Normally, aldosterone enters the nucleus and directs the synthesis of messenger ribonucleic acids that encode specific transport proteins.) Thus, spironolactone inhibits all of the actions of aldosterone: Na$^+$ reabsorption, K$^+$ secretion, and H$^+$ secretion. The drug was expected to decrease Professor Simon's ECF volume and arterial pressure and to correct his hypokalemia and metabolic alkalosis.

Key topics

Aldosterone

α-Intercalated cells

Angiotensin II

Arterial blood pressure (P_a)

Atrial natriuretic peptide, or atrialpeptin (ANP)

Cardiac output

Conn's syndrome

Cortisol

Creatinine clearance

ECF volume expansion

Equilibrium potential

Fractional excretion

Frank–Starling mechanism

Glomerular filtration rate (GFR)

Henderson–Hasselbalch equation

Hyperaldosteronism

Hyperpolarization

Hypokalemia

K^+ balance

Metabolic alkalosis

Mineralocorticoid escape (escape from aldosterone)

Na^+ excretion

Nernst equation

Pheochromocytoma

Plasma renin activity

Principal cells

Renal artery stenosis

Renin

Renin-angiotensin II-aldosterone system

Renovascular hypertension

Respiratory compensation

Resting membrane potential

Spironolactone

Starling forces

Total peripheral resistance (TPR)

Case 33

Central Diabetes Insipidus

Lisa Kim is a 19-year-old prenursing student who works part-time in a pediatrician's office. Recently, Lisa's life seemed to revolve around being close to a bathroom and a drinking fountain. Lisa was urinating every hour (polyuria) and drinking more than 5 L of water daily (polydipsia). She always carried a water bottle with her and drank almost constantly. Lisa's employer, a physician, was concerned, and wondered whether Lisa had either a psychiatric disorder involving compulsive water drinking (primary polydipsia) or diabetes insipidus. He convinced Lisa to make an appointment with her personal physician.

The findings on physical examination were normal. Lisa's blood pressure was 105/70, her heart rate was 85 beats/min, and her visual fields were normal. Blood and urine samples were obtained for evaluation (Table 4–7).

TABLE 4–7	**Lisa's Laboratory Values**	
	Plasma	**Urine**
Na+	147 mEq/L (normal, 140 mEq/L)	
Osmolarity	301 mOsm/L (normal, 290 mOsm/L)	70 mOsm/L
Glucose (fasting)	90 mg/dL (normal, 70–100 mg/dL)	Negative

Because of these initial laboratory findings, Lisa's physician performed a 2-hour water deprivation test. At the end of the test, Lisa's urine osmolarity remained at 70 mOsm/L and her plasma osmolarity increased to 325 mOsm/L. Lisa was then injected subcutaneously with dDAVP (an analogue of arginine vasopressin). After the injection, Lisa's urine osmolarity increased to 500 mOsm/L and her plasma osmolarity decreased to 290 mOsm/L.

Based on the test results and her response to vasopressin (also called antidiuretic hormone [ADH]), Lisa was diagnosed with central diabetes insipidus. Because she had no history of head injury and subsequent magnetic resonance imaging scans ruled out a brain tumor, Lisa's physician concluded that Lisa had developed a form of central diabetes insipidus in which there are circulating antibodies to ADH-secreting neurons.

Lisa started treatment with dDAVP nasal spray. She describes the spray as "amazing." As long as Lisa uses the nasal spray, her urine output is normal, and she is no longer constantly thirsty.

 QUESTIONS

1. What is the normal value for urine osmolarity? Describe the mechanisms that regulate the urine osmolarity.

2. The initial measurements on Lisa's blood and urine (see Table 4–7) suggested that the cause of her polyuria was *not* primary polydipsia. Why not? What additional information, provided by the water deprivation test, confirmed that she did not have primary polydipsia?

3. What important potential diagnosis, associated with polyuria and polydipsia, was ruled out by the absence of glucose in the urine?

4. After the initial blood and urine tests were performed, Lisa's physician suspected that Lisa had *either* central *or* nephrogenic diabetes insipidus. Explain how each of these diagnoses could be consistent with her measured values for plasma and urine osmolarity.

5. How did the physician confirm that Lisa had central (rather than nephrogenic) diabetes insipidus?

6. Although it was not measured, the serum ADH level could also have distinguished between central and nephrogenic diabetes insipidus. How?

7. When Lisa's physician administered the "test" dose of dDAVP, he was surprised that Lisa's urine osmolarity increased to only 500 mOsm/L. He thought that her urine osmolarity would be higher. Then he recalled that her response is typical when exogenous vasopressin is first administered to a person with central diabetes insipidus. Why did he initially think that her urine osmolarity would be higher than 500 mOsm/L? Why wasn't it higher?

8. Why was dDAVP effective in treating Lisa's central diabetes insipidus?

9. The physician explained to Lisa that she is at risk for developing hyposmolarity while she is taking dDAVP. Why? How can she avoid becoming hyposmolar?

10. If Lisa had nephrogenic diabetes insipidus, how would her treatment been different?

ANSWERS AND EXPLANATIONS

1. **Urine osmolarity** has no single "normal" value. It can be as low as 50 mOsm/L, as high as 1,200 mOsm/L, or any value in between. Normal urine osmolarity depends on the person's plasma osmolarity and water status. For example, in a person who is dehydrated, the kidneys should concentrate the urine; in this case, "normal" urine osmolarity is higher than plasma osmolarity (i.e., >300 mOsm/L [hyperosmotic]). In a person who is drinking water, the kidneys should dilute the urine; in this case, "normal" urine osmolarity is lower than plasma osmolarity (i.e., <300 mOsm/L [hyposmotic]).

The question about regulation of urine osmolarity is really asking how plasma osmolarity is maintained constant at a value of 290 mOsm/L. Constant plasma osmolarity is possible because the amount of water reabsorbed by the collecting ducts varies according to the body's need, as follows.

In a person who is **dehydrated**, plasma osmolarity increases. As a result, osmoreceptors in the anterior hypothalamus are stimulated, triggering the release of **antidiuretic hormone (ADH)** from the posterior pituitary. ADH circulates to the kidneys and increases the water permeability of the **principal cells** of the late distal tubule and collecting ducts. As a result, water is reabsorbed into the bloodstream, and the urine is rendered hyperosmotic. The water that is reabsorbed helps to restore plasma osmolarity back to normal (Fig. 4–7).

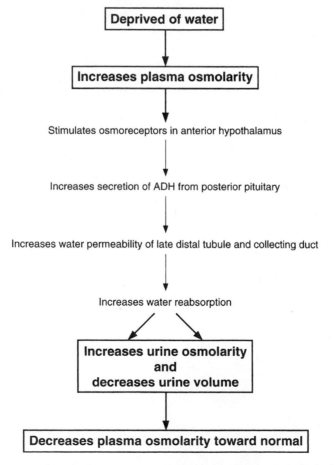

Figure 4–7 Responses to water deprivation. (ADH, antidiuretic hormone.) (Reprinted, with permission, from Costanzo LS: *BRS Physiology*. 4th ed. Baltimore: Lippincott Williams & Wilkins; 2007:172.)

The diagram of a nephron in Figure 4–8 shows how the urine becomes hyperosmotic in a person who is dehydrated. The **proximal tubule** reabsorbs solute and water isosmotically. Two later segments of the nephron are impermeable to water: the **thick ascending limb** and the **early distal tubule (diluting segments).** These segments reabsorb solute, but do not reabsorb water; the water that is "left behind" in the tubular fluid **(free water, or solute-free water)** dilutes the tubular fluid with respect to the plasma. In the presence of **ADH**, this free water is reabsorbed by the **late distal tubule** and **collecting ducts** until the tubular fluid equilibrates osmotically with the surrounding interstitial fluid. In the collecting ducts, which pass through the medulla and papilla of the kidney, the tubular fluid equilibrates with the **corticopapillary osmotic gradient.** The osmolarity of the final urine becomes equal to the osmolarity at the tip of the papilla (1,200 mOsm/L).

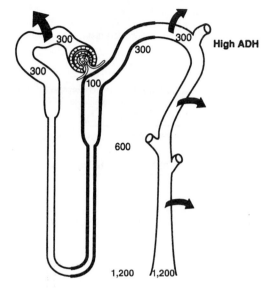

Figure 4–8 Mechanisms for producing hyperosmotic (concentrated) urine in the presence of antidiuretic hormone (ADH). *Numbers* indicate osmolarity. *Heavy arrows* indicate water reabsorption. The *thick outline* shows the water-impermeable segments of the nephron. (Adapted, with permission, from Valtin H. *Renal Function.* 2nd ed. Boston: Little, Brown; 1983:162.)

In a person who is **drinking water,** plasma osmolarity decreases, inhibiting osmoreceptors in the anterior hypothalamus and inhibiting the release of ADH from the posterior pituitary. When circulating levels of ADH are low, the principal cells of the late distal tubule and collecting ducts are impermeable to water. Instead of water being reabsorbed by these segments of the nephron, it is excreted and the urine becomes hyposmotic. The water that was ingested is excreted in the urine and, as a result, plasma osmolarity returns to normal (Fig. 4–9).

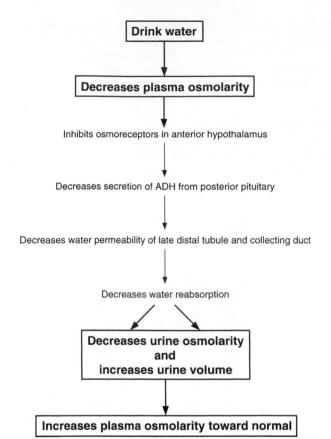

Figure 4–9 Responses to water intake. (ADH, antidiuretic hormone.) (Reprinted, with permission, from Costanzo LS: *BRS Physiology*. 4th ed. Baltimore: Lippincott Williams & Wilkins; 2007:173.)

The diagram of a nephron in Figure 4–10 shows how the urine becomes hyposmotic in a person who is drinking water. The thick ascending limb and early distal tubule dilute the tubular fluid by reabsorbing solute and leaving free water behind in the tubular fluid, as discussed earlier. When ADH is suppressed or is absent, this free water cannot be reabsorbed by the late distal tubule and collecting ducts; as a result, the urine remains dilute, or hyposmotic, with an osmolarity as low as 50 mOsm/L.

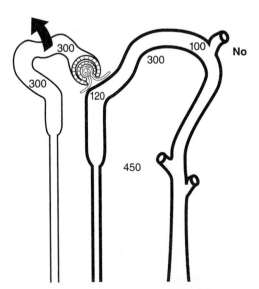

Figure 4–10 Mechanisms for producing hyposmotic (dilute) urine in the absence of antidiuretic hormone (ADH). *Numbers* indicate osmolarity. The *heavy arrow* indicates water reabsorption. The *thick outline* shows the water-impermeable segments of the nephron. (Adapted, with permission, from Valtin H. *Renal Function*. 2nd ed. Boston: Little, Brown; 1983:162.)

2. Lisa's initial plasma and urine values suggested that she did *not* have primary polydipsia. Although her hyposmotic urine (70 mOsm/L) was consistent with excessive water drinking, her plasma osmolarity (301 mOsm/L) was not. If Lisa's *primary* problem was drinking too much water, her plasma osmolarity would have been lower than the normal value of 290 mOsm/L (leading to inhibition of ADH secretion and subsequent water diuresis).

   This conclusion is also supported by the results of the **water deprivation test.** If Lisa had primary polydipsia, her urine would have become hyperosmotic when drinking water was withheld (because ADH would no longer have been suppressed by excessive water intake). Instead, despite 2 hours of water deprivation, Lisa's urine remained hyposmotic (70 mOsm/L). The continued loss of free water in the urine (without replacement by drinking water) caused her plasma osmolarity to rise even further (325 mOsm/L).

3. Untreated **diabetes mellitus** is associated with **polyuria** and **polydipsia.** The polyuria occurs as a result of **osmotic diuresis** that is caused by unreabsorbed glucose (see Case 30). Because no glucose was detected in Lisa's urine, it can be concluded that she was not undergoing a glucose-based osmotic diuresis.

4. In **central diabetes insipidus** (secondary to head injury, a hypothalamic or pituitary tumor, or idiopathic causes), ADH secretion from the posterior pituitary is deficient. In the absence of ADH, the principal cells of the late distal tubule and collecting ducts are impermeable to water. As a result, free water is not reabsorbed in these segments and the urine is rendered hyposmotic. Because excess free water is excreted, the plasma osmolarity increases.

   In **nephrogenic diabetes insipidus** (secondary to lithium toxicity or hypercalcemia), ADH is secreted normally by the posterior pituitary. However, the renal principal cells do not respond to the hormone because of a defect in cell signaling (a defect in the ADH receptor, the G protein, or the adenylyl cyclase). Because the principal cells are "resistant" to ADH, free water is not reabsorbed in the late distal tubule and collecting ducts, and the urine is rendered hyposmotic. Excess free water is excreted, and the plasma osmolarity increases.

   Thus, both forms of diabetes insipidus (central and nephrogenic) are associated with hyposmotic urine and hyperosmotic plasma. The central form is caused by ADH deficiency; the nephrogenic form is caused by ADH resistance.

5. The physician gave Lisa a test dose of **dDAVP,** an analogue of **vasopressin** (ADH). Lisa's kidneys responded to dDAVP and started to produce hyperosmotic urine with an osmolarity of 500 mOsm/L. Because her kidneys responded to ADH, the physician concluded that Lisa had *central* diabetes insipidus. If she had *nephrogenic* diabetes insipidus, exogenous ADH could not have elicited an increase in urine osmolarity.

6. Another way to distinguish central from nephrogenic diabetes insipidus is to measure the serum ADH level. In the central form, by definition, ADH levels are low. In the nephrogenic form, ADH levels are even higher than in a healthy person because plasma hyperosmolarity stimulates ADH secretion from the person's own (normal) posterior pituitary.

7. The physician initially thought that Lisa's urine would become maximally concentrated, or maximally hyperosmotic (1,200 mOsm/L), when she received the test dose of dDAVP. He knew that exogenous ADH should increase the water permeability of the collecting ducts, and that water would be reabsorbed until her urine osmolarity was equal to the osmolarity at the tip of the papilla (which he presumed was 1,200 mOsm/L). Why was Lisa's urine osmolarity only 500 mOsm/L, not 1,200 mOsm/L? Was ADH ineffective?

   Actually, ADH was quite effective, but Lisa's **corticopapillary gradient** was not as large as that of a healthy person. A lesser known consequence of ADH deficiency is that it decreases the corticopapillary gradient. Normally, ADH stimulates two processes that create and maintain the gradient: (i) **countercurrent multiplication** (a function of the loops of Henle) and (ii) **urea recycling** (a function of the inner medullary collecting ducts). During prolonged ADH deficiency, both countercurrent multiplication and urea recycling are reduced. Consequently, the size of the corticopapillary osmotic gradient is reduced. Continuous treatment with dDAVP would eventually restore Lisa's corticopapillary osmotic gradient; at that point, she would be able to produce maximally concentrated urine.

8. Lisa was treated with dDAVP, a vasopressin (ADH) analogue that acts just like the endogenous ADH that Lisa was lacking. Thus, exogenous dDAVP increased the water permeability of the principal cells of the late distal tubule and collecting ducts. As a result, water was reabsorbed from these segments, her urine became hyperosmotic, and her urine flow rate decreased. As this water was reabsorbed into the bloodstream, plasma osmolarity was reduced to normal. As discussed in the previous question, we would also expect dDAVP to eventually restore Lisa's corticopapillary osmotic gradient, by stimulating countercurrent multiplication and urea recycling.

9. The physician warned Lisa that she could become hyposmolar (have decreased plasma osmolarity) while taking dDAVP because the treatment exposes the kidneys to a constant high level of ADH. With dDAVP treatment, her urine would always be hyperosmotic, regardless of how much water she was drinking. In healthy persons, ADH is secreted from the posterior pituitary only when it is needed (during water deprivation). To avoid becoming hyposmolar, Lisa must not drink too much water, thus obviating the need to make hyposmotic urine.

10. The underlying problem in **nephrogenic diabetes insipidus** is resistance to ADH. The kidneys do not respond to exogenous dDAVP, just as they do not respond to endogenous ADH. In some cases, the underlying cause of nephrogenic diabetes insipidus can be treated (e.g., stopping Li^+ therapy, correcting hypercalcemia). In other cases, the treatment is **thiazide diuretics.** The rationale for using thiazide diuretics in nephrogenic diabetes insipidus is three-fold. (i) They prevent dilution of urine in the early distal tubule. Recall that in the early distal tubule, NaCl is normally reabsorbed without water, leaving free water behind in the tubular fluid. In nephrogenic diabetes insipidus, since ADH cannot promote water reabsorption in the collecting ducts, this free water is excreted in the urine. Thiazide diuretics inhibit NaCl reabsorption in the early distal tubule, causing more NaCl to be excreted and making the urine less dilute. (ii) Thiazide diuretics decrease glomerular filtration rate; as less water is filtered, less free water is excreted. (iii) Thiazide diuretics, by increasing Na^+ excretion, can cause ECF volume contraction. In response to volume contraction, proximal tubule reabsorption of solutes and water increases; as more water is reabsorbed, less water is excreted.

Key topics

Antidiuretic hormone (ADH)

Central diabetes insipidus

Corticopapillary osmotic gradient

Countercurrent multiplication

Diabetes mellitus

Diluting segments

Early distal tubule

Free water, or solute-free water

Nephrogenic diabetes insipidus

Osmotic diuresis

Polydipsia

Polyuria

Response to dehydration

Response to water drinking

Thiazide diuretics

Thick ascending limb of the loop of Henle

Urea recycling

Urine osmolarity

Vasopressin

Case 34

Syndrome of Inappropriate Antidiuretic Hormone

Krishna Sharma is a 68-year-old mechanical engineer who retired 1 year ago, when he was diagnosed with oat cell carcinoma of the lung. Always an active person, he has tried to stay busy at home with consulting work, but the disease has sapped his energy. After dinner one evening, his wife noticed that he seemed confused and lethargic. While he was sitting in his recliner watching television, he had a grand mal seizure. His wife called the paramedics, who took him to the emergency department of the local hospital. In the emergency department, the information shown in Table 4–8 was obtained.

TABLE 4–8	Mr. Sharma's Laboratory Values	
Plasma Na⁺	112 mEq/L (normal, 140 mEq/L)	
Plasma osmolarity	230 mOsm/L (normal, 290 mOsm/L)	
Urine osmolarity	950 mOsm/L	

Mr. Sharma's blood pressure was normal, both supine (lying) and upright. He was treated immediately with an infusion of hypertonic (3%) NaCl. He was released from the hospital a few days later, with strict instructions to limit his water intake.

 QUESTIONS

1. Oat cell carcinomas of the lung may secrete antidiuretic hormone (ADH). Unlike ADH secretion from the posterior pituitary, ectopic hormone secretion from the cancer cells is not feedback-regulated. As a result, blood levels of ADH can become extraordinarily high. What is the major effect of these high levels of ADH on the kidney? In light of this effect, explain Mr. Sharma's urine osmolarity.

2. Why was Mr. Sharma's plasma Na⁺ concentration so low? Why was his plasma osmolarity so low?

3. Mr. Sharma's disease is called syndrome of inappropriate antidiuretic hormone (SIADH). What is "inappropriate" about SIADH?

4. Why did Mr. Sharma have a grand mal seizure?

5. Was Mr. Sharma's total body water increased, decreased, or normal? Why was his blood pressure normal?

6. Hypertonic NaCl is 3% NaCl, which corresponds to an NaCl concentration of 517 mEq/L. How did infusion of hypertonic NaCl help to correct Mr. Sharma's low plasma Na⁺ concentration?

7. Why was it so important that Mr. Sharma restrict his water intake when he went home? What would happen if he did not limit his water intake?

8. If Mr. Sharma found water restriction too difficult, his physician planned to treat him with demeclocycline, an ADH antagonist. How would this drug have helped him?

ANSWERS ON NEXT PAGE

ANSWERS AND EXPLANATIONS

1. The major action of **antidiuretic hormone (ADH)** is to increase the **water permeability** of the **principal cells** of the late distal tubule and collecting ducts. As a result, the tubular fluid equilibrates osmotically with the interstitial fluid surrounding the nephron. Because the collecting ducts pass through the **corticopapillary osmotic gradient** of the medulla and papilla, the tubular fluid becomes **hyperosmotic** (see Fig. 4–8). In the presence of high levels of ADH, the final urine osmolarity is equilibrated with the osmolarity at the tip of the papilla, which can be as high as 1,200 mOsm/L.

A urine osmolarity of 950 mOsm/L indicates that Mr. Sharma was, most definitely, concentrating his urine. To concentrate his urine, he needed both a corticopapillary osmotic gradient (for the urine to equilibrate with) and ADH (to increase water permeability and permit that osmotic equilibration). You may wonder why his urine osmolarity was only 950 mOsm/L (rather than 1,200 mOsm/L, as shown in the ideal nephron in Fig. 4–8). In all likelihood, at the time of measurement, the osmolarity at the tip of his renal papilla happened to be 950 mOsm/L. In the presence of high ADH, his collecting ducts equilibrated with *that* osmolarity.

2. It is tempting to say that Mr. Sharma's plasma Na^+ concentration was low **(hyponatremia)** because he lost Na^+ from his body. However, loss of Na^+ is not the only possible reason for a low plasma Na^+ concentration. Remember, the question is about Na^+ *concentration,* which is the amount of Na^+ divided by the volume. Thus, plasma Na^+ concentration can be decreased if the amount of Na^+ in plasma is decreased *or* if the amount of water in plasma is increased. In fact, *decreased plasma Na^+ concentration is almost always the result of water excess, not Na^+ loss.*

In Mr. Sharma's case, SIADH, with its high circulating levels of ADH, caused increased water reabsorption by the collecting ducts. This excess water was retained in the body and diluted the plasma Na^+ concentration. Mr. Sharma's plasma osmolarity was low for the same reason that his plasma Na^+ concentration was low: reabsorption of too much water by the collecting ducts led to dilution of solutes in the plasma.

3. The "inappropriate" aspect of **syndrome of inappropriate antidiuretic hormone (SIADH)** refers to an inappropriately high ADH level and high water reabsorption when there is already too much water in the body. (Evidence of too much water in the body is provided by the low plasma Na^+ concentration and osmolarity.) For example, Mr. Sharma's very low plasma osmolarity (230 mOsm/L) should have completely inhibited ADH secretion by his posterior pituitary. No doubt, it did! However, Mr. Sharma's lung cancer cells secreted their own ADH autonomously, without any feedback control or regulation. This autonomous secretion by the cancer cells was not inhibited by his low plasma osmolarity and was *inappropriate for his plasma osmolarity.*

4. Mr. Sharma had a seizure because of swelling of his brain cells. As discussed earlier, high levels of ADH stimulated water reabsorption by his kidneys. This excess water diluted his extracellular osmolarity, as reflected in his decreased plasma osmolarity. As a result, extracellular osmolarity became transiently lower than intracellular osmolarity. Extracellular osmolarity was lower only *transiently,* however, because water shifted from extracellular fluid (ECF) to intracellular fluid (ICF) to reestablish osmotic equilibrium. This shift of water caused swelling of all cells, including brain cells. Because the brain is contained in a fixed structure (the skull), the swelling of brain cells caused a seizure.

5. Mr. Sharma's total body water was *increased.* High levels of ADH caused increased water reabsorption and net addition of water to the body. This additional water distributed between ECF and ICF in the usual proportions (i.e., one-third to the ECF and two-thirds to the ICF).

One of the puzzling features of SIADH, and one exhibited by Mr. Sharma, is that this addition of water to the body does not usually cause an increase in blood pressure. (One might expect increased ECF volume to be associated with increased blood volume and increased blood pressure.) In SIADH, blood pressure usually does not increase for two reasons. (i) Most (two-thirds) of the excess water retained in the body goes to the ICF rather than to the ECF; thus, ECF volume, blood volume, and blood pressure are not affected as much as you might initially think. (ii) The initial increase in ECF volume activates atrial volume receptors that stimulate secretion of **atrial natriuretic peptide (ANP)**. ANP causes increased Na^+ excretion, which decreases the Na^+ content and volume of the ECF toward normal. In essence, there is an "escape" from the effects of high ADH on ECF volume.

6. Hypertonic NaCl has an Na^+ concentration of 517 mEq/L. Mr. Sharma's ECF (which includes plasma) had an Na^+ concentration of 112 mEq/L. Thus, the infused solution, with its much higher Na^+ concentration, increased Mr. Sharma's plasma Na^+ concentration and osmolarity.

7. The primary treatment for chronic SIADH is water restriction. Mr. Sharma's cancer cells are likely to continue their unrelenting secretion of ADH, which will continue to "force" his urine to be concentrated. If Mr. Sharma restricts his water intake, then hyperosmotic urine is "appropriate." However, if he drinks large quantities of water, his kidneys will not be able to make appropriately dilute urine (because of his permanently high ADH state) and he will become hyponatremic and hyposmolar again.

8. **Demeclocycline**, an ADH antagonist, would be expected to block the action of ADH on the collecting ducts and inhibit ADH-stimulated water reabsorption. Therefore, it is possible that Mr. Sharma would not have to restrict his water intake while taking this drug.

Key topics

Antidiuretic hormone (ADH)

Atrial natriuretic peptide, or atrialpeptin (ANP)

Corticopapillary osmotic gradient

Demeclocycline

Hyperosmotic urine

Hyponatremia

Hyposmolarity

Principal cells

Syndrome of inappropriate antidiuretic hormone (SIADH)

Case 35

Generalized Edema: Nephrotic Syndrome

Roger Mowry is a 66-year-old long-distance truck driver. Ten years ago, he was diagnosed with focal segmental glomerulosclerosis (a glomerular disease that causes nephrotic syndrome). Because he is constantly on the road, Roger found it difficult to have periodic check-ups. Recently, however, his symptoms were alarming—he had gained weight, his face and legs were swollen, and his pants no longer buttoned around the waist. Since these are signs that his physician had warned him about, he called in sick and made an appointment for a check-up. On physical examination, the physician noted periorbital edema, pitting edema of his extremities, ascites, and an S_3 gallop. Plasma and 24-hour urine values are shown in Table 4–9.

TABLE 4–9	Roger's Plasma and Urine Values	
Plasma Concentration		
Na^+	142 mEq/L (Normal, 140 mEq/L)	
Albumin	1 g/dL (Normal, 4.5 g/dL)	
Lipids	Elevated	
24-Hour Urine		
Protein	4 g/24 hr	
Lipids	Positive	

The physician ordered a strict low-Na^+ diet and prescribed a loop diuretic, furosemide. After a few days, Roger called in to report that the furosemide wasn't working—"nothing's happening, doc." The physician increased the dosage of furosemide and prescribed a second diuretic, spironolactone, to be taken at the same time.

 QUESTIONS

1. As a consequence of long-standing focal segmental glomerulosclerosis, Roger developed nephrotic syndrome, a clinical complex characterized, first and foremost, by proteinuria. Why was Roger excreting large amounts of protein in his urine?

2. Why did Roger have hypoalbuminemia, and what is the expected effect on plasma oncotic pressure?

3. What mechanism can you propose for his hyperlipidemia? For his lipiduria?

4. Roger had generalized edema, caused in part by his hypoalbuminemia. How does hypoalbuminemia lead to generalized edema?

5. An additional cause of Roger's edema was retention of Na^+ and water by his kidneys. Propose a mechanism for increased Na^+ and water reabsorption in nephrotic syndrome, and explain how this increase would contribute to edema.

6. What is the meaning of his S_3 gallop?

7. The presence of generalized edema is associated with increased total body Na^+ content. If Roger's total body Na^+ content was increased, why did he have a normal plasma Na^+ concentration?

8. Why did Roger's physician place him on a low-Na^+ diet?

9. Roger needed to receive a diuretic in order to increase his Na^+ and water excretion. Why was the initial dosage of furosemide ineffective? What was the rationale for increasing the dosage?

10. Why was spironolactone added to his treatment?

ANSWERS AND EXPLANATIONS

1. The **glomerular capillary wall** is a three-layered structure, consisting of an endothelial cell layer, a glomerular basement membrane, and an epithelial cell layer. Slits and pores in the layers determine *what* can be filtered on the basis of molecular size—water and the small solutes of plasma are readily filtered, whereas plasma proteins and blood cells are too large to be filtered. In addition to size restrictions, the slits and pores are lined with negatively charged glycoproteins that further restrict the filtration of negatively charged macromolecules such as plasma proteins. In nephrotic syndrome, a defect in the glomerular capillary wall results in increased permeability to plasma proteins. Thus, albumin, which is not normally filtered, can cross the glomerular capillaries and be excreted in the urine.

2. Roger had **hypoalbuminemia** because the albumin that was filtered was then excreted in the urine. Because synthetic processes in the liver could not replace all of the urinary losses, there was a decrease in plasma albumin concentration. The decrease in plasma albumin led to decreased plasma oncotic pressure.

3. The **hyperlipidemia** was due to increased hepatic lipoprotein synthesis, triggered by decreased plasma protein concentration and decreased plasma oncotic pressure. **Lipiduria** occurred because the damaged glomular capillary wall was not only more permeable to plasma proteins, but also more permeable to circulating lipids.

4. Hypoalbumemia caused increased net filtration across systemic capillaries and led to **edema** formation. As shown in Figure 4–11 and also discussed in Case 16, there are four **Starling pressures** in the capillaries. The balance of these pressures determines whether there will be net fluid movement out of the capillaries (filtration) or net fluid movement into the capillary (absorption). In most capillary beds, Starling pressures are such that there is a small net filtration, which is returned to the circulation by the lymphatics. In nephrotic syndrome, the decrease in plasma oncotic pressure alters the balance of the Starling pressures, such that there is an increased force favoring filtration out of capillaries into interstitium. Edema forms when interstitial fluid volume exceeds the ability of the lymphatics to return it to the vascular compartment.

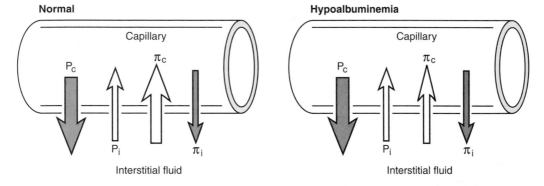

Figure 4–11   Effect of hypoalbuminemia and decreased Π_c to increase net filtration across capillaries.

5. Hypoalbuminemia is not the only cause of edema in nephrotic syndrome. There is also a secondary increase in renal Na^+ reabsorption, which increases extracellular fluid (ECF) volume and causes a further increase in interstitial fluid volume. The increase in Na^+ reabsorption occurs as follows. Initially, **hypoproteinemia**, by decreasing plasma oncotic pressure, leads to increased filtration from plasma into interstitial fluid, as discussed in Question 4. This increased filtration means that interstitial fluid is now a larger-than-usual fraction of the ECF

volume, leaving plasma with a smaller-than-usual fraction of ECF volume. Because plasma volume is decreased, blood volume is also decreased, and there is decreased perfusion of the kidneys. This decrease in renal perfusion is sensed by the juxtaglomerular apparatus and activates the **renin-angiotension II-aldosterone system.** Increased levels of angiotensin II and aldosterone directly stimulate renal Na^+ reabsorption, and consequently there is an increase in body Na^+ content (Fig. 4–12) and **positive Na^+ balance.** Since most of the body's Na^+ content is in the ECF and most of the ECF volume is interstitial fluid, there is an increase in ECF Na^+ content, ECF volume, and interstitial fluid volume. Thus, in Roger, the secondary increase in Na^+ reabsorption led to worsening of his edema.

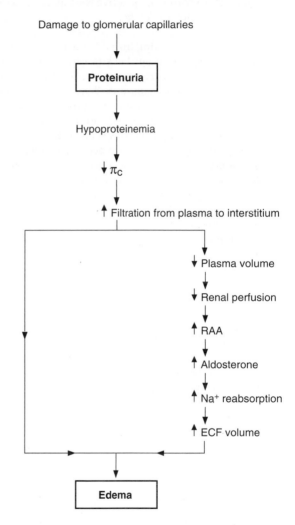

Figure 4–12 Causes of edema in nephrotic syndrome. (π_c, plasma oncotic pressure; RAA, renin–angiotensin II–aldosterone system; ECF, extracellular fluid.)

6. When present in adults, the **third heart sound,** S_3, is abnormal and sometimes is called an **S_3 gallop.** It occurs early in diastole, following opening of the atrioventricular valves and during the period of rapid ventricular filling. The S_3 gallop is associated with volume overload, and in Roger, would be consistent with the increase in ECF volume that occurred secondary to increased renal Na^+ reabsorption, as discussed in Question 5.

7. We concluded that Roger's generalized edema was associated with increased total body Na^+ content. If this is true, shouldn't the increase in body Na^+ content have been reflected in increased in plasma Na^+ concentration? Not necessarily! In fact, we cannot use the plasma Na^+ concentration to conclude the state of body Na^+ content, since one can have increased

body Na⁺ content with increased, decreased, or normal plasma Na⁺ concentration, depending on accompanying changes in body water content. In Roger's case, because Na⁺ content was increased and Na⁺ concentration was normal, we can conclude that he had a proportional increase in body water content. The extra water was added by increased water reabsorption in the kidneys (in the presence of antidiuretic hormone) and increased water-drinking (secondary to increased thirst).

8. Because Roger reabsorbed excess Na⁺, he excreted less Na⁺. When a person excretes less Na⁺ than he ingests, there is a net increase in body Na⁺ content, or positive Na⁺ balance. One approach to correcting positive Na⁺ balance is to attempt to match the low urinary Na⁺ excretion with a low Na⁺ intake.

9. In addition to lowering his Na⁺ intake, Roger needed a diuretic to increase Na⁺ excretion and bring body Na⁺ content back toward normal. **Furosemide** is a potent diuretic that inhibits the **Na⁺-K⁺-2Cl⁻ cotransporter** in the thick ascending limb and leads to increased Na⁺ and water excretion, i.e., diuresis. Why, in Roger, did "nothing happen?" Did he have so-called **refractory edema**, or **diuretic resistance?** To answer this question, recall that Na⁺-K⁺-2Cl⁻ cotransporters are localized on the *luminal* membrane of thick ascending limb cells. Therefore, for **loop diuretics** such as furosemide to act, they must have access to the luminal membrane. Furosemide gains access to luminal fluid in two ways: it is filtered across glomerular capillaries and it is secreted by an organic acid transporter in the proximal tubule. Normally, all of the furosemide present in luminal fluid is in the free form (not protein-bound) and is available to inhibit the Na⁺-K⁺-2Cl⁻ cotransporter. However, Roger's nephrotic syndrome caused him to filter large quantities of plasma proteins, which bound furosemide in luminal fluid. In the bound form, furosemide cannot inhibit the cotransporter and is, therefore, ineffective as a diuretic. By increasing the dosage of furosemide, more drug was filtered and secreted into the lumen, there was a higher total drug level in the lumen, and there was also a higher level of free, unbound drug to inhibit the cotransporter.

10. **Spironolactone**, a diuretic, is an aldosterone-antagonist that inhibits Na⁺ reabsorption in the principal cells of the late distal tubule and collecting duct. There were two advantages to giving Roger spironolactone along with furosemide. First, spironolactone enters principal cells from the basolateral side and competitively inhibits aldosterone from binding to its intracellular receptor. Therefore, for its action, spironolactone does not need to be present in luminal fluid, and the problem of inactivation by binding to urinary proteins is avoided. Second, since Roger was retaining excess Na⁺ because of increased levels of aldosterone, spironolactone would specifically inhibit that pathway.

Key topics

Diuretic resistance

Edema

Furosemide

Glomerular capillaries

Hyperlipidemia

Hypoalbuminemia

Hypoproteinemia

Loop diuretics

Na^+-K^+-$2Cl^-$ cotransporter

Positive Na^+ balance

Renin–angiotensin II–aldosterone system

Refractory edema

S_3 gallop

Spironolactone

Starling pressures

Case 36

Metabolic Acidosis: Diabetic Ketoacidosis

David Mandel, who was diagnosed with type I diabetes mellitus when he was 12 years old (see Case 31), is now a third-year medical student. David's diabetes remained in control throughout middle and high school, college, and the first 2 years of medical school. However, when David started his surgery clerkship, his regular schedule of meals and insulin injections was completely disrupted. One morning, after a very late night in trauma surgery, David completely forgot to take his insulin! At 5 AM, before rounds, he drank orange juice and ate two doughnuts. At 7 AM, he drank more juice because he was very thirsty. He mentioned to the student next to him that he felt "strange" and that his heart was racing. At 9 AM, he excused himself from the operating room because he thought he was going to faint. Later that morning, he was found unconscious in the call room. He was transferred immediately to the emergency department, where the information shown in Table 4–10 was obtained.

TABLE 4–10	David's Physical Examination and Laboratory Values
Blood pressure	90/40
Pulse rate	130/min
Respirations	32/min, deep and rapid
Plasma Concentration	
Glucose	560 mg/dL (normal fasting, 70-110 mg/dL)
Na^+	132 mEq/L (normal, 140 mEq/L)
K^+	5.8 mEq/L (normal, 4.5 mEq/L)
Cl^-	96 mEq/L (normal, 105 mEq/L)
HCO_3^-	8 mEq/L (normal, 24 mEq/L)
Ketones	++ (normal, none)
Arterial Blood	
P_{O_2}	112 mm Hg (normal, 100 mm Hg)
P_{CO_2}	20 mm Hg (normal, 40 mm Hg)
pH	7.22 (normal, 7.4)

Based on the information shown in Table 4–10, it was determined that David was in diabetic ketoacidosis. He was given an intravenous infusion of saline and insulin. Later, after his blood glucose had decreased to 175 mg/dL and his plasma K^+ had decreased to 4 mEq/L, glucose and K^+ were added to the infusion. David stayed in the hospital overnight. By the next morning, his blood glucose, electrolytes, and blood gas values were normal.

 QUESTIONS

1. What acid–base disorder did David have? What was its etiology?

2. Did David's lungs provide the expected degree of "respiratory compensation"?

3. Why was his breathing rate so rapid and deep? What is this type of breathing called?

4. How did David's failure to take insulin cause his acid–base disorder?

5. What was David's serum anion gap, and what is its significance?

6. Why was David so thirsty at 7 AM?

7. Why was his pulse rate increased?

8. What factors contributed to David's elevated plasma K^+ concentration (hyperkalemia)? Was his K^+ balance positive, negative, or normal?

9. How did the initial treatment with insulin and saline help to correct David's fluid and electrolyte disturbances?

10. Why were glucose and K^+ added to the infusion after his plasma glucose and K^+ levels were corrected to normal?

ANSWERS AND EXPLANATIONS

1. David's pH, HCO_3^-, and P_{CO_2} values are consistent with metabolic acidosis: decreased pH, decreased HCO_3^-, and decreased P_{CO_2} (Table 4–11).

TABLE 4–11	*Summary of Acid–Base Disorders*				
Disorder	$CO_2 + H_2O$	$\leftrightarrow H^+$	$+ \ HCO_3^-$	Respiratory Compensation	Renal Compensation
Metabolic Acidosis	↓ (Respiratory compensation)	↑	↓	Hyperventilation	
Metabolic Alkalosis	↑ (Respiratory compensation)	↓	↑	Hypoventilation	
Respiratory Acidosis	↑	↑	↑		↑H^+ excretion ↑HCO_3^- reabsorption
Respiratory Alkalosis	↓	↓	↓		↓ H^+ excretion ↓ HCO_3^- reabsorption

Heavy arrows indicate primary disturbance. (Reprinted, with permission, from Costanzo LS. *BRS Physiology*. 4th ed. Baltimore: Lippincott Williams & Wilkins; 2007:182.)

David had **metabolic acidosis** (diabetic ketoacidosis, or DKA) secondary to overproduction of the ketoacids β-OH-butyric acid and acetoacetic acid. Metabolic acidosis is usually caused by an increase in the amount of fixed acid in the body, as a result of either ingestion or overproduction of acid. The excess fixed acid is buffered by extracellular HCO_3^-, and as a result, the HCO_3^- concentration in blood decreases. This decrease in blood HCO_3^- concentration causes the pH of the blood to decrease (acidemia), as described by the **Henderson–Hasselbalch equation** (see Case 30):

$$pH = 6.1 + \log \frac{HCO_3^-}{P_{CO_2}}$$

The acidemia then causes an increase in breathing rate, or **hyperventilation**, by stimulating **peripheral chemoreceptors.** As a result, arterial P_{CO_2} decreases. This decrease in arterial P_{CO_2} is the **respiratory compensation** for metabolic acidosis. Essentially, the lungs are attempting to decrease the denominator (CO_2) of the Henderson–Hasselbalch equation as much as the numerator (HCO_3^-) is decreased, which tends to normalize the ratio of HCO_3^- to CO_2 and to normalize the pH.

2. The expected degree of **respiratory compensation** can be calculated from the **"renal rules."** These rules predict the appropriate compensatory responses for simple acid–base disorders (see Appendix). For example, in simple metabolic acidosis, the renal rules can determine whether the lungs are hyperventilating to the extent expected for a given decrease in HCO_3^- concentration. David's HCO_3^- concentration is decreased to 8 mEq/L (normal, 24 mEq/L). The rules can be used to predict the expected decrease in P_{CO_2} for this decrease in HCO_3^-. If David's actual P_{CO_2} is the same as the predicted P_{CO_2}, the respiratory compensation is considered to be appropriate, and no other acid–base abnormality is present. If David's actual P_{CO_2} is different from the predicted value, then another acid–base disorder is present (in addition to the metabolic acidosis).

The renal rules shown in the Appendix tell us that in simple metabolic acidosis, the expected change in P_{CO_2} (from the normal value of 40 mm Hg) is 1.3 times the change in HCO_3^- concentration (from the normal value of 24 mEq/L). Thus, in David's case:

Decrease in HCO_3^- (from normal) = 24 mEq/L – 8 mEq/L
= 16 mEq/L

$$\text{Predicted decrease in } P_{CO_2} \text{ (from normal)} = 1.3 \times 16 \text{ mEq/L}$$
$$= 20.8 \text{ mm Hg}$$
$$\text{Predicted } P_{CO_2} = 40 \text{ mm Hg} - 20.8 \text{ mm Hg}$$
$$= 19.2 \text{ mm Hg}$$

The predicted P_{CO_2} is 19.2 mm Hg. David's actual P_{CO_2} was 20 mm Hg. Thus, his degree of respiratory compensation was both appropriate and expected for a person with an HCO_3^- concentration of 8 mEq/L; no additional acid–base disorders were present.

3. David's rapid, deep breathing is the respiratory compensation for his metabolic acidosis. This hyperventilation, typically seen in diabetic ketoacidosis, is called **Kussmaul respiration.**

4. David has type I diabetes mellitus. The beta cells of his endocrine pancreas do not secrete enough insulin, which is absolutely required for storage of ingested nutrients (see below). Ever since David developed type I diabetes mellitus in middle school, he has depended on injections of exogenous insulin to store the nutrients he ingests. When David forgot to take his insulin in the morning and then ate a high-carbohydrate meal (orange juice and dough-nuts), he was in trouble!

   If you have not yet studied endocrine physiology, briefly, the major **actions of** insulin **are coordinated for** storage of nutrients. They include uptake of glucose into cells and increased synthesis of glycogen, protein, and fat. Therefore, **insulin deficiency** has the following effects: (i) decreased glucose uptake into cells, resulting in **hyperglycemia;** (ii) increased pro-tein catabolism, resulting in increased blood levels of amino acids, which serve as gluco-neogenic substrates; (iii) increased lipolysis, resulting in increased blood levels of free fatty acids; and (iv) increased hepatic **ketogenesis** from the fatty acid substrates. The resulting **ketoacids** are the fixed acids **β-OII-butyric acid** and **acetoacetic acid.** Overproduction of these fixed acids causes **diabetic ketoacidosis** (discussed in Question 1).

5. The serum anion gap is "about" electroneutrality, which is an absolute requirement for every body fluid compartment (e.g., serum). That is, in every compartment, the concentration of cations must be exactly balanced by an equal concentration of anions. In the serum compart-ment, we usually measure Na^+ (a cation) and Cl^- and HCO_3^- (anions). When the concentration of Na^+ is compared with the sum of the concentrations of Cl^- and HCO_3^-, there is a "gap." This gap, the **anion gap,** is comprised of unmeasured anions and includes plasma albumin, phos-phate, sulfate, citrate, and lactate (Fig. 4–13).

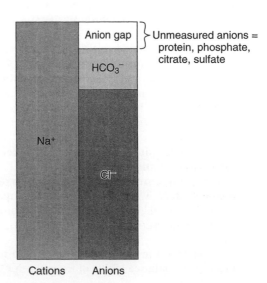

Figure 4–13 Serum anion gap. (Reprinted, with per-mission, from Costanzo LS: *BRS Physiology.* 4th ed. Baltimore: Lippincott Williams & Wilkins; 2007:1985.)

The anion gap is calculated as follows:

$$\text{Anion gap} = [Na^+] - ([Cl^-] + [HCO_3^-])$$

where

Anion gap = unmeasured anions in serum or plasma
$[Na^+]$ = plasma Na^+ concentration (mEq/L)
$[Cl^-]$ = plasma Cl^- concentration (mEq/L)
$[HCO_3^-]$ = plasma HCO_3^- concentration (mEq/L)

The normal range for the serum anion gap is 8 to 16 mEq/L (**average value, 12 mEq/L**). David's serum anion gap is:

$$\text{Anion gap} = 132\ \text{mEq/L} - (96\ \text{mEq/L} + 8\ \text{mEq/L})$$
$$= 28\ \text{mEq/L}$$

A calculated anion gap of 28 mEq/L is much higher than the normal value of 12 mEq/L. Why would the anion gap be increased? Since the anion gap represents unmeasured anions, a logical conclusion is that the concentration of unmeasured anions in David's plasma was increased because of the presence of ketoanions. Thus, David had **metabolic acidosis with an increased anion gap.** To maintain electroneutrality, the decrease in HCO_3^- concentration (a *measured* anion) was offset by the increase in ketoanions (*unmeasured* anions).

Did you notice that the anion gap was *increased* exactly to the same extent that the HCO_3^- was *decreased?* In other words, the anion gap of 28 mEq/L was *16 mEq/L* above the normal value of 12 mEq/L, and the HCO_3^- of 8 mEq/L was *16 mEq/L* below the normal value of 24 mEq/L. This comparison, called "Δ/Δ" (Δ anion gap/Δ HCO_3^-), is used when metabolic acidosis is associated with an increased anion gap. Δ/Δ is used to determine whether metabolic acidosis is the only acid–base disorder that is affecting the HCO_3^- concentration. In David's case, we can conclude that metabolic acidosis was the only disorder present—to preserve electroneutrality, the decrease in HCO_3^- was offset exactly by the increase in unmeasured anions. Therefore, no process, other than the increased anion gap metabolic acidosis, was affecting David's HCO_3^- concentration.

6. David was extremely **thirsty** at 7 AM because he was hyperglycemic. He forgot to take his insulin, but ate a high-carbohydrate meal. Without insulin, the glucose he ingested could not be taken up into his cells, and his blood glucose concentration became elevated. At its normal plasma concentration, glucose contributes little to total plasma osmolarity. However, in **hyperglycemia**, the contribution of glucose to the total plasma osmolarity becomes more significant. Thus, David's plasma osmolarity was probably elevated secondary to hyperglycemia, and this **hyperosmolarity** stimulated thirst centers in the hypothalamus.

In addition, David lost Na^+ and water from his body secondary to the osmotic diuresis that was caused by unreabsorbed glucose (see Case 31). **Extracellular fluid (ECF) volume contraction** stimulates the **renin–angiotensin II–aldosterone system** (through decreases in renal perfusion pressure); angiotensin II is a powerful thirst stimulant (dypsogen). Other evidence for ECF volume contraction was David's hypotension in the emergency room (blood pressure of 90/40).

7. David's **pulse rate** was increased secondary to his decreased blood pressure. Recall from cardiovascular physiology that decreased arterial pressure activates baroreceptors in the carotid sinus **(baroreceptor reflex)**, which relay this information to cardiovascular centers in the brain stem. These centers increase sympathetic outflow to the heart and blood vessels in an attempt to increase blood pressure toward normal. An increase in heart rate is one of these sympathetic responses.

8. To determine the factors that contributed to David's hyperkalemia, we must consider both **internal K^+ balance** (shifts of K^+ between extracellular and intracellular fluid) and **external**

K⁺ balance (e.g., renal mechanisms). Thus, hyperkalemia can be caused by a shift of K⁺ from intracellular to extracellular fluid, by a decrease in K⁺ excretion, or by a combination of the two.

The major factors that cause a **K⁺ shift** from intracellular to extracellular fluid are shown in Table 4–12. They include insulin deficiency, -adrenergic antagonists, acidosis (in which extracellular H⁺ exchanges for intracellular K⁺), hyperosmolarity, exercise, and cell lysis. In David's case, the likely contributors were insulin deficiency (surely!) and hyperosmolarity (secondary to hyperglycemia). It might seem that acidosis would also cause a K⁺ shift, but this effect is less likely in ketoacidosis. The ketoanions (with their negative charge) accompany H⁺ (with its positive charge) into the cells, thereby preserving electroneutrality. Thus, when an organic anion such as the ketoanion is available to enter cells with H⁺, an H⁺–K⁺ shift is not needed (Table 4–12).

TABLE 4–12 *Shifts of K⁺ Between Extracellular Fluid and Intracellular Fluid*	
Causes of Shift of K⁺ out of Cells → Hyperkalemia	**Causes of Shift of K⁺ into Cells → Hypokalemia**
Insulin deficiency	Insulin
β-Adrenergic antagonists	β-Adrenergic agonists
Acidosis (exchange of extracellular H⁺ for intracellular K⁺)	Alkalosis (exchange of intracellular H⁺ for extracellular K⁺)
Hyperosmolarity (H₂O flows out of the cell; K⁺ diffuses out with H₂O)	Hypoosmolarity (H₂O flows into the cell; K⁺ diffuses in with H₂O)
Inhibitors of Na⁺– K⁺ pump (e.g., digitalis) when pump is blocked, K⁺ is not taken up into cells)	
Exercise	
Cell lysis	

(Reprinted, with permission, from Costanzo LS: BRS Physiology. 4th ed. Baltimore: Lippinocott Williams & Wilkins; 2007:167.)

Recall that the major mechanism for K⁺ excretion by the kidney involves **K⁺ secretion** by the **principal cells** of the late distal tubule and collecting ducts. Table 4–13 shows the factors that *decrease* K⁺ secretion by the principal cells. Other than acidosis (which is probably not a factor, for the reason discussed earlier for K⁺ shifts), nothing stands out as a possibility. In other words, decreased K⁺ secretion does not seem to be contributing to David's hyperkalemia. In fact, there are reasons to believe that David had *increased* K⁺ secretion, which brings us to the question of whether David's K⁺ balance was positive, negative, or normal.

TABLE 4–13 *Changes in Distal K⁺ Secretion*	
Causes of Increased Distal K⁺ Secretion	**Causes of Decreased Distal K⁺ Secretion**
High-K⁺ diet	Low-K⁺ diet
Hyperaldosteronism	Hypoaldosteronism
Alkalosis	Acidosis
Thiazide diuretics	K⁺-sparing diuretics
Loop diuretics	
Luminal anions	

(Reprinted, with permission, from Costanzo LS: *BRS Physiology*. 4th ed. Baltimore: Lippincott Williams & Wilkins; 2007:169.)

K⁺ balance refers to whether the renal excretion of K⁺ exactly matches K⁺ intake. Perfect K⁺ balance occurs when excretion equals intake. If excretion is less than intake, K⁺ balance is positive. If excretion is greater than intake, K⁺ balance is negative. It is likely that David was in *negative* K⁺ balance for two reasons: (i) increased flow rate to the distal tubule (secondary to osmotic diuresis) and (ii) hyperaldosteronism secondary to ECF volume contraction. Both increased urine flow rate and hyperaldosteronism increase K⁺ secretion by the principal cells and may lead to **negative K⁺ balance.**

If you're feeling confused, join the crowd! Yes, hyperkalemia can coexist with negative K⁺ balance. While David had a net loss of K⁺ in the urine (which caused negative K⁺ balance), he simultaneously had a shift of K⁺ from his cells (which caused hyperkalemia). In his case, the cellular shift "won"—it had a larger overall effect on plasma K⁺ concentration.

9. The initial treatment with insulin and saline was intended to correct the insulin deficiency (which caused hyperglycemia, diabetic ketoacidosis, and hyperkalemia) and the volume contraction (which occurred secondary to osmotic diuresis).

10. Once the blood glucose and K⁺ concentrations were in the normal range, glucose and K⁺ were added to the infusion to prevent David from becoming *hypo*glycemic and *hypo*kalemic. Without the addition of glucose to the infusion, David would have become hypoglycemic as insulin shifted glucose into his cells. And, without the addition of K⁺ to the infusion, he would have become hypokalemic as insulin shifted K⁺ into his cells. Remember, because David was in negative K⁺ balance, he needed exogenous K⁺ repletion.

Key topics

Acidemia

Anion gap

Baroreceptor reflex

Peripheral chemoreceptors

Control of breathing

Diabetic ketoacidosis

External K⁺ balance

Henderson–Hasselbalch equation

Hyperglycemia

Insulin deficiency

Internal K⁺ balance

K⁺ secretion

K⁺ shifts

Ketoacids (β-OH butyric acid and acetoacetic acid)

Kussmaul respiration

Metabolic acidosis

Principal cells

Renin–angiotensin II–aldosterone system

Respiratory compensation

Type I diabetes mellitus

Volume contraction, or extracellular volume contraction

Case 37

Metabolic Acidosis: Diarrhea

Melanie Peterson's wedding to the man of her dreams was perfect in every respect. However, while on her honeymoon in Mexico, Melanie had severe "traveler's diarrhea." Despite attempts to control the diarrhea with over-the-counter medications, she continued to have 8 to 10 watery stools daily. She became progressively weaker, and on the third day, she was taken to the local emergency department. On physical examination, Melanie's eyes were sunken, her mucous membranes were dry, and her jugular veins were flat. She was pale, and her skin was cool and clammy. Her blood pressure was 90/60 when she was supine (lying) and 60/40 when she was upright. Her pulse rate was elevated at 120/min when she was supine. Her respirations were deep and rapid (24 breaths/min). Table 4–14 shows the results of laboratory tests that were performed.

TABLE 4–14	*Melanie's Laboratory Values*

Arterial Blood

pH	7.25 (normal, 7.4)
P_{CO_2}	24 mm Hg (normal, 40 mm Hg)

Venous Blood

Na^+	132 mEq/L (normal, 140 mEq/L)
K^+	2.3 mEq/L (normal, 4.5 mEq/L)
Cl^-	111 mEq/L (normal, 105 mEq/L)

Melanie was admitted to the hospital, where she was treated with strong antidiarrheal medications and an infusion of NaCl and $KHCO_3$. Within 24 hours, she felt well enough to be released from the hospital and enjoy the rest of her honeymoon.

 QUESTIONS

1. What acid–base disorder did Melanie have?

2. How did diarrhea cause this acid–base disorder?

3. What explanation can you offer for the increased depth and frequency of Melanie's breathing?

4. What is the value for Melanie's anion gap? Is it increased, decreased, or normal? What is the significance of the anion gap in this case?

5. Why was Melanie's blood pressure lower than normal?

6. Why was her pulse rate so high while she was supine? Why was her skin cool and clammy? If her pulse rate had been measured while she was upright, would it have been higher, lower, or the same as when she was supine?

7. How would you expect Melanie's renin–angiotensin II–aldosterone system to be affected?

8. Why was Melanie's blood K^+ concentration so low?

9. What was the rationale for treating Melanie with an infusion of NaCl and $KHCO_3$?

ANSWERS AND EXPLANATIONS

1. To correctly analyze the acid–base disorder, we need to know the values for arterial pH, P_{CO_2}, and HCO_3^-. The values for pH and P_{CO_2} are given, and the HCO_3^- concentration can be calculated with the **Henderson–Hasselbalch equation** (see Case 30).

$$pH = 6.1 + \log \frac{HCO_3^-}{P_{CO_2} \times 0.03}$$

$$7.25 = 6.1 + \log \frac{HCO_3^-}{24 \text{ mm Hg} \times 0.03}$$

$$1.15 = \log \frac{HCO_3^-}{0.72}$$

Taking the antilog of both sides:

$$14.13 = \frac{HCO_3^-}{0.72}$$

$$HCO_3^- = 10.2 \text{ mEq/L (normal, 24 mEq/L)}$$

The arterial blood values (acidic pH of 7.25, decreased HCO_3^- concentration of 10.2 mEq/L, and decreased P_{CO_2} of 24 mm Hg) are consistent with **metabolic acidosis.** Recall that the initiating event in metabolic acidosis is a decrease in HCO_3^- concentration; this decrease can be caused *either* by a gain of fixed acid (fixed acid is buffered by extracellular HCO_3^-, leading to a decreased HCO_3^- concentration) *or* by loss of HCO_3^- from the body. Melanie's P_{CO_2} was decreased because peripheral chemoreceptors sensed the acidemia (decreased blood pH) and directed an increase in breathing rate **(hyperventilation).** Hyperventilation drove off extra CO_2 and led to the decrease in arterial P_{CO_2}.

2. Melanie's metabolic acidosis was caused by the severe **diarrhea.** You may recall that several gastrointestinal secretions, including **saliva** and **pancreatic secretions**, have a very high HCO_3^- content. If the transit rate through the gastrointestinal tract is increased (e.g., in diarrhea), there is excessive loss of this HCO_3^--rich fluid. Loss of HCO_3^- leads to decreased HCO_3^- concentration in the blood (metabolic acidosis).

3. Melanie was breathing deeply and rapidly (hyperventilating) because of the **respiratory compensation** for metabolic acidosis. As explained earlier, the acidemia (secondary to loss of HCO_3^-) stimulated peripheral chemoreceptors, which directed an increase in breathing rate.

4. The anion gap was discussed in Case 36. Briefly, the **anion gap** represents unmeasured anions in serum or plasma. Unmeasured anions include albumin, phosphate, citrate, sulfate, and lactate. The average normal value for the serum anion gap is **12 mEq/L.**

   The anion gap is calculated whenever a metabolic acidosis is present to aid in diagnosing the *cause* of the disorder. In metabolic acidosis, the HCO_3^- concentration is always decreased and to maintain electroneutrality, this "lost" HCO_3^- must be replaced by another anion. If HCO_3^- is replaced by an unmeasured anion (e.g., lactate, ketoanions, phosphate), the anion gap is increased. If HCO_3^- is replaced by a measured anion (e.g., Cl^-), the anion gap is normal.

   The anion gap is calculated as the difference between the concentration of measured cations (Na^+) and measured anions (Cl^- and HCO_3^-). Melanie's anion gap was:

$$\text{Anion gap} = [Na^+] - ([Cl^-] + [HCO_3^-])$$
$$= 132 \text{ mEq/L} - (111 \text{ mEq/L} + 10.2 \text{ mEq/L})$$
$$= 10.8 \text{ mEq/L}$$

Melanie's calculated anion gap was *normal*. Thus, she had metabolic acidosis with a normal anion gap, whose significance is explained as follows. In her metabolic acidosis, the decrease in HCO_3^- concentration was offset by an increase in Cl^- concentration, not by an increase in unmeasured anions. One measured anion (HCO_3^-) was replaced by another measured anion (Cl^-), and the anion gap was unchanged from normal. (Indeed, the Cl^- concentration in Melanie's blood of 111 mEq/L is higher than the normal value of 105 mEq/L.) Thus, the complete (and rather impressive) name of her acid–base disorder is **hyperchloremic metabolic acidosis with a normal anion gap.**

Finally, how did the Cl^- concentration in Melanie's blood become elevated? We discussed the fact that an HCO_3^--rich solution was lost from the gastrointestinal tract in diarrheal fluid. Thus, relatively speaking, Cl^- was "left behind" in the body in a smaller volume (i.e., Cl^- became concentrated).

5. Melanie's blood pressure was decreased because she lost large volumes of an extracellular-type fluid in diarrhea. Loss of extracellular fluid (ECF) caused a decrease in blood volume and interstitial fluid volume (i.e., **ECF volume contraction**). The loss of interstitial fluid was evident in her sunken eyes and dry mucous membranes. The loss of blood volume was evident in her decreased blood pressure and flat jugular veins. (When blood volume decreases, venous return decreases, leading to decreased cardiac output and arterial pressure.)

6. Melanie's pulse rate was elevated secondary to the response of the carotid sinus **baroreceptors** to decreased arterial pressure. When the baroreceptors detected a decrease in arterial pressure, they initiated reflexes that increased sympathetic outflow to the heart and blood vessels to increase arterial pressure toward normal. Among these sympathetic responses is an increase in heart rate (through β_1 receptors in the sinoatrial node). Another sympathetic response is activation of α_1 receptors on arterioles, which leads to vasoconstriction in several vascular beds, including renal, splanchnic, and skin. Constriction of cutaneous blood vessels made Melanie's skin pale and clammy.

When Melanie was upright, her blood pressure was even lower than when she was supine (**orthostatic hypotension**). The reason for her orthostatic hypotension was ECF volume contraction. When she was upright, venous blood pooled in her lower extremities, further compromising her venous return and further decreasing her cardiac output and arterial pressure. Thus, if her pulse rate had been measured in the upright position, it would have been *even higher* than when she was supine (because the baroreceptors would have been more strongly stimulated by the lower blood pressure).

7. You should have predicted that Melanie's **renin–angiotensin II–aldosterone system** was *activated* by the decreased arterial pressure. Decreased arterial pressure (through decreased renal perfusion pressure) stimulates renin secretion and results in increased production of angiotensin II and aldosterone.

8. Recall from the earlier discussions of K^+ homeostasis (Cases 32 and 36) that two potential mechanisms can lead to decreased blood K^+ concentration. These mechanisms are a shift of K^+ from extracellular to intracellular fluid and increased loss of K^+ from the body. Melanie's **hypokalemia** had two likely causes, both related to K^+ loss from the body. (i) Significant amounts of K^+ were lost in diarrheal fluid secondary to flow-dependent **K^+ secretion** in the colon. (The colonic secretory mechanism is similar to the K^+ secretory mechanism in the renal principal cells.) When the flow rate through the colon increases (diarrhea), the amount of K^+ secreted into the lumen of the gastrointestinal tract increases. (ii) The renin–angiotensin II–aldosterone system was activated by ECF volume contraction, as discussed earlier. One of the major actions of aldosterone is to increase K^+ secretion by the renal principal cells. Thus, the combined effects of increased colonic and renal K^+ secretion led to gastrointestinal and renal K^+ losses, producing hypokalemia.

Did a K^+ shift into cells contribute to Melanie's hypokalemia? The major factors that cause a K^+ shift into cells are insulin, β-adrenergic agonists, and alkalosis (see Table 4–12 in Case 36). None appears to play a role here. It is interesting that Melanie's acidosis *might* have caused a K^+ shift *out* of her cells, which would have produced hyperkalemia. Clearly, she did not have hyperkalemia; therefore, if this K^+ shift mechanism was present, it was overridden by the large K^+ losses in the stool and urine.

9. The rationale behind giving Melanie an infusion of NaCl and $KHCO_3$ was to replace the substances she lost by the gastrointestinal tract and kidney (water, Na^+, Cl^-, K^+, and HCO_3^-). It was particularly critical to replace ECF volume with an infusion of NaCl. ECF volume contraction had activated the renin–angiotensin II–aldosterone system, which led to urinary K^+ loss and compounded the hypokalemia caused by the original gastrointestinal K^+ loss.

Key topics

Anion gap

Baroreceptors

Diarrhea

Extracellular fluid (ECF) volume contraction

Hyperchloremic metabolic acidosis

Hyperventilation

Hypokalemia

K^+ secretion (renal)

K^+ shifts

Metabolic acidosis

Metabolic acidosis with normal anion gap

Orthostatic hypotension

Pancreatic secretions

Principal cells

Renin–angiotensin II–aldosterone system

Saliva

Case 38

Metabolic Acidosis: Methanol Poisoning

Lester Grimes, aged 59, has had a rough time lately. He lost his job because of "corporate reorganization." (He thinks it was because of his age.) His wife left him, and the children blame him for the break-up. Lester was starting to think that the world would be better off without him. One evening, he went into his garage and drank a bottle of paint remover. He started vomiting, and then he passed out. Fortunately, his son found him in time. In the emergency department, Lester was hyperventilating, and the blood values shown in Table 4–15 were obtained.

TABLE 4–15	Lester's Laboratory Values
Arterial Blood	
pH	7.30 (normal, 7.4)
P_{CO_2}	25 mm Hg (normal, 40 mm Hg)
Venous Blood	
Na^+	141 mEq/L (normal, 140 mEq/L)
K^+	4.6 mEq/L (normal, 4.5 mEq/L)
Total CO_2 (HCO_3^-)	12 mEq/L (normal, 24 mEq/L)
Cl^-	102 mEq/L (normal, 105 mEq/L)
Glucose	90 mg/dL (normal fasting, 70–110 mg/dL)
Blood urea nitrogen (BUN)	20 mg/dL (normal, 9-18 mg/dL)
Osmolarity	330 mOsm/L (normal, 290 mOsm/L)

Methanol poisoning was confirmed by blood analysis. Lester's stomach was pumped, and he was given an infusion of saline, HCO_3^-, and ethanol. He recovered, and his wife drove him home from the hospital. She said, "We can work it out—I can't imagine life without Lester."

 QUESTIONS

1. What acid–base disorder did Lester have?

2. Why was Lester hyperventilating?

3. Did he have the expected degree of respiratory compensation?

4. Methanol poisoning caused Lester's acid–base disorder. How did methanol cause this disorder, and what is the rationale for treating him with ethanol?

5. What was Lester's serum anion gap, and what is its significance?

6. What was Lester's osmolar gap, and what is its significance?

7. When HCO_3^- was administered to correct his metabolic acidosis, it also increased the excretion of formic acid. How?

ANSWERS AND EXPLANATIONS

1. Lester's pH, HCO_3^-, and P_{CO_2} are consistent with **metabolic acidosis** (see Table 4–11).

2. Lester was hyperventilating as the **respiratory compensation** for metabolic acidosis. Metabolic acidosis is associated with a decrease in blood HCO_3^- concentration, which decreases the blood pH (acidemia). The decrease in blood pH stimulates **peripheral chemoreceptors**, which then drive an increase in breathing, or hyperventilation. Hyperventilation lowers the P_{CO_2}, which is the respiratory compensation for metabolic acidosis.

3. The expected degree of respiratory compensation is calculated from the **"renal rules"** given in the Appendix. The renal rules allow us to determine whether Lester's hyperventilation is to the extent expected for the severity of his metabolic acidosis (i.e., for the extent that his HCO_3^- is decreased below normal). Lester's HCO_3^- was 12 mEq/L, which is 12 mEq/L below normal. Renal rules allow us to calculate the expected P_{CO_2} for this decrease in HCO_3^- concentration as follows:

$$\text{Decrease in } HCO_3^- \text{(from normal)} = 24 \text{ mEq/L} - 12 \text{ mEq/L} = 12 \text{ mEq/L}$$
$$\text{Predicted decrease in } P_{CO_2} \text{ (from normal)} = 1.3 \times 12 \text{ mEq/L} = 15.6 \text{ mm Hg}$$
$$\text{Predicted } P_{CO_2} = 40 \text{ mm Hg} - 15.6 \text{ mm Hg} = 24.4 \text{ mm Hg}$$

The predicted P_{CO_2} is 24.4 mm Hg, which is almost identical to Lester's actual P_{CO_2} of 25 mm Hg. Thus, his respiratory compensation was appropriate and expected for a person with *simple* **metabolic acidosis** and no additional acid–base disorders.

4. **Methanol**, or wood alcohol, is a component of paint remover, shellac, varnish, canned fuel (Sterno), and windshield wiper fluid. As shown in Figure 4–14, methanol is metabolized by alcohol dehydrogenase to formaldehyde, which is then converted by aldehyde dehydrogenase to **formic acid**. Formic acid is a fixed acid, which causes metabolic acidosis. Formic acid also causes retinal toxicity and blindness, and thus prompt treatment is required. Intravenous **ethanol** is an effective therapy for methanol poisoning because **alcohol dehydrogenase** has a much higher affinity for ethanol than for methanol. Thus, ethanol competes with methanol for metabolism, preventing the further conversion of methanol to its toxic metabolites.

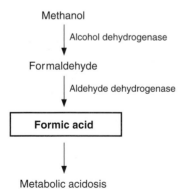

Figure 4–14   Metabolism of methanol to formaldehyde and formic acid.

5. The **anion gap** was discussed in Case 36. Briefly, the anion gap represents unmeasured anions in serum or plasma. The average normal value for serum anion gap is 12 mEq/L. Lester's anion gap was:

$$\text{Anion gap} = [Na^+] - ([Cl^-] + [HCO_3^-])$$
$$= 141 \text{ mEq/L} - (102 \text{ mEq/L} + 12 \text{ mEq/L})$$
$$= 27 \text{ mEq/L}$$

His anion gap of 27 mEq/L is increased. Thus, Lester had metabolic acidosis with **increased anion gap**, which is explained as follows. To maintain the electroneutrality of serum, the decrease in HCO_3^- concentration (responsible for his metabolic acidosis) was offset by an increase in unmeasured anions, in this case **formate.**

6. The major solutes of plasma are Na^+ (with accompanying anions, Cl^- and HCO_3^-), glucose, and urea (blood urea nitrogen, BUN). Since osmolarity is total solute concentration, the plasma osmolarity can be estimated, as described in Case 31, by taking the sum of the Na^+ concentration (multiplied by 2 to account for the balancing anions), the plasma glucose concentration, and the BUN. Using this method, Lester's estimated plasma osmolarity (P_{osm}) was:

$$\text{Estimated } P_{osm} = 2 \times \text{plasma } [Na^+] + \frac{\text{glucose}}{18} + \frac{\text{BUN}}{2.8}$$

$$= 2 \times 141 \text{ mEq/L} + \frac{90 \text{ mg/dL}}{18} + \frac{20 \text{ mg/dL}}{2.8}$$

$$= 282 + 5 + 7.1$$

$$= 294 \text{ mOsm/L}$$

Lester's measured P_{osm} of 330 mOsm/L was much higher than his estimated P_{osm}. What could account for this discrepancy, or "osmolar gap?" **Osmolar gap** is the difference between estimated P_{osm} and measured P_{osm}. Normally, there is little or no difference between the two values because estimated P_{osm} takes into account almost all solutes usually present in plasma. In Lester's case, the presence of a significant osmolar gap of 36 mOsm/L (330 mOsm/L – 294 mOsm/L) means that a solute that is not counted in the estimate (because it is not usually present) contributed to his measured osmolarity. In Lester's case, that solute is methanol. Because methanol is a small molecule with low molecular weight (32 g/mole), poisonous levels can achieve high molar concentrations in the plasma and thereby contribute significantly to the measured plasma osmolarity.

In metabolic acidosis with an increased anion gap, the presence of an osmolar gap is suggestive, although not diagnostic, of methanol or ethylene glycol poisoning. (**Ethylene glycol**, a component of antifreeze, is metabolized to glycolic and oxalic acids, which are fixed acids that cause metabolic acidosis with increased anion gap. Ethylene glycol, like methanol, has a relatively low molecular weight [62 g/mole], and therefore, at poisonous concentrations, raises the measured osmolarity of plasma.)

Do other substances that cause increased anion gap metabolic acidosis (e.g., ketoacids, lactic acid, salicylic acid) also produce an osmolar gap? Potentially, yes. However, ketoacids, lactic acid, and salicylic acid are large molecules, and toxic concentrations do not raise the osmolarity of plasma as much as low-molecular weight substances like methanol and ethylene glycol.

7. The infusion of HCO_3^- raised Lester's blood HCO_3^- concentration and corrected his metabolic acidosis. The HCO_3^- infusion was also helpful in facilitating formic acid excretion in the urine. In the urine, formic acid (the non-ionized form) is in equilibrium with formate (the ionized form); the relative amount of each form depends on the urine pH. Because formic acid is uncharged, it can diffuse from the urine, across the renal tubular cells, and into the blood (called **non-ionic diffusion**); any formic acid that back-diffuses into the blood is not excreted. Formate, with its negative charge, cannot diffuse back into the blood, and is excreted. The HCO_3^- infusion alkalinized Lester's urine, which favored formation of formate relative to formic acid, lessened back-diffusion, and increased excretion of formic acid.

Key topics

Alcohol dehydrogenase

Anion gap

Ethanol

Formic acid

Metabolic acidosis

Methanol

Non-ionic diffusion

Osmolar gap

Respiratory compensation

Case 39

Metabolic Alkalosis: Vomiting

Maria Cuervo is a 20-year-old philosophy major at a state university. When the "24-hour" stomach flu went around campus during final exams, she was one of the unlucky students to become ill. However, instead of 24 hours, Maria vomited for 3 days. During that time, she was unable to keep anything down, and she sucked on ice chips to relieve her thirst. By the time she was seen in the student health center, the vomiting had stopped, but she could barely hold her head up. On physical examination, Maria's blood pressure was 100/60, and she had decreased skin turgor and dry mucous membranes. The blood values shown in Table 4–16 were obtained.

TABLE 4–16	*Maria's Laboratory Values*
Arterial Blood	
pH	7.53 (normal, 7.4)
HCO_3^-	37 mEq/L (normal, 24 mEq/L)
P_{CO_2}	45 mm Hg (normal, 40 mm Hg)
Venous Blood	
Na^+	137 mEq/L (normal, 140 mEq/L)
Cl^-	82 mEq/L (normal, 105 mEq/L)
K^+	2.8 mEq/L (normal, 4.5 mEq/L)

Maria was admitted to the infirmary, where she received an infusion of isotonic saline and K^+. She was released the next day, after her fluid and electrolyte status had returned to normal.

 QUESTIONS

1. What acid–base disorder did Maria have after vomiting for 3 days?

2. How does vomiting cause this acid–base disorder? Or, posing the question differently, why does vomiting lead to an increase in the blood HCO_3^- concentration?

3. Why was Maria's blood Cl^- concentration decreased?

4. Compared with a healthy person, was Maria's breathing rate increased, decreased, or the same?

5. Why was Maria's blood pressure decreased? Why did she have decreased skin turgor and dry mucous membranes?

6. What effect would her decreased blood pressure be expected to have on the renin–angiotensin II–aldosterone system?

7. Why was Maria's blood K^+ concentration so low? (Hint: Identify three separate mechanisms that might have contributed to her hypokalemia.)

8. What effect did Maria's extracellular fluid (ECF) volume contraction have on her acid–base status? What acid–base disorder is caused by ECF volume contraction?

9. What was the value for Maria's anion gap? Was it normal, increased, or decreased? What is the significance of her anion gap?

10. Why was it important for Maria to receive an infusion of saline?

11. Why was K^+ included in the infusion?

ANSWERS ON NEXT PAGE

ANSWERS AND EXPLANATIONS

1. Maria's arterial blood values are consistent with **metabolic alkalosis:** alkaline pH (7.53), increased HCO_3^- concentration (37 mEq/L), and increased P_{CO_2} (45 mm Hg). The primary disturbance in metabolic alkalosis is an increase in the blood HCO_3^- concentration, which increases the pH (according to the Henderson–Hasselbalch equation). The alkalemia is sensed by peripheral chemoreceptors, which direct a decrease in breathing rate (hypoventilation) that causes an increase in P_{CO_2}. This hypoventilation is the **respiratory compensation** for metabolic alkalosis.

$$pH = 6.1 + \log \frac{HCO_3^-}{P_{CO_2}}$$

Thus, Maria's arterial pH was alkaline because her HCO_3^- concentration (in the numerator) was increased. By hypoventilating, Maria's lungs attempted to increase the P_{CO_2} in the denominator, correcting the ratio of HCO_3^- to CO_2 and the pH toward normal.

2. The question of how vomiting causes metabolic alkalosis (or, how vomiting causes an increase in the blood concentration of HCO_3^-) leads us to a discussion of fundamental mechanisms of the gastrointestinal tract.

   Gastric **parietal cells** produce H^+ and HCO_3^- from CO_2 and water, using the enzyme carbonic anhydrase. The H^+ is secreted into the lumen of the stomach to aid protein digestion, and the HCO_3^- enters the blood. After a meal, gastric venous blood pH becomes alkaline because of this addition of HCO_3^- **(alkaline tide).** In healthy persons, the acidic chyme moves from the stomach to the small intestine, where the H^+ stimulates secretion of pancreatic HCO_3^-. (Pancreatic HCO_3^- then neutralizes the H^+.) Thus, in healthy persons, HCO_3^- that was added to the blood by gastric parietal cells does not remain in the blood; it is secreted into the intestinal lumen via pancreatic secretions.

   In persons who are vomiting, the H^+ that was secreted in the stomach never reaches the small intestine and therefore never stimulates **pancreatic HCO_3^- secretion.** Therefore, HCO_3^- that was generated by gastric parietal cells remains in the blood, and, as a result, the blood HCO_3^- concentration increases.

3. Maria's blood Cl^- concentration was decreased because gastric parietal cells secrete Cl^- along with H^+ (HCl). When Maria vomited, both H^+ and Cl^- were lost from her body, and her blood Cl^- concentration decreased.

4. Maria's breathing rate must have been *decreased* **(hypoventilation)** because her arterial P_{CO_2} was increased. (Recall, from respiratory physiology, the inverse relationship between alveolar ventilation and P_{CO_2}.) As discussed earlier, Maria was hypoventilating because peripheral chemoreceptors sensed the alkalemia that was caused by her increased HCO_3^- concentration.

5. Maria's blood pressure was decreased because she lost **extracellular fluid (ECF) volume** when she vomited. Decreased ECF volume led to decreased blood volume and decreased venous return to the heart. Decreased venous return caused a decrease in cardiac output (through the Frank–Starling mechanism) and decreased arterial pressure. Maria's decreased skin turgor and dry mucous membranes were further signs of decreased ECF volume (specifically, of decreased interstitial fluid volume).

6. Decreased arterial pressure should have activated Maria's **renin–angiotensin II–aldosterone system** as follows. Decreased arterial pressure leads to decreased renal perfusion pressure, which stimulates renin secretion. Renin catalyzes the conversion of angiotensinogen

to angiotensin I. Angiotensin-converting enzyme catalyzes the conversion of angiotensin I to angiotensin II. Angiotensin II causes vasoconstriction of arterioles and secretion of aldosterone.

7. Maria had severe **hypokalemia.** Recall, from our previous discussions of K^+ homeostasis in Cases 32, 36, and 37, that hypokalemia can result either from a shift of K^+ into cells or from increased K^+ loss from the body.

First, consider the major factors that cause a **K^+ shift** from ECF to ICF: **insulin, β-adrenergic agonists,** and alkalosis. Of these factors, metabolic alkalosis could have contributed to Maria's hypokalemia; as H^+ left her cells, K^+ entered her cells to maintain electroneutrality.

Next, consider the factors that might result in increased **K^+ loss from the body,** through either the gastrointestinal tract or the kidneys. Certainly, some K^+ was lost in **gastric juice** when Maria vomited. In addition, and most importantly, Maria's renin-angiotensin II-aldosterone system was activated by ECF volume contraction. A major action of **aldosterone** is to increase **K^+ secretion** by the **principal cells** of the late distal tubule and collecting ducts, resulting in increased K^+ loss in urine.

8. In Question 5, we discussed the fact that vomiting causes ECF volume contraction. However, we have not considered the possibility that this ECF volume contraction might cause its own acid–base disturbance. Maria had metabolic alkalosis because she lost H^+ by vomiting. To compound the problem, ECF volume contraction caused its own metabolic alkalosis (called **contraction alkalosis** Fig. 4–15).

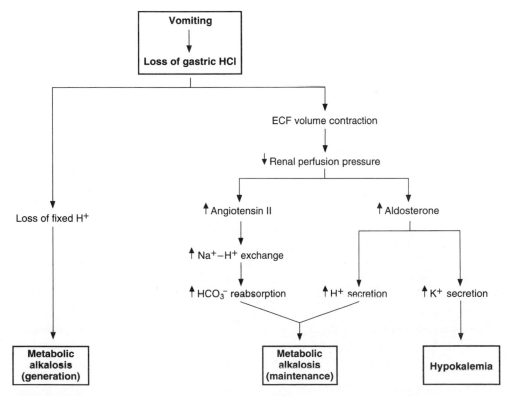

Figure 4–15 Metabolic alkalosis caused by vomiting. (ECF, extracellular fluid.) (Reprinted, with permission, from Costanzo LS: *BRS Physiology.* 4th ed. Baltimore: Lippincott Williams & Wilkins; 2007:188.)

As Figure 4–15 shows, the metabolic alkalosis produced by vomiting has two components. The first component, or the "generation phase," is due to the initial loss of gastric HCl. The second component is due to ECF volume contraction, which causes a "maintenance phase," as follows. Vomiting causes ECF volume contraction, which activates the renin-angiotensin II-aldosterone system (as discussed earlier). Activation of the **renin-angiotensin II-aldosterone** system causes an increase in blood HCO_3^- concentration (metabolic alkalosis) in two ways. (i) Angiotensin II stimulates Na^+–H^+ exchange in the proximal tubule and leads to an increase in the reabsorption of filtered HCO_3^- (Fig. 4–16).

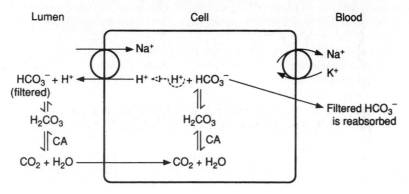

Figure 4–16 Mechanism for reabsorption of filtered HCO_3^- in the proximal tubule. *CA,* carbonic anhydrase. (Reprinted, with permission, from Costanzo LS: *BRS Physiology.* 4th ed. Baltimore: Lippincott Williams & Wilkins; 2007:179.)

(ii) Aldosterone stimulates the H^+ pump **(H^+ ATPase)** of the **intercalated cells** of the late distal tubule and collecting ducts. Increased secretion of H^+ by this pump is accompanied by reabsorption of "new" HCO_3^-, which leads to a further increase in the blood HCO_3^- concentration (Fig. 4–17).

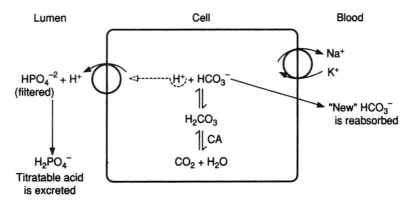

Figure 4–17 Mechanism for excretion of H^+ as titratable acid. (CA, carbonic anhydrase.) (Reprinted, with permission, from Costanzo LS: *BRS Physiology.* 4th ed. Baltimore: Lippincott Williams & Wilkins; 2007:180.)

9. Maria's **anion gap** was:

$$\text{Anion gap} = [Na^+] - ([Cl^-] + [HCO_3^-])$$
$$= 137 \text{ mEq/L} - (37 \text{ mEq/L} + 82 \text{ mEq/L})$$
$$= 18 \text{ mEq/L}$$

As discussed in Cases 36 and 37, the normal range for the anion gap is 8 to 16 mEq/L, with an average value of 12 mEq/L. Maria's anion gap was elevated at 18 mEq/L. You have learned that an increased anion gap accompanies some forms of *metabolic acidosis*. Since Maria's overriding acid–base disorder was *metabolic alkalosis*, how can an increased anion gap be explained? It is likely that a second acid–base disorder (metabolic acidosis) was probably developing. For 3 days, she could not keep any food down; during this period of starvation, she was hydrolyzing fat and generating fatty acids. The fatty acids were metabolized to ketoacids and caused a metabolic acidosis that was superimposed on Maria's metabolic alkalosis.

10. It was important to correct Maria's ECF volume contraction with a saline infusion. Recall that activation of her renin–angiotensin II–aldosterone system secondary to volume **contraction** had two very detrimental effects. (i) It maintained her metabolic alkalosis (contraction alkalosis), and (ii) it contributed to her hypokalemia. Even if the vomiting stopped, the metabolic alkalosis and hypokalemia would have persisted until her ECF volume was returned to normal.

11. K^+ was included in the infusion solution because Maria was in **negative K^+ balance.** Recall from the earlier discussion that two of the three etiologies of her hypokalemia involved K^+ loss from the body (gastric secretions and urine). Thus, to restore K^+ balance, Maria needed to replace the K^+ that she lost.

Key topics

β-adrenergic agonist

Aldosterone

Alkaline tide

Contraction alkalosis

Extracellular fluid (ECF) volume contraction

H^+-K^+ ATPase

Hypokalemia

Insulin

Intercalated cells

K^+ shifts

Metabolic alkalosis

Negative K^+ balance

Pancreatic HCO_3^- secretion

Parietal cells

Principal cells

Renin–angiotensin II–aldosterone system

Case 40

Respiratory Acidosis: Chronic Obstructive Pulmonary Disease

Bernice Betweiler was a 73-year-old retired seamstress who had chronic obstructive pulmonary disease secondary to a long history of smoking (see Case 25). Six months before her death, she was examined by her physician. Her blood values at that time are shown in Table 4–17.

TABLE 4–17	Bernice's Laboratory Values 6 Months Before Her Terminal Admission
P_{O_2}	48 mm Hg (normal, 100 mm Hg)
P_{CO_2}	69 mm Hg (normal, 40 mm Hg)
HCO_3^-	34 mEq/L (normal, 24 mEq/L)
pH	7.32 (normal, 7.4)

Against her physician's warnings, Bernice adamantly refused to stop smoking. Six months later, Bernice was desperately ill and was taken to the emergency department by her sister. Her blood values at that time are shown in Table 4–18.

TABLE 4–18	Bernice's Laboratory Values at Her Terminal Admission
P_{O_2}	35 mm Hg (normal, 100 mm Hg)
P_{CO_2}	69 mm Hg (normal, 40 mm Hg)
HCO_3^-	20 mEq/L (normal, 24 mEq/L)
pH	7.09 (normal, 7.4)

She remained in the hospital and died 2 weeks later.

 QUESTIONS

1. When Bernice visited her physician 6 months before her death, what acid–base disorder did she have? What was the cause of this disorder?

2. Why was her HCO_3^- concentration increased at that visit?

3. At that visit, was the degree of renal compensation appropriate for her P_{CO_2}?

4. At the terminal admission to the hospital, why was Bernice's pH so much lower than it had been 6 months earlier? Propose a mechanism to explain how her HCO_3^- concentration had become lower than normal at the terminal admission (when it had previously been higher than normal).

5. Given your conclusions about Bernice's condition at the terminal admission, would you expect her anion gap to have been increased, decreased, or normal?

ANSWERS ON NEXT PAGE

ANSWERS AND EXPLANATIONS

1. At the initial visit to her physician, Bernice had **respiratory acidosis.** Decreased alveolar ventilation, secondary to her obstructive lung disease, led to an increase in P_{CO_2} because perfused regions of her lungs were not ventilated **(ventilation–perfusion defect).** In those poorly ventilated regions of the lungs, CO_2 could not be expired. The increase in P_{CO_2} caused a decrease in her arterial pH.

2. The HCO_3^- concentration is always increased to some extent in simple respiratory acidosis. The extent of this increase depends on whether the disorder is acute or chronic. In *acute* **respiratory acidosis**, the HCO_3^- concentration is *modestly* increased secondary to mass action effects that are explained by the following reactions. As CO_2 is retained and P_{CO_2} increases, the reactions are driven to the right, causing an increase in HCO_3^- concentration.

$$CO_2 + H_2O \rightleftarrows H_2CO_3 \rightleftarrows H^+ + HCO_3^-$$

In *chronic* **respiratory acidosis**, the increase in HCO_3^- concentration is much greater because, in addition to mass action effects, the kidney increases the synthesis and reabsorption of "new" HCO_3^- **(renal compensation).** This compensation for respiratory acidosis occurs in the **intercalated cells** of the late distal tubule and collecting ducts, where H^+ is secreted and new (i.e., newly synthesized) HCO_3^- is reabsorbed. When arterial P_{CO_2} is chronically elevated, renal intracellular P_{CO_2} is elevated as well. This increased intracellular P_{CO_2} supplies more H^+ for urinary secretion and more HCO_3^- for reabsorption (see Fig. 4–17).

Why is this renal response, which causes an increase in the blood HCO_3^- concentration, called a compensation? Compensation for what? The increase in HCO_3^- concentration is "compensating for," or bringing, the pH toward normal, as shown in the Henderson-Hasselbalch equation:

$$pH = 6.1 + \log \frac{HCO_3^-}{P_{CO_2}}$$

In respiratory acidosis, CO_2 (the denominator of the ratio) is increased secondary to hypoventilation. This increase in P_{CO_2} causes a decrease in arterial pH. In the chronic phase of respiratory acidosis, the kidneys increase the HCO_3^- concentration (the numerator). This increase tends to normalize the ratio of HCO_3^- to CO_2 and the pH. Although Bernice had retained significant amounts of CO_2 (her P_{CO_2} was 69 mm Hg), her pH was only modestly acidic (7.32) 6 months prior to her death. Bernice "lived" at an elevated P_{CO_2} of 69 mm Hg because her kidneys compensated, or brought, her pH almost to normal. (Incidentally, healthy persons "live" at a P_{CO_2} of 40 mm Hg.)

3. The question asks whether the degree of renal compensation (for her elevated P_{CO_2}) was appropriate. In other words, did Bernice's kidneys increase her HCO_3^- concentration to the extent expected? The Appendix shows the rules for calculating the expected compensatory responses for simple acid–base disorders. For simple **chronic respiratory acidosis**, HCO_3^- is expected to increase by 0.4 mEq/L for every 1-mm Hg increase in P_{CO_2}. To calculate the expected, or predicted, increase in HCO_3^-, we determine how much the P_{CO_2} was increased above the normal value of 40 mm Hg, then multiply this increase by 0.4. The predicted change in HCO_3^- is added to the normal value of HCO_3^- to determine the predicted HCO_3^- concentration.

$$\text{Increase in } P_{CO_2} = 69 \text{ mm Hg} - 40 \text{ mm Hg}$$
$$= 29 \text{ mm Hg}$$
$$\text{Predicted increase in } HCO_3^- = 29 \text{ mm Hg} \times 0.4 \text{ mEq/L per mm Hg}$$
$$= 11.6 \text{ mEq/L}$$
$$\text{Predicted } HCO_3^- \text{ concentration} = 24 \text{ mEq/L} + 11.6 \text{ mEq/L}$$
$$= 35.6 \text{ mEq/L}$$

In other words, if Bernice had simple chronic respiratory acidosis, her HCO_3^- concentration should have been 35.6 mEq/L, based on the expected renal compensation. At the initial visit, her actual HCO_3^- concentration was 34 mEq/L, which is very close to the predicted value. Therefore, we can conclude that Bernice had only one acid–base disorder at the earlier visit: simple chronic respiratory acidosis.

4. At the terminal admission, three changes in Bernice's blood values were noted. (i) Her P_{O_2} was lower than it had been previously (hypoxemia), (ii) her HCO_3^- concentration had switched from being higher than normal to being lower than normal, and (iii) her pH had become much more acidic. Her P_{CO_2} was unchanged (still elevated, at 69 mm Hg).

   Bernice's pH was more acidic at the time of her terminal admission because her HCO_3^- concentration had decreased. Recall from our earlier discussion that Bernice had "lived" with an elevated P_{CO_2} because renal compensation elevated her HCO_3^- concentration, which brought her pH almost to normal. At the terminal admission, her HCO_3^- was no longer elevated; in fact, it was decreased to less than normal. Referring back to the **Henderson–Hasselbalch equation**, you can appreciate that either a decrease in the numerator (HCO_3^-) or an increase in the denominator (P_{CO_2}) causes a decrease in pH; if both changes occur simultaneously, the pH can become devastatingly low!

   An important issue we must address is *why* Bernice's HCO_3^- was decreased at the terminal admission when it had been increased (by renal compensation) earlier. What process decreased her HCO_3^- concentration? The answer is that Bernice had developed a **metabolic acidosis** that was superimposed on her chronic respiratory acidosis. (In metabolic acidosis, excess fixed acid is buffered by extracellular HCO_3^-, which lowers the HCO_3^- concentration.) Although it is difficult to know with certainty the cause of this metabolic acidosis, one possibility is that **lactic acidosis** developed secondary to **hypoxia**. At the terminal admission, Bernice's P_{O_2} was even lower (35 mm Hg) than it was at the earlier visit. As a result, O_2 delivery to the tissues was more severely compromised. As the tissues switched to anaerobic metabolism, lactic acid (a fixed acid) was produced, causing metabolic acidosis.

5. If the superimposed metabolic acidosis resulted from accumulation of lactic acid, Bernice's **anion gap** would have been *increased*. Lactic acid causes a type of metabolic acidosis that is accompanied by an increased concentration of unmeasured anions (lactate), which increases the anion gap.

Key topics

Anion gap

Chronic obstructive pulmonary disease

HCO_3^- reabsorption

Henderson–Hasselbalch equation

Hypoxemia

Hypoxia

Intercalated cells

Lactic acidosis

Metabolic acidosis

Renal compensation for respiratory acidosis

Respiratory acidosis

Ventilation-perfusion ($\dot{V}/\dot{Q}$) defect

Case 41

Respiratory Alkalosis: Hysterical Hyperventilation

Charlotte Lind, a 55-year-old interior designer, has been terrified of flying ever since she had a "bad" experience on a commuter flight. Nevertheless, she and her husband planned a trip to Paris to celebrate their 30th wedding anniversary. As the time for the trip approached, Charlotte had what she called "anxiety attacks." One evening, a few days before the scheduled flight to Paris, Charlotte started hyperventilating uncontrollably. She became light-headed, and her hands and feet were numb and tingling. She thought she was having a stroke. Her husband rushed her to the local emergency department, where a blood sample was drawn immediately (Table 4–19). The emergency department staff asked Charlotte to breathe into and out of a paper bag. A second blood sample was drawn (Table 4–20), Charlotte was pronounced "well," and she returned home that evening.

TABLE 4–19	*Charlotte's Laboratory Values on Arrival in the Emergency Department*
pH	7.56 (normal, 7.4)
P_{CO_2}	23 mm Hg (normal, 40 mm Hg)
HCO_3^-	20 mEq/L (normal, 24 mEq/L)

TABLE 4–20	*Charlotte's Laboratory Values after Breathing into and out of a Paper Bag*
pH	7.41 (normal, 7.4)
P_{CO_2}	41 mm Hg (normal, 40 mm Hg)
HCO_3^-	25 mEq/L (normal, 24 mEq/L)

 QUESTIONS

1. When Charlotte arrived in the emergency department, what acid–base disorder did she have? What was its cause?

2. Why was her HCO_3^- concentration decreased? Was her HCO_3^- concentration decreased to an extent that was consistent with an acute or chronic acid–base disorder?

3. Why was Charlotte light-headed?

4. Why did Charlotte experience tingling and numbness of her feet and hands?

5. How did breathing into and out of a paper bag correct Charlotte's acid–base disorder?

ANSWERS ON NEXT PAGE

ANSWERS AND EXPLANATIONS

1. When Charlotte arrived at the emergency department, she had an alkaline pH, a decreased P_{CO_2}, and a slightly decreased HCO_3^- concentration. These findings are consistent with **respiratory alkalosis.** Respiratory alkalosis is caused by hyperventilation, which drives off extra CO_2, decreases arterial P_{CO_2}, and increases pH. (Refer to the **Henderson–Hasselbalch equation** to appreciate why a decrease in P_{CO_2} increases the pH.)

2. Charlotte's HCO_3^- concentration was decreased because of mass action effects that occur secondary to decreased P_{CO_2}, as shown in the following reactions. The decreased P_{CO_2} (caused by hyperventilation) acted like a "sink," pulling the reactions to the left by mass action and decreasing the HCO_3^- concentration.

$$CO_2 + H_2O \rightleftarrows H_2CO_3 \rightleftarrows H^+ + HCO_3^-$$

The extent of decrease in the HCO_3^- concentration was consistent with *acute* **respiratory alkalosis,** as can be demonstrated by calculating the predicted change in HCO_3^- concentration for a given decrease in P_{CO_2}. As shown in the Appendix, when respiratory alkalosis is *acute*, the HCO_3^- concentration is expected to decrease by 0.2 mEq/L for every 1-mm Hg decrease in P_{CO_2}. If Charlotte's respiratory alkalosis was acute, the predicted HCO_3^- concentration was:

$$\text{Decrease in } P_{CO_2} = 40 \text{ mm Hg} - 23 \text{ mm Hg}$$
$$= 17 \text{ mm Hg}$$
$$\text{Predicted decrease in } HCO_3^- = 17 \text{ mm Hg} \times 0.2 \text{ mEq/L per mm Hg}$$
$$= 3.4 \text{ mEq/L}$$
$$\text{Predicted } HCO_3^- \text{ concentration} = 24 \text{ mEq/L} - 3.4 \text{ mEq/L}$$
$$= 20.6 \text{ mEq/L}$$

Charlotte's measured HCO_3^- of 20 mEq/L was entirely consistent with the HCO_3^- concentration predicted for acute respiratory alkalosis.

If Charlotte had *chronic* respiratory alkalosis with the same P_{CO_2} of 23 mm Hg, her HCO_3^- should have been even lower. According to the Appendix, her HCO_3^- would have decreased by 0.4 mEq/L for every 1-mm Hg decrease in P_{CO_2}, or 17 mm Hg $\times$ 0.4, or 6.8 mEq/L. (The greater predicted decrease in HCO_3^- concentration in chronic respiratory alkalosis is explained by renal compensation, which is decreased reabsorption of HCO_3^-.)

3. Charlotte was light-headed because her decreased P_{CO_2} caused vasoconstriction of cerebral blood vessels, resulting in a decrease in **cerebral blood flow.** CO_2 is the major local metabolite that regulates cerebral blood flow; decreases in P_{CO_2} cause vasoconstriction of cerebral arterioles.

4. Charlotte experienced tingling and numbness of her hands and feet because respiratory alkalosis can produce a decrease in the ionized Ca^{2+} concentration in blood. To understand this effect, remember that normally 40% of the total Ca^{2+} in blood is bound to plasma albumin, 10% is bound to anions (e.g., phosphate), and 50 is free, ionized Ca^{2+}. Only the free, ionized form of Ca^{2+} is physiologically active. When the *ionized* Ca^{2+} concentration decreases, symptoms of **hypocalcemia** occur. Because H^+ and Ca^{2+} ions compete for negatively charged binding sites on plasma albumin, logically, a change in H^+ concentration (or pH) of the blood would cause a change in the fraction of bound Ca^{2+}. For example, when the H^+ concentration of blood decreases (e.g., in respiratory alkalosis), less H^+ is available to bind to albumin; therefore, more Ca^{2+} binds. As more Ca^{2+} binds to albumin, less Ca^{2+} is present in the free, ionized

form. Decreases in ionized Ca^{2+} concentration cause increased neuronal excitability and tingling and numbness (Fig. 4–18).

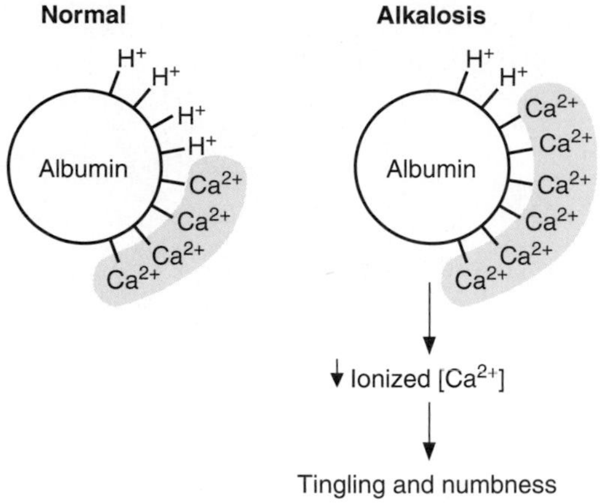

Figure 4–18 Effect of alkalosis on ionized Ca^{2+} concentration in blood.

5. When Charlotte breathed into and out of a paper bag, she rebreathed her own (expired) CO_2 and restored her P_{CO_2} to normal. By returning her P_{CO_2} to normal, she eliminated her respiratory alkalosis.

Key topics

Cerebral blood flow

Henderson–Hasselbalch equation

Hypocalcemia

Renal compensation for respiratory alkalosis

Respiratory alkalosis

Gastrointestinal Physiology

Case 42

Difficulty in Swallowing: Achalasia

Jim Booker, a 49-year-old insurance broker, is having digestive problems. He has difficulty swallowing both solid foods and liquids, and occasionally he regurgitates. The problem is most noticeable when he is under stress, especially when he eats too fast. Jim says that it feels like food is "stuck" in his esophagus and won't go down. Without intending to, he lost 10 pounds in the past 2 months. His wife was especially worried about the weight loss and insisted that Jim see a physician. After doing a complete physical examination, the physician ordered several tests, including a barium swallow and esophageal manometry. After the testing, he was diagnosed with achalasia, a disease characterized by impaired peristalsis in the distal two-thirds of the esophagus and failure of the lower esophageal sphincter to relax during swallowing. The physician recommended that Jim be treated with a procedure that physically dilates the lower esophageal sphincter.

 QUESTIONS

1. What is the role of esophageal peristalsis in normal swallowing?

2. In a normal swallow, what events occur in the lower esophageal sphincter (LES), and what is the timing of these events? What is the innervation of the LES, and what transmitters are involved in its function?

3. How is Jim's achalasia responsible for his difficulty swallowing and regurgitation? How does it explain the feeling of food stuck in the esophagus?

4. On barium swallow testing, the radiologist noted dilation of the esophagus. How can you explain this finding?

5. Results of Jim's esophageal manometry (pressure measurements) are shown in Figure 5–1 and compared to results in normal persons. What major differences are seen in achalasia as compared to normal, and what is the explanation for these differences?

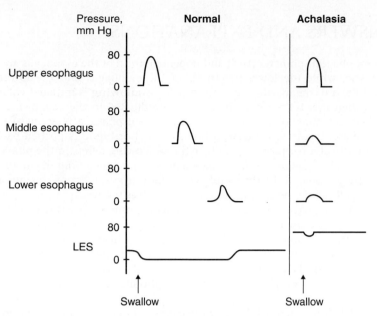

Figure 5–1 Esophageal pressures following a swallow in normal persons and in patients with achalasia. (LES, lower esophageal sphincter.)

ANSWERS AND EXPLANATIONS

1. The upper esophageal sphincter (UES) and upper one-third of the esophagus are comprised of skeletal muscle, while the lower two-thirds of the esophagus and the **lower esophageal sphincter (LES)** are comprised of smooth muscle. **Swallowing** is initiated voluntarily in the mouth, and thereafter is controlled by a reflex coordinated in the swallowing center in the medulla. There are three phases in swallowing: an oral phase, a pharyngeal phase, and an esophageal phase. In the **oral phase**, a bolus of food or liquid is pushed back toward the pharynx and activates receptors that initiate the swallowing reflex. In the **pharyngeal phase**, which includes relaxation of the UES, the food bolus is propelled from the mouth through the pharynx to the esophagus. In the **esophageal phase** (the subject of this question), food is propelled caudally along the esophagus to the stomach as follows. A **primary peristaltic wave** travels down the esophagus, propelling the food along; primary **peristalsis** is mediated by the swallowing reflex and involves a series of coordinated sequential contractions—a region of esophagus contracts behind the food, creating an area of high pressure behind the bolus and pushing it along the esophagus. If the primary peristaltic wave does not clear the esophagus of food, then a **secondary peristaltic wave**, initiated by distention of the esophagus and mediated by the enteric nervous system, begins at the site of distention.

2. At rest, the LES is contracted and has a positive pressure to ensure that gastric contents do not reflux into the esophagus. During swallowing, however, the LES must relax and dilate in a timely fashion so that the bolus of food or liquid can move from the esophagus into the stomach. When the peristaltic wave is initiated in the esophagus, the LES simultaneously relaxes, its pressure decreases to zero (atmospheric), and the LES opens. The LES remains open until the peristaltic wave reaches the terminal portion of the esophagus. Relaxation of the LES is mediated by **inhibitory neurons** in the vagus nerve that release the neurotransmitters **vasoactive intestinal peptide (VIP)** and **nitric oxide (NO).**

3. In achalasia, the symptoms of difficulty swallowing, regurgitation, and feeling of food being stuck in the esophagus are present because: (i) there is impaired peristalsis in the lower two-thirds of the esophagus, such that food and liquids are not propelled caudally; and (ii) there is selective loss of inhibitory neurons innervating the LES, such that the LES fails to relax and dilate during swallowing. Consequently, food and liquids cannot progress normally from the esophagus into the stomach.

4. On barium swallow testing, dilation of the esophagus occurred because of the high resting tone of the LES.

5. Following a swallow in **normal persons,** a peristaltic wave begins in the upper esophagus and proceeds sequentially in the caudad direction. Prior to contraction, the pressure in the esophagus is zero (i.e., equal to atmospheric pressure). When each segment of esophagus contracts, its pressure increases and then decreases back to zero; each sequential contraction moves the bolus along the esophagus. At the same time the peristaltic wave is initiated, the LES relaxes and pressure in the LES falls to zero (i.e., atmospheric); LES pressure remains at zero until the peristaltic wave has proceeded through the esophagus. Thus, the LES remains open until the bolus can be pushed into the stomach.

In persons with **achalasia,** the patterns of esophageal pressures show two major differences following a swallow. First, esophageal peristalsis is impaired so that each segment of esophagus contracts at the same time; consequently there is no sequential peristaltic wave to move the bolus along. Second, there is loss of inhibitory innervation of the LES, so that pressure in the LES is elevated at rest and remains elevated throughout the swallow; because the LES does not relax, the bolus cannot pass easily from the esophagus to the stomach.

Key topics

Achalasia

Lower esophageal sphincter

Nitric oxide

Peristalsis

Primary peristaltic wave

Secondary peristaltic wave

Swallowing

Vasoactive intestinal peptide

Case 43

Malabsorption of Carbohydrates: Lactose Intolerance

Candice Nguyen is a 21-year-old student at a prestigious engineering school. During the past 6 months, she experienced several bouts of severe abdominal bloating and cramps, followed by diarrhea. At first, she thought these episodes were caused by the stress of her demanding academic program. However, she noticed that the symptoms occurred approximately 1 hour after she drank milk or ate ice cream. On a visit home, Candice mentioned the symptoms to her mother, who exclaimed, "Don't you know that your father and I have never been able to drink milk?"

Candice was examined by her primary care physician, who found her to be in excellent health. Because Candice's symptoms were temporally related to ingestion of dairy products, the physician ordered a lactose-H_2 breath test, which confirmed that Candice has lactose intolerance. Her fecal osmolar gap was measured and was elevated. As further confirmation of the diagnosis, Candice abstained from dairy products for 1 week and had *no* episodes of bloating, cramping, or diarrhea.

 QUESTIONS

1. How are dietary carbohydrates *digested* in the gastrointestinal tract? What are the roles of salivary, pancreatic, and intestinal mucosal brush border enzymes in carbohydrate digestion? What three monosaccharides are the final products of these digestive steps?

2. How are dietary carbohydrates *absorbed* from the lumen of the gastrointestinal tract into the blood? Draw a small intestinal epithelial cell that shows the appropriate transporters in the apical and basolateral membranes.

3. Describe the steps involved in the digestion and absorption of lactose.

4. Propose a mechanism for Candice's lactose intolerance.

5. Why did her lactose intolerance cause diarrhea?

6. Candice's lactose-H_2 breath test (which involves measuring H_2 gas in the breath after ingesting 50 g lactose) was *positive*. Why?

7. What is the fecal osmolar gap? Why was Candice's fecal osmolar gap elevated?

8. What treatment was recommended?

ANSWERS ON NEXT PAGE

ANSWERS AND EXPLANATIONS

1. Dietary carbohydrates include starch, disaccharides, monosaccharides, and cellulose (which is indigestible). Of these, only monosaccharides (glucose, galactose, and fructose) are absorbable. Thus, to be absorbed, starches and disaccharides must first be digested to glucose, galactose, or fructose (Fig. 5–2).

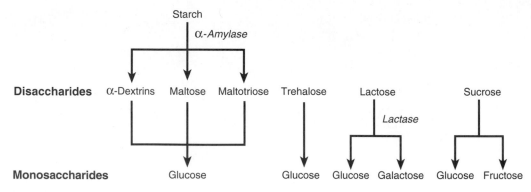

Figure 5–2   Digestion of carbohydrates in the gastrointestinal tract.

Starch is digested to disaccharides (α-dextrins, maltose, and maltotriose) by α-amylase in saliva and pancreatic secretions. Other disaccharides, present in the diet, include trehalose, lactose, and sucrose. Thus, disaccharides are either produced from the digestion of starch or are ingested in food. These disaccharides are then digested to monosaccharides by enzymes located in the brush border of intestinal mucosal cells. α-Dextrins, maltose, and maltotriose are digested to glucose by α-dextrinase, maltase, and sucrase, respectively. Trehalose is digested to glucose by trehelase. Lactose is digested to glucose and galactose by lactase. Sucrose is digested to glucose and fructose by sucrase. Thus, the three monosaccharide products of all these digestive steps are **glucose, galactose**, and **fructose.**

2. Monosaccharides are the only absorbable form of carbohydrates. Figure 5–3 shows a small intestinal epithelial cell with its apical membrane facing the lumen of the intestine and its basolateral membrane facing the blood. Absorption of monosaccharides is a two-step process involving (i) transport first across the apical membrane and (ii) subsequent transport across the basolateral membrane. In this regard, glucose and galactose are processed somewhat differently from fructose, as follows. Glucose and galactose enter the cell across the apical membrane by **Na⁺-dependent cotransport** mechanisms (Na⁺-glucose and Na⁺-galactose cotransporters). These Na⁺-dependent cotransporters, which are **secondary active transport**, are energized (driven) by the Na⁺ gradient across the apical cell membrane. (This Na⁺ gradient is maintained by Na⁺-K⁺ ATPase that is located in the basolateral membrane.) Glucose and galactose then exit the cell across the basolateral membrane by **facilitated diffusion**. In contrast, fructose enters and exits the cell by facilitated diffusion.

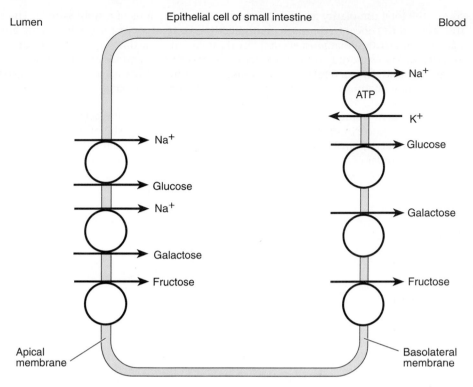

Lumen   Epithelial cell of small intestine   Blood

Figure 5–3   Absorption of monosaccharides by epithelial cells in the small intestine.

3. The steps in the digestion and absorption of lactose are given in the answers to the previous questions. **Lactose** (a dietary disaccharide that is present in dairy products) is digested by **lactase** (a brush border enzyme) to glucose and galactose. Glucose and galactose are then absorbed by the two-step process described in Question 2: Na^+-dependent cotransport across the apical membrane followed by facilitated diffusion across the basolateral membrane.

4. Lactose cannot be absorbed by intestinal epithelial cells. As a disaccharide, it must first be digested to the absorbable monosaccharides glucose and galactose. Thus, **lactose intolerance** can result from a defect in lactose digestion to monosaccharides (e.g., lactase deficiency) or from a defect in one of the monosaccharide transporters. Note, however, that a defect in the glucose or galactose transporter would create nonspecific intolerance to di- and monosaccharides. Candice has **lactase deficiency** (either too little lactase or none at all). Because of this deficiency, she cannot digest dietary lactose in milk products to the absorbable monosaccharides glucose and galactose.

5. Lactose intolerance causes diarrhea because undigested lactose is not absorbed. Some of the lactose is fermented by colonic bacteria to lactic acid, methane, and H_2 gas. Undigested lactose and lactic acid then behave as osmotically active solutes in the lumen of the gastrointestinal tract. These solutes draw water isosmotically into the intestinal lumen and produce **osmotic diarrhea.** (When lactose is digested normally to glucose and galactose, these osmotically active monosaccharides are absorbed, and thus do not remain in the lumen of the gastrointestinal tract.)

6. Candice's **lactose-H₂ breath test** was positive because undigested lactose in the lumen of the gastrointestinal tract was fermented by colonic bacteria. A byproduct of this fermentation (H_2 gas) was absorbed into the bloodstream, expired by the lungs, and then detected in the test.

7. The **fecal osmolar gap** may be an unfamiliar term that refers to unmeasured solutes in the feces. The concept can be useful in understanding the pathophysiology of diarrhea. The test

measures the total osmolarity and the Na^+ and K^+ concentrations of a stool sample. The sum of the Na^+ and K^+ concentrations are multiplied by two to account for the balancing anions (usually Cl^- and HCO_3^-) that must accompany these cations. The difference between total fecal osmolarity and the sum of two times the fecal Na^+ and K^+ concentrations is the fecal osmolar gap. The fecal osmolar gap represents *unmeasured* fecal solutes. Candice's fecal osmolar gap was elevated because unabsorbed lactose contributed to the total osmolarity of the stool.

8. Candice's treatment is simple. If she avoids dairy products that contain lactose, no unabsorbed lactose will accumulate in the lumen of her gastrointestinal tract. If she does not want to eliminate dairy products from her diet, she can take lactase tablets, which will substitute for the missing brush border enzyme.

Key topics

Digestion of carbohydrates

Facilitated diffusion

Fecal osmolar gap

Lactase

Lactase deficiency

Lactose intolerance

Na^+-galactose cotransport

Na^+-glucose cotransport

Osmotic diarrhea

Secondary active transport

Case 44

Peptic Ulcer Disease: Zollinger–Ellison Syndrome

Abe Rosenfeld, who is 47 years old, owns a house painting business with his brothers. The brothers pride themselves on maintaining high standards and satisfying their customers. For several months, Abe had a number of symptoms, including indigestion, loss of appetite, abdominal pain, and diarrhea. One day, he remarked to his brothers that his diarrhea looked "oily." The abdominal pain was relieved temporarily by eating and by taking over-the-counter antacids. Finally, he saw his physician, who referred him to a gastroenterologist. Abe underwent fiberoptic endoscopy, which showed an ulcer in the duodenal bulb. To determine the cause of the ulcer, additional tests were performed, including a serum gastrin level, analysis of gastric contents, a pentagastrin stimulation test, and a secretin stimulation test (Table 5–1).

TABLE 5–1	*Abe's Laboratory Values and Results of Laboratory Tests*
Serum gastrin level	800 pg/mL (normal, 0–130 pg/mL)
Basal gastric H^+ secretion	100 mEq/hr (normal, 10 mEq/hr)
Pentagastrin stimulation test	No increase in H^+ secretion
Secretin stimulation test	Serum gastrin increased to 1,100 pg/mL

A computed tomography scan showed a 3-cm mass on the head of the pancreas. The mass was thought to be a gastrinoma (gastrin-secreting tumor). While awaiting surgery to remove the mass, Abe was treated with a drug called omeprazole. Abe underwent laparoscopic surgery, during which the tumor was localized and removed. Abe's ulcer subsequently healed, and his symptoms disappeared.

 QUESTIONS

1. Abe had peptic ulcer disease, which is caused by digestion of the gastrointestinal mucosa by H^+ and pepsin. What is the mechanism of H^+ secretion by gastric parietal cells? What are the major factors that regulate H^+ secretion?

2. The gastroenterologist diagnosed Abe with Zollinger–Ellison syndrome, or gastrinoma (a gastrin-secreting tumor). Abe had two important laboratory findings that were consistent with this diagnosis: (i) an elevated serum gastrin level and (ii) an elevated basal level of gastric H^+ secretion. How does Zollinger–Ellison syndrome increase gastric H^+ secretion?

3. Why did Abe have a duodenal ulcer?

4. In Abe, pentagastrin, a gastrin analogue, did *not* stimulate gastric H^+ secretion. How is this finding consistent with the diagnosis of Zollinger–Ellison syndrome? How would a healthy person respond to the pentagastrin stimulation test?

5. In the secretin stimulation test, Abe's serum gastrin level increased from his basal level of 800 pg/mL (already very elevated!) to 1,100 pg/mL. In healthy persons, the secretin stimulation test causes no change, or a decrease, in the serum gastrin level. Propose a mechanism to explain Abe's response to secretin.

6. Why did Abe have diarrhea?

7. The oily appearance of Abe's stools was caused by fat in the stool (steatorrhea). Why did Abe have steatorrhea?

8. Abe felt better when he ate. Why?

9. What is the mechanism of action of omeprazole? Why was Abe treated with this drug while he awaited surgery?

ANSWERS AND EXPLANATIONS

1. Causative factors in **peptic ulcer disease** include (but are not limited to) increased H⁺ secretion by gastric parietal cells, *Helicobacter pylori* infection, use of **nonsteroidal anti-inflammatory drugs (NSAIDs)** such as aspirin, and smoking. The common factor in each etiology is digestion of the gastrointestinal mucosa by H⁺; hence the dictum, **"no acid, no ulcer."** As is typical, Abe's ulcer was located in the duodenal bulb. Excess H⁺, delivered from the stomach to the upper duodenum, exceeded the neutralizing capacity of pancreatic and intestinal secretions and digested a portion of his duodenal mucosa.

Figure 5–4 shows the mechanism of H⁺ secretion by gastric **parietal cells.** The apical membrane of the cell, which faces the lumen of the stomach, contains an **H⁺-K⁺ ATPase.** The basolateral membrane, which faces the blood, contains the Na⁺-K⁺ ATPase and a Cl⁻-HCO₃⁻ exchanger. Inside the parietal cell, CO_2 and H_2O combine to form H_2CO_3, which dissociates into H⁺ and HCO_3^-. The H⁺ is secreted into the lumen of the stomach by the H⁺-K⁺ ATPase, acidifying the stomach contents to help with digestion of dietary proteins; an acidic gastric pH is required to convert inactive pepsinogen to its active form, pepsin (a proteolytic enzyme). The HCO_3^- is exchanged for Cl⁻ across the basolateral membrane and thus is absorbed into gastric venous blood. Eventually, this HCO_3^- is secreted into the lumen of the small intestine (through pancreatic secretions), where it neutralizes the acidic chyme delivered from the stomach.

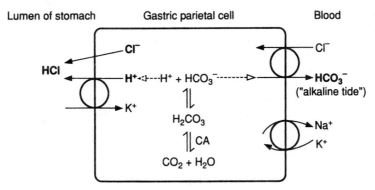

Figure 5–4 Simplified mechanism of H⁺ secretion by gastric parietal cells. (Reprinted, with permission, from Costanzo LS. *BRS Physiology*. 4th ed. Baltimore: Lippincott Williams & Wilkins; 2007:215.)

The major factors that stimulate H⁺ secretion by the parietal cells are the parasympathetic nervous system (vagus nerve), gastrin, and **histamine** (Fig. 5–5). (i) Postganglionic parasympathetic nerve fibers (**vagus nerve**) stimulate H⁺ secretion both directly and indirectly. The parietal cells are *directly* innervated by postganglionic neurons that release **acetylcholine**, which activates a **muscarinic (M_3) receptor** and stimulates H⁺ secretion. The G (gastrin-secreting) cells also have parasympathetic innervation. These postganglionic neurons release bombesin or gastrin-releasing peptide, thus *indirectly* stimulating H⁺ secretion by increasing gastrin secretion. (ii) **G cells** in the gastric antrum release **gastrin**, which enters the circulation and stimulates H⁺ secretion by the parietal cells through the **cholecystokinin-B (CCK_B) receptor.** (iii) Finally, **histamine** is released from enterochromaffin-like cells located near the parietal cells. Histamine diffuses to the parietal cells and activates **H_2 receptors**, stimulating H⁺ secretion.

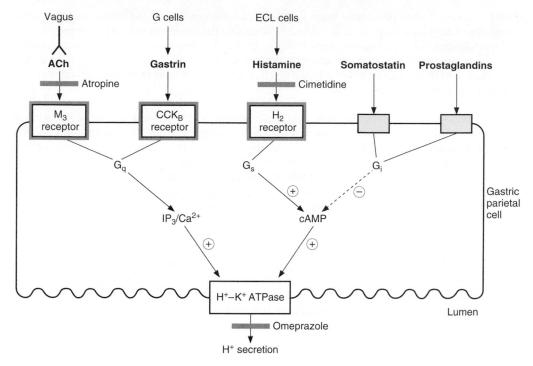

Figure 5–5 Agents that stimulate and inhibit H^+ secretion by gastric parietal cells. (ACh, acetylcholine; cAMP, cyclic adenosine monophosphate; IP_3, inositol 1,4,5-triphosphate; M, muscarinic; ECL, enterochromaffin-like; CCK, cholecystokinin.)

In addition to these stimulatory factors, **somatostatin**, which is released from D cells of the gastrointestinal tract, *inhibits* H^+ secretion in three ways. (i) Somatostatin directly inhibits H^+ secretion by parietal cells via a G_i protein. (ii) Somatostatin inhibits the release of gastrin from G cells, thus diminishing the stimulatory effect of gastrin. (iii) Finally, somatostatin inhibits the release of histamine from enterochromaffin-like cells, thus diminishing the stimulatory effect of histamine. **Prostaglandins** also *inhibit* H^+ secretion via a G_i protein.

2. In **Zollinger–Ellison syndrome**, or **gastrinoma** (a tumor often located in the pancreas), large amounts of gastrin are secreted into the circulation. Gastrin travels to its target tissue, the gastric parietal cells, where it stimulates H^+ secretion and causes hypertrophy of the gastric mucosa. Abe had very high circulating levels of gastrin; consequently, he had very high basal levels of gastric H^+ secretion.

   Physiologic gastrin secretion by the antral G cells can be compared with *nonphysiologic* gastrin secretion by a gastrinoma. The physiologic secretion of gastrin and, consequently, the physiologic secretion of H^+ are regulated by negative feedback. In other words, when the contents of the stomach are sufficiently acidified, the low gastric pH directly inhibits further gastrin secretion. With gastrinoma, the situation is different. The secretion of gastrin by the gastrinoma is *not* feedback-regulated; therefore, even when the stomach contents are very acidic, gastrin secretion continues unabated.

3. Abe's duodenal ulcer developed because the H^+ load delivered from the stomach to the small intestine was greater than could be buffered. Normally, the duodenal mucosa is protected from the acidic stomach contents by neutralizing (high HCO_3^-) secretions from the pancreas, liver, and intestine. In Abe's case, unrelenting gastrin secretion led to unrelenting H^+ secretion (in excess of what could be buffered). As a result, the acidic contents of the duodenum digested a portion of the duodenal mucosa.

4. In the **pentagastrin stimulation test,** a gastrin analogue is infused while gastric H^+ secretion is monitored. (Gastric contents are sampled through a nasogastric tube.) In healthy persons, the gastrin analogue acts just like endogenous gastrin: it stimulates H^+ secretion by gastric parietal cells (usually to a level about threefold higher than basal secretory rates). In Abe, the gastrin analogue did *nothing*—Abe had such high circulating levels of gastrin from the tumor that H^+ secretion was already maximally stimulated. The small additional amount of gastrin that was administered as pentagastrin in the test could not further stimulate H^+ secretion.

5. You may have had difficulty with this question. It was included to introduce you to an important diagnostic test for Zollinger–Ellison syndrome. For reasons that are not understood, secretin directly stimulates gastrin secretion by gastrinoma cells, but not by antral G cells. Therefore, when a person with Zollinger–Ellison syndrome is challenged with the **secretin stimulation test,** the serum gastrin level increases further. When a healthy person is challenged with secretin, the serum gastrin level is decreased or is unchanged.

6. Abe had **diarrhea** because a large volume of gastric juice was secreted along with H^+. When the volume of gastrointestinal secretions exceeds the absorptive capacity of the intestine, diarrhea occurs. (Another feature of the diarrhea in Zollinger–Ellison syndrome is steatorrhea, which is discussed in the next question.)

7. Abe had fat in his stool **(steatorrhea)** because he did not adequately absorb dietary lipids. To understand how steatorrhea can occur, it is helpful to review the steps involved in normal fat digestion and absorption (Fig. 5–6). Dietary lipids are digested by three **pancreatic enzymes:** pancreatic lipase digests triglycerides; cholesterol ester hydrolase digests cholesterol esters; and phospholipase A_2 digests phospholipids. (i) The products of lipid digestion (i.e., monoglycerides, fatty acids, cholesterol, and lysolecithin) are solubilized in **micelles** in the intestinal lumen. The outer layer of the micelles is composed of **bile salts,** which have amphipathic properties. "Amphipathic" means that the molecules have both hydrophilic and hydrophobic regions and are, accordingly, soluble in both water and oil. The hydrophilic portion of the bile salts is dissolved in the aqueous solution of the intestinal lumen. The hydrophobic portion of the bile salts is dissolved in the center of the micelle, which contains the products of lipid digestion. In this way, hydrophobic dietary lipids can be solubilized in the "unfriendly" aqueous environment of the intestinal lumen. (ii) At the apical membrane of the intestinal cells, the products of lipid digestion are released from the micelles and diffuse into the cell. (iii) Inside the intestinal cells, the lipids are re-esterified, packaged in **chylomicrons,** and (iv) transported into lymphatic vessels. Each step in the process of lipid digestion and absorption is essential; if any step is defective, lipid absorption is impaired.

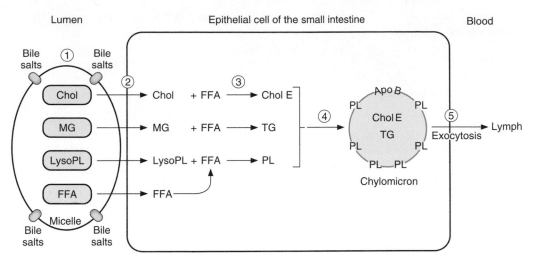

Figure 5–6 Absorption of lipids in small intestine. The *numbers* show the sequence of events described in the text. (ApoB, β-lipoprotein; Chol, cholesterol; CholE, cholesterol ester; FFA, free fatty acids; LysoPL, lysolecithin; MG, monoglycerides; PL, phospholipids; TG, triglycerides.)

We can now determine which step in Abe's lipid digestion and absorption was impaired. Abe had three major defects in lipid digestion and absorption, all related to the acidic pH of his intestinal contents. (i) Pancreatic enzymes are inactivated at acidic pH (the optimal pH for pancreatic lipase is 6). Thus, *digestion* of dietary lipids to absorbable compounds was impaired. (ii) Bile salts are weak acids that exist primarily in their nonionized (HA) form at acidic pH. In this nonionized form, the bile salts are lipid-soluble and are absorbed "too early" in the small intestine (before micelle formation and lipid absorption are complete). Normally, bile acids are absorbed in the terminal portion of the small intestine (the ileum) via the **enterohepatic circulation** (after they have completed their absorptive work for the dietary lipids). (iii) Acid damages the mucosa of the small intestine, thereby reducing the surface area for absorption of lipids. Thus, for all of these reasons, the "oil" that Abe saw in his stool was undigested, unabsorbed triglycerides, cholesterol esters, and phospholipids.

8. Abe felt better when he ate because food is a buffer for H^+. Some of the excess H^+ was "mopped up" by the food in his stomach, reducing the load of free H^+ that was delivered to the small intestine.

9. **Omeprazole** inhibits the **H^+-K^+ ATPase** in gastric parietal cells. This class of drugs is sometimes called the "**proton pump inhibitors**." Recall that H^+-K^+ ATPase secretes H^+ from the parietal cell into the lumen of the stomach. While awaiting surgery to remove the gastrinoma, Abe was treated with this drug, which reduced the amount of H^+ secreted.

Key topics

Acetylcholine

Bile salts

Cholecystokinin-B receptor

Chylomicrons

Diarrhea

Enterohepatic circulation

Gastrin

Gastrinoma

G cells

H^+-K^+ ATPase

H_2 receptors

Helicobacter pylori

Histamine

Micelles

Muscarinic (M_3) receptor

Nonsteroidal anti-inflammatory drugs (NSAIDs)

Omeprazole

Pancreatic lipase

Parietal cells

Peptic ulcer disease

Proton pump inhibitors

Somatostatin

Steatorrhea

Vagus nerve

Zollinger–Ellison syndrome

Case 45

Peptic Ulcer Disease: *Helicobacter pylori* Infection

Dolly Spector is a 59-year-old real estate agent who had frequent bouts of "acid indigestion." She described burning and a dull ache in her stomach, which improved when she ate food or took over-the-counter antacid medication. A client mentioned that she had an ulcer that started with the same symptoms, which prompted Dolly to see her physician.

On physical examination, Dolly had epigastric tenderness. A serologic test and a ^{13}C-urea breath test were both positive, consistent with *Helicobacter pylori* infection. Endoscopy confirmed the presence of a duodenal ulcer. Dolly was treated with an antibiotic (to eradicate *H. pylori*) and omeprazole.

 QUESTIONS

1. What is the mechanism of gastric H^+ secretion, and what factors regulate it?

2. Normally, why isn't the gastric mucosa eroded and digested by the H^+ and pepsin that are present in the gastric lumen?

3. What causes peptic ulcer disease, and what are the major causative factors?

4. *H. pylori* colonizes the *gastric* mucus. How does this lead to *duodenal* ulcer?

5. *H. pylori* contains the enzyme urease, which permits the bacterium to colonize gastric mucus. What is the permissive role of urease?

6. What is the ^{13}C-urea breath test, and why is it positive in *H. pylori* infection?

7. What is the basis for Dolly's treatment with omeprazole?

ANSWERS AND EXPLANATIONS

1. The mechanism of gastric H^+ secretion was discussed in Case 44 and illustrated in Figure 5–5. Briefly, the apical membrane of parietal cells contains an **H^+-K^+ ATPase** that pumps H^+ from the cell into the lumen of the stomach. The major factors that stimulate H^+ secretion by parietal cells are **acetylcholine** (muscarinic [M_3] receptors), **gastrin** (CCK_B receptors), and **histamine** (H_2 receptors). The major factors that inhibit H^+ secretion are **somatostatin** and **prostaglandins**.

2. The gastric mucosal epithelium would seem to be in direct contact with the gastric luminal contents, which are very acidic and contain the digestive enzyme pepsin. What prevents the gastric luminal contents from eroding and digesting the mucosal epithelial cells? First, mucous neck glands secrete **mucus**, which forms a gel-like protective barrier between the cells and the gastric lumen. Second, gastric epithelial cells secrete HCO_3^-, which is trapped in the mucus. Should any H^+ penetrate the mucus, it is neutralized by HCO_3^- before it reaches the epithelial cells. Should any pepsin penetrate the mucus, it is inactivated in the relatively alkaline environment.

3. **Peptic ulcer disease** is an ulcerative lesion of the gastric or duodenal mucosa. The ulceration is caused by the erosive and digestive action of **H^+** and **pepsin** on the mucosa, which is normally protected by the layer of mucus and HCO_3^-. Thus, for a peptic ulcer to be created, there must be: (i) loss of the protective mucus barrier, (ii) excessive H^+ and pepsin secretion, or (iii) a combination of the two. Stated differently, peptic ulcer disease is caused by an imbalance between the factors that protect the gastroduodenal mucosa and the factors that damage it; these factors are summarized in Figure 5–7. **Protective factors**, in addition to mucus and HCO_3^-, are prostaglandins, mucosal blood flow, and growth factors. **Damaging factors**, in addition to H^+ and pepsin, are **Helicobacter Pylori** (*H. pylori*) infection, nonsteroidal anti-inflammatory drugs (NSAIDs), stress, smoking, and alcohol consumption.

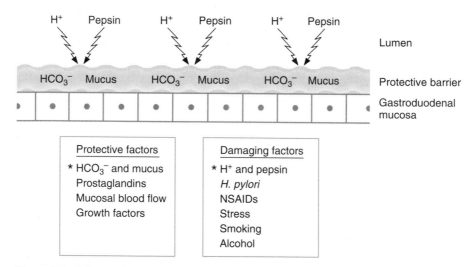

Figure 5–7   Balance of protective and damaging factors on gastroduodenal mucosa.

4. *H. pylori* is a **gram-negative bacterium** that colonizes the gastric mucus. The infection can lead to gastric or duodenal ulcer.

   In producing **gastric ulcer**, the causation is fairly direct: *H. pylori* colonizes the gastric mucus (often in the antrum), attaches to the gastric epithelium, and releases cytotoxins (e.g., cagA toxin) and other factors that break down the protective mucus barrier and the underlying cells.

In producing **duodenal ulcer,** as in Dolly's case, the causation is indirect. If the bacterium colonizes *gastric* mucus, how does it cause *duodenal* ulcer? The sequence of events is illustrated in Figure 5–8. (i) *H. pylori* colonizes gastric mucus and **inhibits somatostatin** secretion from D cells in the gastric antrum. Somatostatin normally inhibits gastrin secretion from G cells in the gastric antrum; thus, the reduction in somatostatin-inhibition results in **increased gastrin secretion,** which leads to **increased H⁺ secretion** by gastric parietal cells. In this way, an increased H⁺ load is delivered to the duodenum. (ii) The gastric *H. pylori* infection spreads to the duodenum and **inhibits duodenal HCO₃⁻ secretion.** Normally, duodenal HCO₃⁻ secretion is sufficient to neutralize the H⁺ that is delivered from the stomach. However, in this case, not only is excess H⁺ delivered to the duodenum, but less HCO₃⁻ is secreted to neutralize it. The bottom line is: neutralization is insufficient and the duodenal contents are abnormally acidic, which leads to the erosive action of H⁺ and pepsin on the duodenal mucosa.

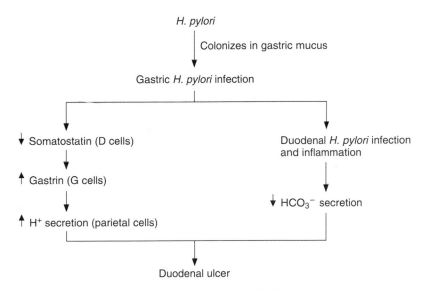

Figure 5–8   Gastric *H. pylori* infection causes duodenal ulcer.

5. *H. pylori* contains **urease,** which permits the bacterium to colonize the gastric mucus. The action of urease is to **convert urea to NH₃.** The NH₃ generated then **alkalinizes** the local environment, allowing the bacterium to survive in the otherwise acidic gastric lumen. By making the environment more hospitable, the bacterium can bind to gastric epithelium and not be shed. Furthermore, the NH₄⁺ that is in equilibrium with NH₃ damages the gastric epithelium.

6. Dolly had a positive ¹³C-urea breath test. For the test, she drank a solution containing ¹³C-urea. The *H. pylori* present in her gastrointestinal tract contained urease, which converted ingested ¹³C-urea to ¹³CO₂ and NH₃. The ¹³CO₂ **was expired** and measured in the breath test.

7. In addition to receiving antibiotics to eradicate the *H. pylori* infection, Dolly was treated with **omeprazole,** an inhibitor of gastric **H⁺-K⁺ ATPase** (a so-called proton pump inhibitor). By reducing gastric H⁺ secretion, less H⁺ was delivered to the duodenum, thus reducing its damaging effect on the duodenal mucosa.

Key topics

^{13}C-urea breath test

Duodenal ulcer

Gastric ulcer

Gastrin

Helicobacter pylori

Histamine

H$^+$-K$^+$ ATPase

Omeprazole

Peptic ulcer disease

Somatostatin

Urease

Case 46

Secretory Diarrhea: *Escherichia coli* Infection

Holly Hudson, a 22-year-old college graduate, works for a nonprofit organization in Central America that is building a school for 80 children. Before she left for Central America, Holly received all of the required vaccinations. While in Central America, she heeded warnings about boiling the drinking water. Despite these precautions, she became infected with a strain of *Escherichia coli* that causes secretory diarrhea. Holly became acutely ill and was producing 10 L of watery stools daily. Her stool did not contain pus or blood. Holly was transported to the nearest clinic, where she was examined (Table 5–2).

TABLE 5-2	*Results of Holly's Physical Examination and Laboratory Tests*	
Blood pressure		80/40 (normal, 120/80)
Heart rate		120 beats/min
Serum K^+		2.3 mEq/L (normal, 4.5 mEq/L)

A stool culture confirmed the presence of enterotoxigenic *E. coli*. Holly was treated with antibiotics, an opiate antidiarrheal medication, and the World Health Organization's oral rehydration solution that contains electrolytes and glucose. The diarrhea subsided, and Holly's blood pressure, heart rate, and electrolytes returned to normal.

 QUESTIONS

1. What is the total volume of fluid that is ingested and secreted in the gastrointestinal tract daily in healthy persons? If the average volume of fluid in feces is 200 mL/day, how much fluid is absorbed by the gastrointestinal tract daily?

2. What is the definition of diarrhea? Discuss the major mechanisms for diarrhea: osmotic, secretory, inflammatory, and motor.

3. Holly was infected with enterotoxigenic *E. coli*. Like *Vibrio cholerae,* this strain of *E. coli* produces an endotoxin that causes secretory diarrhea. What cells of the gastrointestinal tract are affected by cholera toxin (and by the endotoxin of this *E. coli*)? How do these toxins cause diarrhea?

4. Would you expect Holly to have an increased fecal osmolar gap? Why or why not?

5. Why was Holly's serum K^+ concentration so low?

6. Why was Holly's blood pressure decreased? Why was her heart rate increased?

7. Holly might have received *intravenous* fluid "resuscitation" to replace the fluid and electrolytes she lost in diarrhea. Instead, she received *oral* fluid resuscitation. What was the rationale for oral treatment?

ANSWERS AND EXPLANATIONS

1. Each day, the gastrointestinal tract secretes, and subsequently absorbs, large volumes of fluid. Typically, the diet provides approximately 2 L fluid; in addition, 1 L is secreted in saliva, 2 L is secreted in gastric juice, 3 L is secreted in pancreatic juice and bile, and 1 L is secreted by the small intestine, for a grand total of 9 L. Clearly, we do not excrete 9 L in the feces every day! In fact, the average volume of fluid excreted daily in the feces is 200 mL. Therefore, the logical conclusion is that approximately 8.8 L fluid must be absorbed by the gastrointestinal tract; most of this absorption occurs in the small intestine.

2. **Diarrhea** comes from the Greek word *diarrhoia,* meaning to "flow through." In practice, diarrhea describes the excretion of excess water in the feces. Diarrhea can occur either because too much fluid is secreted (in excess of what can be absorbed) or because too little fluid is absorbed. Thus, each of the four mechanisms of diarrhea mentioned in the question must be caused by increased secretion, decreased absorption, or a combination of the two.

   In **osmotic diarrhea** (e.g., lactose in lactase-deficient persons; sorbitol in chewing gum; magnesium in milk of magnesia), poorly absorbed solutes cause osmotic flow of water into the lumen of the gastrointestinal tract. In **secretory diarrhea** (e.g., *Vibrio cholerae,* enterotoxigenic *E. coli,* VIPoma, stimulant laxatives), increased volumes of fluid are secreted by the intestine, overwhelming the absorptive capacity of the gastrointestinal tract. In **inflammatory diarrhea** (e.g., dysentery, ulcerative colitis), damage to the intestinal mucosa interferes with absorption, creating an osmotic effect from the nonabsorbed solutes. Also, various chemical mediators, released in response to inflammation, stimulate intestinal secretion. In **rapid transit (motor) diarrhea** (e.g., pathologic hypermotility, intestinal bypass), fluid passes through the intestine too quickly for normal absorption to occur.

3. Holly's diarrhea was caused by activation of secretory epithelial cells that line the intestinal crypts. These **intestinal crypt cells** (Fig. 5–9) are different from the absorptive cells that line the intestinal villi. The apical membrane of the crypt cells contains **Cl⁻ channels.** The basolateral membrane contains Na⁺-K⁺ ATPase and an Na⁺-K⁺-2Cl⁻ cotransporter similar to that found in the thick ascending limb of the loop of Henle. This "three-ion" cotransporter brings Na⁺, K⁺, and Cl⁻ into the cell from the blood. Cl⁻ is then secreted into the lumen of the intestine through apical membrane Cl⁻ channels. Na⁺ passively follows Cl⁻, moving between the cells and, finally, water is secreted into the lumen, following the movement of NaCl.

   Usually, the Cl⁻ channels of the apical membrane of the crypt cells are closed, but they may open in response to hormones or neurotransmitters, including **vasoactive intestinal peptide (VIP).** The receptors for these hormones and neurotransmitters (e.g., for VIP) are located in the basolateral membrane and are coupled to **adenylyl cyclase.** When activated, adenylyl cyclase generates intracellular **cyclic adenosine monophosphate (cAMP).** Cyclic AMP opens the apical Cl⁻ channels, initiating secretion of Cl⁻, followed by secretion of Na⁺ and water. Normally, electrolytes and water secreted by the deeper crypt cells are subsequently absorbed by the more superficial villar cells. However, if intestinal crypt cell secretion is excessive (as in Holly's case), the absorptive mechanism is overwhelmed, and diarrhea occurs.

Epithelial cell of intestinal crypt

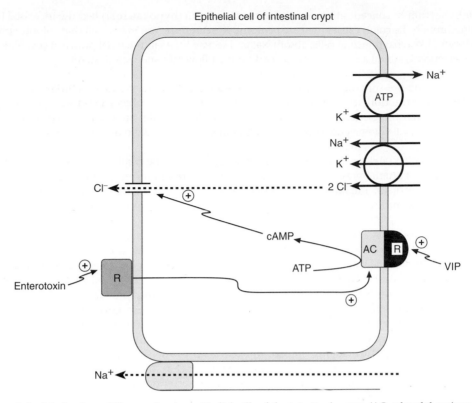

Figure 5–9 Mechanism of Cl⁻ secretion by epithelial cells of the intestinal crypts. (AC, adenylyl cyclase; ATP, adenosine triphosphate; cAMP, cyclic adenosine monophosphate; R, receptor; VIP, vasoactive intestinal peptide.)

With infection by **Vibrio cholerae** or **enterotoxigenic E. coli,** the bacterial toxins (e. g. cholera toxin) bind to receptors on the apical membranes of the crypt cells. Activation of these receptors leads to intense, irreversible stimulation of **adenylyl cyclase**, generation of cyclic AMP, and opening of Cl⁻ channels in the apical membrane. The **Cl⁻ channels** are held open, and Cl⁻ secretion is intensely stimulated, followed by secretion of Na⁺ and water.

You may wonder whether it is true that the toxin receptor is located on the *apical* membrane of the crypt cells, even though the adenylyl cyclase it activates is located on the *basolateral* membrane. Yes, it is true, although it is not clear which intracellular messenger relays information from the apical membrane to the basolateral membrane. (On the other hand, we know that the step between activation of adenylyl cyclase and opening of Cl⁻ channels is mediated by cyclic AMP.)

Since adenylyl cyclase is *irreversibly* stimulated, you may wonder how someone can recover from an infection with *V. cholerae* or enterotoxigenic *E. coli*. The answer is that adenylyl cyclase and Cl⁻ secretion are irreversibly stimulated only for the *life of the intestinal crypt cell*. Fortunately, intestinal mucosal cells turn over rapidly and, with appropriate antibiotic treatment and fluid resuscitation, the person can recover.

4. The **fecal osmolar gap** estimates *unmeasured solutes* in the stool. This test measures total osmolarity and the Na⁺ and K⁺ concentrations of stool. The sum of the Na⁺ and K⁺ concentrations is multiplied by two, accounting for the anions that must accompany these cations. The fecal osmolar gap is the difference between total osmolarity and two times the sum of the Na⁺ and K⁺ concentrations.

Holly would *not* be expected to have an increased fecal osmolar gap because her diarrhea was caused by excess secretion of electrolytes. In other words, all of the excess solute in her stool was in the form of electrolytes that are measured and accounted for, not in the form of unmeasured solutes (e.g., lactose, sorbitol; see Case 43).

5. Holly's serum K^+ concentration was very low (2.3 mEq/L) **(hypokalemia)** because increased flow rate through the colon causes increased **colonic K^+ secretion.** You may recall that colonic epithelial cells, like renal principal cells, absorb Na^+ and secrete K^+. As in the renal principal cells, colonic K^+ secretion is stimulated both by increased luminal flow rate and by aldosterone.

6. Holly's blood pressure was decreased (80/40) because she had severe **extracellular fluid (ECF) volume contraction** secondary to diarrhea. Her secretory diarrhea caused loss of NaCl and water through the gastrointestinal tract. Because NaCl and water are the major constituents of ECF, Holly's ECF volume and, consequently, her blood volume and blood pressure were reduced.

   Holly's heart rate was increased because baroreceptors in the carotid sinus were activated by the decreased arterial pressure. Activation of these baroreceptors led to increased sympathetic outflow to the heart and blood vessels. One of these actions of the sympathetic nervous system is an increase in heart rate (through activation of β_1 receptors in the sinoatrial node).

7. Certainly, Holly's ECF volume could have been restored by *intravenous* infusion of a solution containing the electrolytes that were lost in diarrhea. However, the alternative and highly effective approach was to give her an oral rehydration solution. The World Health Organization's **oral rehydration solution** contains water, Na^+, K^+, Cl^-, HCO_3^-, and significantly, glucose. An *oral* solution that contains glucose (in addition to water and electrolytes) is given because the glucose stimulates **Na^+-dependent glucose cotransport** in the small intestine. For every glucose absorbed by this transporter, one Na^+ is absorbed, and to maintain electroneutrality, one Cl^- is also absorbed. Water absorption follows solute absorption to maintain isosmolarity. Thus, adding glucose to the lumen of the gastrointestinal tract stimulates electrolyte and water absorption by the intestinal villar cells, offsetting the high secretory rate in the crypt cells. (Picture a battle between intestinal secretion and absorption! Even if intestinal secretion is very high, if absorption can be increased, less fluid will remain in the intestinal lumen to cause diarrhea.) Incidentally, the introduction of oral rehydration solutions has greatly reduced the number of diarrhea-related deaths in children worldwide.

Key topics

Adenylyl cyclase

Cholera toxin

Cl^- channels

Cyclic adenosine monophosphate (cAMP)

Diarrhea

Enterotoxigenic *Escherichia coli*

Extracellular fluid volume contraction

Fecal osmolar gap

Hypokalemia

Intestinal crypt cells

K^+ secretion by the colon

Na^+-glucose cotransport

Oral rehydration solution

Secretory diarrhea

Vasoactive intestinal peptide (VIP)

Vibrio cholerae

Case 47

Bile Acid Deficiency: Ileal Resection

Paul Bostian is a 39-year-old high school guidance counselor who was diagnosed with Crohn's disease (an inflammatory bowel disease) when he was a teenager. For 20 years, he was treated medically with antidiarrheal agents and strong anti-inflammatory drugs, including glucocorticoids. During that time, Paul had two spontaneous remissions. However, after these remissions, his disease always returned "with a vengeance." Last year, he had a small bowel obstruction that could not be relieved with nonsurgical approaches, and he underwent emergency surgery that removed 80% of his ileum.

Since the surgery, Paul has had diarrhea. His stools are oily, pale, and foul-smelling. He takes the drug cholestyramine to control his diarrhea. However, he continues to have steatorrhea. Paul also receives monthly injections of vitamin B_{12}.

 QUESTIONS

1. What steps are involved in the biosynthesis of bile acids? What is a primary bile acid? What is a secondary bile acid? What are bile salts? What purpose is served by converting bile acids to bile salts?

2. Describe the enterohepatic circulation of bile salts.

3. What role do bile salts play in the absorption of dietary lipids?

4. Why did Paul have oily stools (steatorrhea) after his ileal resection?

5. Paul has "bile acid diarrhea." Why do bile acids cause diarrhea? (Big hint: They stimulate colonic Cl^- secretion.) Why don't healthy persons have bile acid diarrhea?

6. Cholestyramine is a cationic resin that binds bile salts. Propose a mechanism that explains its effectiveness in treating Paul's diarrhea.

7. Why did Paul need monthly injections of vitamin B_{12}? What conditions can lead to vitamin B_{12} deficiency?

ANSWERS AND EXPLANATIONS

1. The **primary bile acids** (cholic acid and chenodeoxycholic acid) are synthesized from cholesterol in the liver. The rate-limiting enzyme in this biosynthetic pathway is cholesterol 7α-hydroxylase, which is feedback-inhibited by cholic acid. These primary bile acids are secreted in bile into the intestinal lumen, where they are dehydroxylated by intestinal bacteria to form the **secondary bile acids** deoxycholic acid and lithocholic acid. In the intestine, a portion of each primary bile acid is dehydroxylated to form a secondary bile acid, and a portion is left unchanged (Fig. 5–10).

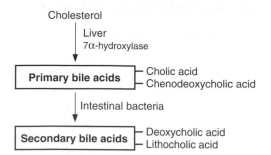

Figure 5–10 Biosynthetic pathways for bile acids.

Bile salts are conjugated forms of bile acids. Each primary bile acid may be conjugated in the liver with the amino acid glycine or taurine, yielding a total of *eight bile salts*. The bile salts are named for the parent bile acid and the conjugating amino acid (e.g., taurocholic acid, glycolithocholic acid).

The purpose of conjugating bile acids to bile salts is to decrease the pK of the compounds, thus making them more soluble in the aqueous solution of the intestinal lumen (where bile salts act). The reasoning is as follows. The duodenal contents have a pH of 3 to 5. The bile acids have a pK of approximately 7. Therefore, in the range of duodenal pH, most bile acids are present in their nonionized (HA) forms, which are *water-insoluble*. The bile salts have a pK of 1 to 4. Consequently, at duodenal pH, most bile salts are present in their ionized (A⁻) forms, which are *water-soluble*. Therefore, in the intestinal lumen, bile salts are more soluble than bile acids. The discussion of Question 3 explains why the solubility of bile salts is very important.

2. **Enterohepatic circulation of bile salts** refers to their circulation between the intestine and the liver. But we need to back up in the story. How did the bile salts reach the intestine in the first place? Recall from the previous question that two primary bile acids are synthesized in the liver and conjugated with glycine or taurine to form their respective bile salts. The hepatocytes continuously produce bile, approximately 50% of which is bile salts. Bile flows through the bile ducts to the **gallbladder**, where it is concentrated (by absorption of ions and water) and stored. Within 30 minutes of ingestion of a meal, the gastrointestinal hormone **cholecystokinin (CCK)** is secreted. CCK simultaneously causes the gallbladder to contract and the **sphincter of Oddi** to relax. As a result, bile is ejected from the gallbladder into the lumen of the intestine. In the intestinal lumen (as discussed earlier), the four bile salts become eight bile salts as a result of bacterial dehydroxylation. Now the bile salts are ready to assist in the process of absorbing dietary lipids (discussed in the next question). (Incidentally, a portion of each bile salt is converted back to its bile acid by bacterial deconjugation. Hence, when we speak of enterohepatic circulation of bile salts, we mean bile salts *plus* bile acids.)

When the bile salts finish their **lipid absorption** work in the duodenum and jejunum, they are *recirculated* to the liver instead of being excreted in the feces. This process (enterohepatic circulation of bile salts) occurs as follows (Fig. 5–11). Bile salts are transported from the lumen of the intestine into the portal blood on an **Na⁺-bile salt cotransporter** located in the terminal small intestine **(ileum)**. This portal blood supplies the liver, which extracts the bile salts and adds them to the total hepatic bile salt pool. In this way, 95% of the bile salts secreted in each circulation are returned to the liver (rather than being excreted). Twenty-five percent of the total bile salt pool is excreted daily and must be replaced.

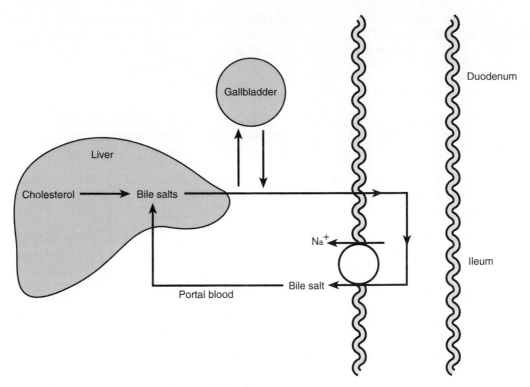

Figure 5–11 Enterohepatic circulation of bile salts.

3. The function of bile salts in the intestinal lumen is to emulsify and solubilize dietary lipids so that the lipids can be digested and absorbed by intestinal epithelial cells. Why do the dietary lipids need this help? Because lipids, which are hydrophobic, are insoluble in aqueous solutions such as that present in the lumen of the small intestine.

The first role of the bile salts is to **emulsify** dietary lipids. The negatively charged bile salts surround the lipids, creating small lipid droplets in the aqueous solution of the small intestinal lumen. The negative charges on the bile salts repel each other so that the droplets disperse, rather than coalesce. In this way, the surface area available for pancreatic digestive enzymes is increased. If emulsification did not occur, dietary lipids would coalesce into large lipid "blobs," with relatively little total surface area for digestion.

The second role of the bile salts is to form **micelles** with the products of **lipid digestion** (cholesterol, monoglycerides, lysolecithin, and fatty acids). The micellar core contains the products of lipid digestion. The micellar surface is composed of bile salts, which are amphipathic (soluble in both lipid and water). The hydrophobic portions of the bile salt molecules point toward the lipid center of the micelle. The hydrophilic portions of the bile salt molecules are dissolved in the aqueous solution in the intestinal lumen. In this way, hydrophobic lipids are dissolved in an otherwise "unfriendly" aqueous environment.

To complete the process of lipid absorption, the micelles diffuse to the apical membrane of the epithelial cells of the intestinal mucosa. There, they release the lipids, which diffuse across the apical membranes into the cell. (The bile salts remain in the intestinal lumen and are normally recirculated to the liver.) Inside the intestinal cells, the lipids are re-esterified, packaged in **chylomicrons**, and transported into the lymph for absorption.

4. Paul had **steatorrhea** (fat in the stool) because his *bile salt pool was depleted* following the ileal resection. Thus, his biliary secretions contained insufficient bile salts to ensure that all dietary lipid was digested and absorbed. Any nonabsorbed lipid was excreted in the feces, where it appeared as lipid droplets or oil.

Why did Paul have this apparent bile salt deficiency? Recall that, normally, the liver must replace only 25% of the bile salt pool daily. Because most of Paul's ileum was removed, he lost this recirculatory feature, and most of his bile salt pool was excreted in feces. As a result, Paul's liver had to synthesize nearly 100% of the secreted bile salts daily, compared with 25% in healthy persons. Simply, his liver could not keep up with this large synthetic demand, and as a result, his bile salt pool decreased.

5. Paul's diarrhea was caused in part by the presence of bile salts in the lumen of the colon (so-called **bile acid diarrhea**). These bile salts stimulate colonic Cl^- secretion; Na^+ and water follow Cl^- into the intestinal lumen, producing a secretory diarrhea.

   Bile acid diarrhea doesn't occur in healthy persons because, normally, bile salts aren't present in the lumen of the colon. They are recirculated from the ileum to the liver before they reach the colon.

6. **Cholestyramine** is a water-insoluble **cationic resin** that binds bile salts in the intestinal lumen. When bile salts are bound to the resin, they cannot stimulate colonic Cl^- secretion or cause secretory diarrhea. (Incidentally, because cholestyramine binds bile salts in the intestinal lumen, it is also useful as a lipid-lowering agent in persons with hypertriglyceridemia.) When bile salts are bound to the resin, they are not absorbable and therefore are not recirculated to the liver. Thus, cholestyramine treatment depletes the bile salt pool, which impairs lipid absorption from the gastrointestinal tract.

7. In addition to recirculating bile salts to the liver, the **ileum** has another essential function, absorption of **vitamin B_{12}**. Recall the steps involved in vitamin B_{12} absorption. Dietary vitamin B_{12} binds to **R proteins** that are secreted in saliva. In the duodenum, pancreatic proteases degrade the R protein, releasing vitamin B_{12}, which forms a stable complex with **intrinsic factor** that is secreted by the gastric parietal cells. The intrinsic factor–vitamin B_{12} complex, which is resistant to proteolytic degradation, travels to the ileum, where it is absorbed into the blood by transporters in the ileal cells. Vitamin B_{12} then circulates in the blood bound to a specific plasma protein **(transcobalamin II)**. Paul received monthly *injections* of vitamin B_{12} because, in the absence of an ileum, he could not absorb vitamin B_{12} that he ingested *orally*.

   In addition to ileal resection, other conditions that cause vitamin B_{12} deficiency can be understood by considering the steps in vitamin B_{12} absorption from the gastrointestinal tract. **Deficiency of intrinsic factor** (secondary to gastrectomy or to atrophy of the gastric parietal cells) results in inability to form the intrinsic factor–vitamin B_{12} complex that is absorbed in the ileum. Also, one subtle manifestation of **pancreatic enzyme deficiency** is the inability to hydrolyze the R protein from the R protein–vitamin B_{12} complex. In this case, vitamin B_{12} is not "free" to complex with intrinsic factor; therefore, it cannot be absorbed. In these conditions, as with **ileectomy**, vitamin B_{12} must be administered by injection.

Key topics

Bile acid diarrhea
Bile acids
Bile salts
Cholecystokinin (CCK)
Cholestyramine
Chylomicrons
Enterohepatic circulation of bile salts
Gallbladder
Ileectomy
Ileum
Intrinsic factor
Lipid absorption
Lipid digestion
Micelles
Na^+-bile salt cotransporter
R proteins
Sphincter of Oddi
Steatorrhea
Transcobalamin II
Vitamin B_{12}

Endocrine and Reproductive Physiology

Case 48

Growth Hormone-Secreting Tumor: Acromegaly

Mavis Trippe is a 41-year-old woman who has worked at the cosmetics counter of the local department store for many years. Mavis' colleagues in cosmetics noted that her physical appearance had changed—her features had become coarse, her lower jaw was protruding, and her teeth had separated. They were concerned that Mavis might have a health problem, and one of the colleagues volunteered to have a talk with her. Mavis was a little hurt at their observations, but then opened up and expressed concerns of her own. She disclosed that her menstrual periods had suddenly stopped 5 years ago; that her hat, shoe, and glove size had increased; and that her fingers had enlarged so much that her rings no longer fit. Every night, she had been getting up several times to urinate. Mavis decided to see a physician for evaluation of these strange symptoms.

Physical examination revealed a woman with coarse facial features, a prominent jaw, and large hands and feet. Her blood pressure was elevated at 170/110. The results of laboratory studies are shown in Table 6–1.

TABLE 6–1	*Mavis' Laboratory Values*	
Glucose, fasting	250 mg/dL	(Normal, 70–100 mg/dL)
Growth hormone, fasting	90 ng/mL	(Normal, 2–6 ng/mL)
IGF-1	Elevated	
FSH	Decreased	
TSH	Normal	
T_4	Normal	
Prolactin	Elevated	

During administration of glucose in a glucose tolerance test, Mavis' growth hormone levels remained elevated. Magnetic resonance imaging (MRI) of Mavis' brain showed a large intrasellar mass that was pushing upward on the roof of the sella turcica. The physician diagnosed her with acromegaly, caused by a pituitary adenoma that was secreting growth hormone.

Transsphenoidal surgery was performed to remove a large pituitary adenoma. Postoperatively, Mavis' growth hormone and blood glucose levels fell into the normal range. Although her menstrual cycles did not return, the physicians told Mavis that, over time, she could expect improvement in her facial features and reduction in the swelling of her feet and hands.

 QUESTIONS

1. A significant feature of acromegaly, and one exhibited by Mavis, is widening of bones in the skull, hands, and feet. What is responsible for this widening?

2. Mavis did not exhibit increased *linear* growth of her long bones. Why not?

3. What explanation can you provide for the increased fasting blood glucose level?

4. Why did she have increased urination?

5. Although Mavis' pituitary adenoma secreted growth hormone, her serum prolactin level was also elevated. What explanation can you offer for the increased prolactin level?

6. What was responsible for Mavis' amenorrhea?

7. Based on your knowledge of the feedback control of growth hormone secretion, propose a drug treatment that could have lowered Mavis' growth hormone level prior to surgery?

ANSWERS AND EXPLANATIONS

1. Mavis' pituitary adenoma secreted excessive amounts of **growth hormone.** Growth hormone itself does not have growth-promoting effects on bone. Rather, growth hormone stimulates the production of **insulin-like growth factor I (IGF-I),** or somatomedin, which mediates its growth-promoting effects on bone and soft tissues. IGF-I is synthesized in the target tissues of growth hormone, including liver, kidney, muscle, cartilage, and bone. IGF-I then acts on its target tissues via a tyrosine kinase receptor that is structurally homologous with the insulin receptor.

2. When growth hormone excess occurs *after* puberty, it produces the clinical syndrome of **acromegaly,** which includes progressive thickening of bones and soft tissues; however, because the epiphyseal plates are already closed, the syndrome does not include lengthening of the long bones. When growth hormone excess occurs *before* puberty, it causes a syndrome called **gigantism,** which, because of intense hormonal stimulation of the epiphyseal plates, includes increased linear growth.

3. One of the metabolic actions of growth hormone is inhibition of glucose uptake into muscle and stimulation of gluconeogenesis in liver. These actions are opposite to those of insulin and, consequently, have been termed the "anti-insulin" or **"diabetogenic" effects of growth hormone.** Mavis' high circulating levels of growth hormone resulted in her elevated blood glucose level, in insulin resistance, and could have led to development of diabetes mellitus.

4. Mavis' polyuria was due to **osmotic diuresis** secondary to her high blood glucose concentration. The high blood glucose led to an increased filtered load of glucose, which exceeded the reabsorptive capacity of the proximal tubule; unreabsorbed glucose was excreted in the urine and acted osmotically to increase Na^+ and water excretion.

5. Normally, **prolactin** secretion by the lactotrophs of the anterior pituitary is under tonic inhibition by **dopamine** secreted from the hypothalamus into hypothalamic-hypophysial portal blood. One explanation for Mavis' high circulating level of prolactin is that the large pituitary adenoma pushed on the lactotrophs and physically disconnected them from the inhibitory effects of hypothalamic dopamine. Without tonic inhibition by dopamine, prolactin secretion was increased. It is also possible that the pituitary adenoma, in addition to secreting growth hormone, was also secreting prolactin.

6. One reason for Mavis' amenorrhea was, again, encroachment of the pituitary adenoma on other hormone-secreting cells of the anterior pituitary, in this case the gonadotrophs. The gonadotrophs are particularly susceptible to the effects of an expanding intrasellar mass, and as a result, there was decreased secretion of follicle-stimulating hormone (FSH) and luteinizing hormone (LH). The decreased levels of FSH and LH caused decreased secretion of estrogen by the ovaries. Another factor contributing to Mavis' amenorrhea was her elevated serum prolactin; when elevated, prolactin inhibits secretion of gonadotropin-releasing hormone (GnRH), leading to further suppression of secretion of FSH and LH.

7. Growth hormone secretion by the anterior pituitary is regulated by two pathways from the hypothalamus, one stimulatory (via **growth hormone-releasing hormone [GHRH]**) and one inhibitory (via **somatostatin).** Growth hormone secretion is controlled by negative feedback as follows (Fig. 6–1). GHRH inhibits its own secretion from the hypothalamus. IGF-I, which is a by-product of growth hormone action on target tissues, inhibits secretion of growth hormone. And, finally, both growth hormone and IGF-I stimulate the secretion of somatostatin, which then inhibits growth hormone secretion.

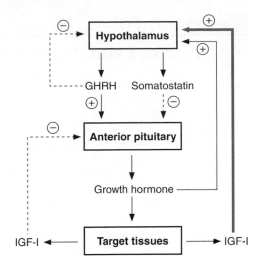

Figure 6–1   Regulation of growth hormone secretion. (GHRH, growth hormone-releasing hormone; IGF-I, insulin-like growth factor I.)

Prior to surgery, Mavis could have been treated with a somatostatin analogue, such as **octreotide,** which, like endogenous somatostatin, inhibits growth hormone secretion.

Key topics

Acromegaly

Dopamine

Gigantism

Growth hormone

Growth hormone-releasing hormone (GHRH)

Insulin-like growth factor I (IGF-I)

Osmotic diuresis

Octreotide

Prolactin

Somatostatin

Case 49

Galactorrhea and Amenorrhea: Prolactinoma

Meghan Fabrizio is a 39-year-old vice president of an Internet company. She has been married for 10 years and has always used barrier methods for birth control. Meghan's menstrual periods started when she was 12 years old and were regular until 18 months ago. At that time, her periods became irregular and then ceased altogether (amenorrhea). Meghan was very concerned because she and her husband had been talking about trying to have a child. Not only had her periods stopped, but a milky substance was leaking from her breasts.

Meghan made an appointment to see her gynecologist. Findings of the pelvic examination were normal, but the gynecologist was able to express milk from her breasts (galactorrhea). Results of a pregnancy test were negative. Other laboratory results are shown in Table 6–2.

TABLE 6–2	*Meghan's Laboratory Values*
Luteinizing hormone, midcycle	5 IU/L (normal, 1–18 IU/L, follicular; 24–100 IU/L, midcycle
Prolactin	86 ng/mL (normal, 5–25 ng/mL)

The laboratory results suggested that Meghan had a prolactinoma. The physician ordered a magnetic resonance imaging scan of her brain. The scan showed a 1.5-cm mass on her pituitary that was believed to be secreting prolactin. While Meghan was awaiting surgery to remove the mass (an adenoma), drug treatment was initiated, which decreased Meghan's serum prolactin level to 20 ng/mL. After the adenoma was removed, Meghan's galactorrhea abated, her menstrual periods resumed, and she is now pregnant with her first child.

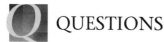 QUESTIONS

1. How is prolactin secretion regulated?

2. What factors increase prolactin secretion and lead to an increase in the serum prolactin level (hyperprolactinemia)? Which of these factors can be ruled in or ruled out in Meghan's case?

3. Why did Meghan have galactorrhea (increased milk production)?

4. Why were her menstrual cycles irregular? What was the significance of her luteinizing hormone (LH) level?

5. What drug was Meghan given to lower her serum prolactin level? What is its mechanism of action?

6. If Meghan's serum prolactin level had remained elevated, it is unlikely that she could have become pregnant. Why?

ANSWERS ON NEXT PAGE

ANSWERS AND EXPLANATIONS

1. **Prolactin** is synthesized and secreted by the **lactotrophs** of the anterior lobe of the pituitary. Its secretion is controlled by the **hypothalamus** (Fig. 6–2) via two regulatory pathways: (i) an inhibitory pathway (through dopamine) and (ii) a stimulatory pathway (through thyrotropin-releasing hormone [TRH]). In persons who are not pregnant or lactating, prolactin secretion by the **anterior pituitary** is **tonically inhibited by dopamine.** In other words, serum prolactin is normally maintained at a low level because inhibition of prolactin secretion by dopamine overrides stimulation of prolactin secretion by TRH.

How does this inhibitory dopamine reach the lactotrophs of the anterior pituitary? Dopaminergic neurons secrete dopamine into the median eminence of the hypothalamus. Capillaries in the median eminence drain into **hypothalamic-hypophysial portal vessels** (the direct blood supply from the hypothalamus to the anterior pituitary). These vessels deliver dopamine directly, and in high concentration, to the lactotrophs of the anterior pituitary.

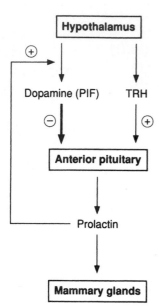

Figure 6–2 Control of prolactin secretion. (PIF, prolactin-inhibiting factor; TRH, thyrotropin-releasing hormone.) (Reprinted, with permission, from Costanzo LS. *BRS Physiology* 4th ed. Baltimore: Lippincott Williams & Wilkins; 2007:243.)

2. Figure 6–2 shows two mechanisms that potentially could result in increased prolactin secretion: (i) increased TRH secretion and (ii) decreased dopamine secretion. The second possibility, decreased dopamine secretion, suggests an important and intriguing cause of hyperprolactinemia: severing of the hypothalamic-hypophysial tract (e.g., after traumatic head injury). If the connection between the hypothalamus and the anterior pituitary is disrupted, the normal inhibitory control of prolactin secretion by hypothalamic dopamine is lost, and hyperprolactinemia occurs. Other factors that increase prolactin secretion are pregnancy (through increased estrogen levels) and breast-feeding (possibly through increased oxytocin secretion).

As for potential causes of Meghan's hyperprolactinemia, pregnancy was ruled out, she was not breast-feeding, and she had no history of traumatic head injury that might have disrupted the blood supply between the hypothalamus and the pituitary. In the absence of other plausible explanations for hyperprolactinemia, it was concluded that the pituitary mass (adenoma) seen on the magnetic resonance imaging scan was probably secreting prolactin.

3. Meghan had **galactorrhea** because she was hyperprolactinemic. The major action of prolactin is lactogenesis (milk production). Prolactin induces the synthesis of lactose (the carbohydrate

of milk), casein (the protein of milk), and lipids. It also promotes the secretion of fluid and electrolytes by the mammary ducts.

4. Meghan's menstrual cycles became irregular and then ceased altogether **(amenorrhea)**. In addition to stimulating milk production, prolactin inhibits the secretion of **gonadotropin-releasing hormone (GnRH)** by the hypothalamus. Inhibition of GnRH secretion leads to decreased secretion of **luteinizing hormone (LH)**, which normally initiates ovulation at the midpoint of the menstrual cycle. Meghan's LH level was low-normal, even for the preovulatory portion of the menstrual cycle, and much lower than the levels expected at the midcycle surge.

5. Dopamine or **dopamine agonists** (e.g., **bromocriptine**) inhibit prolactin secretion by the anterior pituitary (see Fig. 6–2). Given systemically, bromocriptine acts just like dopamine: it inhibits prolactin secretion. When Meghan was treated with bromocriptine, her serum prolactin level decreased from 86 ng/mL to 20 ng/mL.

6. It is unlikely that Meghan could have become pregnant in her hyperprolactinemic state because prolactin inhibits GnRH secretion (and, consequently, LH secretion). Without an ovulatory surge of LH, ovulation does not occur **(anovulation)**; without ovulation, fertilization and pregnancy are impossible. As an aside, fertility is significantly reduced during breast-feeding because the high serum prolactin levels inhibit GnRH and LH secretion. In some parts of the world, breast-feeding is an important mechanism for family spacing, although it is not 100% effective.

Key topics

Amenorrhea

Anovulation

Anterior pituitary

Bromocriptine

Dopamine

Galactorrhea

Gonadotropin-releasing hormone (GnRH)

Hypothalamic-hypophysial portal vessels

Hypothalamus

Lactogenesis

Lactotrophs

Leutinizing hormone (LH)

Prolactin

Case 50

Hyperthyroidism: Graves' Disease

Natasha Schick is a 19-year-old aspiring model who has always dieted to keep her weight in an "acceptable" range. However, within the past 3 months, she has lost 20 lb despite a voracious appetite. She complains of nervousness, sleeplessness, heart palpitations, and irregular menstrual periods. She notes that she is "always hot" and wants the thermostat set lower than her apartment mates.

On physical examination, Natasha was restless and had a noticeable tremor in her hands. At 5 feet, 8 inches tall, she weighed only 110 lb. Her arterial blood pressure was 160/85, and her heart rate was 110 beats/min. She had a wide-eyed stare, and her lower neck appeared full; these characteristics were not present in photographs taken 1 year earlier.

Based on her symptoms, the physician suspected that Natasha had thyrotoxicosis, or increased circulating levels of thyroid hormones. However, it was unclear from the available information *why* her thyroid hormone levels were elevated. Laboratory tests were performed to determine the etiology of her condition (Table 6–3).

TABLE 6–3	*Natasha's Laboratory Results*
Total T_4	Increased
Free T_4	Increased
TSH	Decreased (undetectable)

T_4, thyroxine; TSH, thyroid-stimulating hormone.

 QUESTIONS

1. Based on her symptoms, Natasha's physician suspected thyrotoxicosis (elevated levels of thyroid hormone). Why is each of the following symptoms consistent with increased levels of thyroid hormones?
   a. Weight loss
   b. Heat intolerance
   c. Increased heart rate
   d. Increased pulse pressure
   e. Increased arterial blood pressure

2. The physician considered the following possible causes of thyrotoxicosis, based on his understanding of the hypothalamic–anterior pituitary–thyroid axis: (i) increased secretion of thyrotropin-releasing hormone (TRH) from the hypothalamus; (ii) increased secretion of thyroid-stimulating hormone (TSH) from the anterior pituitary; (iii) primary hyperactivity of the thyroid gland (e.g., Graves' disease); and (iv) ingestion of exogenous thyroid hormones (factitious hyperthyroidism). Using the laboratory findings and your knowledge of the regulation of thyroid hormone secretion, include or exclude each of the four potential causes of Natasha's thyrotoxicosis.

3. Natasha's physician performed a radioactive I⁻ uptake test to measure the activity of her thyroid gland. When her thyroid was scanned for radioactivity, I⁻ uptake was increased uniformly throughout the gland. How did this additional information help refine the diagnosis? Which potential cause of thyrotoxicosis discussed in Question 2 was ruled out by this result?

4. The triiodothyronine (T_3) resin uptake test measures the binding of radioactive T_3 to a synthetic resin. In the test, a standard amount of radioactive T_3 is added to an assay system that contains a sample of the patient's serum and a T_3-binding resin. The rationale is that radioactive T_3 will first bind to unoccupied sites on the patient's thyroid-binding globulin (TBG) and any remaining, or "leftover," radioactive T_3 will bind to the resin. Thus, T_3 resin uptake is increased when circulating TBG levels are decreased (e.g., liver disease; fewer TBG binding sites are available) or when endogenous free T_3 levels are increased (endogenous hormone occupies more sites on TBG). Conversely, resin uptake is decreased when circulating TBG levels are increased (e.g., pregnancy) or when endogenous T_3 levels are decreased.

   Natasha's T_3 resin uptake was increased. Using all of the information you have been given thus far, explain this finding.

5. Based on Natasha's symptoms and laboratory findings, Natasha's physicians concluded that she had Graves' disease. Why? Describe the etiology and pathophysiology of this disease.

6. Surgery was scheduled to remove Natasha's thyroid gland (thyroidectomy). While awaiting surgery, Natasha was given two drugs, propylthiouracil (PTU) and propranolol. What was the rationale for giving each of these drugs?

7. Natasha's thyroidectomy was successful, and she was recovering well. Her nervousness and palpitations disappeared, she was gaining weight, and her blood pressure returned to normal. However, she began to experience alarming new symptoms, including muscle cramps, tingling in her fingers and toes, and numbness around her mouth. She returned to her endocrinologist, who noted a positive Chvostek sign (in which tapping on the facial nerve elicits a spasm of the facial muscles). Her total blood Ca^{2+} concentration was 7.8 mg/dL, and her ionized Ca^{2+} concentration was 3.8 mg/dL, both of which were lower than normal (hypocalcemia). What caused Natasha to become hypocalcemic? How did hypocalcemia cause her new symptoms?

8. How was this new problem treated?

ANSWERS AND EXPLANATIONS

1. **Thyrotoxicosis** is a pathophysiologic state caused by elevated circulating levels of free **thyroid hormones.** Natasha's symptoms and physical findings were consistent with thyrotoxicosis. (a) Thyroid hormones **increase basal metabolic rate (BMR)**, O_2 consumption, and nutrient consumption. Thus, Natasha was in a hypermetabolic state and had a voracious appetite. (b) The increased O_2 consumption resulted in **increased heat production.** The body's normal cooling mechanisms were insufficient to dissipate the extra heat, and Natasha always felt hot. (c) Thyroid hormones induce the synthesis of a number of proteins, including β_1 **receptors** in the heart. Up-regulation of β_1 receptors in the sinoatrial node produced an increased heart rate, or a positive **chronotropic effect.** (d) Up-regulation of β_1 receptors in ventricular muscle produced an increase in **contractility** and **stroke volume**, which was seen as an increase in **pulse pressure.** (e) Both heart rate and contractility were increased; as a consequence, **cardiac output** was increased. The increase in cardiac output produced an **increase in arterial pressure** (arterial pressure [P_a] = cardiac output × total peripheral resistance).

2. Figure 6–3 shows the hypothalamic–anterior pituitary–thyroid axis and the feedback system that regulates secretion of thyroid hormones. Natasha's laboratory data showed increased levels of free T_4 and total T_4 and decreased levels of TSH. (Total T_4 includes the free and protein-bound components in plasma.)

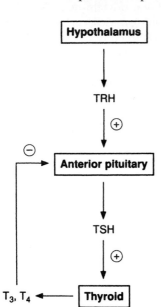

Figure 6–3 Control of thyroid hormone secretion. (T_3, triiodothyronine; T_4, thyroxine; TRH, thyrotropin-releasing hormone; TSH, thyroid-stimulating hormone.) (Reprinted, with permission, from Costanzo LS. *BRS Physiology* 4th ed. Baltimore: Lippincott Williams & Wilkins; 2007:247.)

(i) Theoretically, but rarely, a hypothalamic tumor can secrete increased levels of TRH. As a result, secretion of TSH by the anterior pituitary is increased, leading to increased secretion of thyroid hormones from the thyroid gland. However, this diagnosis was ruled out by the decreased (undetectable) level of TSH in the blood. If the primary defect was in the hypothalamus, TSH levels would have been increased, not decreased. (ii) By similar reasoning, the anterior pituitary can secrete too much TSH (e.g., from a **pituitary adenoma**), driving increased secretion of thyroid hormones. However, this diagnosis was also ruled out by the finding of undetectable levels of TSH. (iii) If there was primary hyperactivity in the thyroid gland itself, either because the thyroid gland was secreting its hormones autonomously or because a substance with TSH-like actions was driving the thyroid gland, then the laboratory data were consistent. Levels of both free T_4 (the primary secretory product of the gland) and total T_4 (which includes both free and protein-bound forms in plasma) would be increased. Importantly, TSH levels would be decreased because of negative feedback inhibition of thyroid hormones on the anterior pituitary gland. (iv) If Natasha had ingested synthetic thyroid hormone **(factitious hyperthyroidism)**, her levels of free T_4 and total T_4 would have been increased and her TSH level would have been decreased. (Like endogenous thyroid hormone, exogenous thyroid hormone inhibits TSH secretion.)

Thus, on the basis of T_4 and TSH levels alone, primary hyperactivity of the thyroid gland looks just like factitious hyperthyroidism. The physicians were left with the question of whether Natasha had a hyperactive thyroid gland or whether she was ingesting exogenous thyroid hormone (e.g., for weight control). The fullness in her neck suggested an enlarged thyroid gland **(goiter)**, but the physicians wanted a more scientific measure of thyroid gland activity (e.g., radioactive I^- scan, as discussed in the next question).

3. The thyroid gland is unique in its requirement for I^-. I^- is taken into the gland by an **Na^+-I^- pump** (or trap), and thyroid hormones are synthesized by the iodination of tyrosines on thyroglobulin (Fig. 6–4).

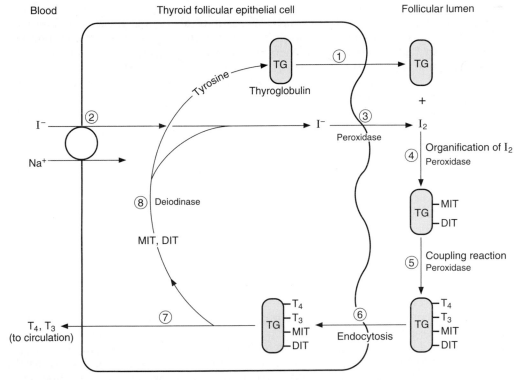

Figure 6–4   Steps in the synthesis of thyroid hormones in thyroid follicular cells. (DIT, diiodotyrosine; MIT, monoiodotyrosine; TG, thyroglobulin; T_3, triiodothyronine; T_4, thyroxine.)

One way to assess thyroid gland activity is to measure **radioactive I^- uptake.** A functional scan of the thyroid can show which areas of the gland are most active, or "hot." In Natasha's case, I^- uptake was increased throughout the gland, suggesting uniform hyperactivity. The functional hyperactivity of the thyroid gland, as demonstrated by the I^- uptake study, ruled out the diagnosis of factitious hyperthyroidism. If Natasha were ingesting exogenous thyroid hormones, her thyroid gland would *not* have shown increased functional activity; in fact, I^- uptake would have been *decreased* because the high levels of thyroid hormone would have suppressed thyroid gland activity (through negative feedback on the anterior pituitary).

4. A finding of increased T_3 **resin uptake** has two possible explanations: (i) TBG levels are decreased or (ii) endogenous levels of thyroid hormones are increased. In Natasha's case, it was

the latter: increased endogenous thyroid hormones (from the hyperactive gland) occupied relatively more binding sites on TBG; thus, fewer TBG binding sites were available to bind radioactive T_3. As a result, uptake of radioactive T_3 by the resin was increased.

5. **Graves' disease,** the most common cause of hyperthyroidism, is an autoimmune disorder caused by the production of abnormal circulating antibodies to TSH receptors on the thyroid gland. These antibodies, called **thyroid-stimulating immunoglobulins,** stimulate the thyroid gland, just like **thyroid-stimulating hormone (TSH)** does. The result is increased synthesis and secretion of thyroid hormones. All of Natasha's symptoms and laboratory findings were consistent with the diagnosis of Graves' disease: increased radioactive I^- uptake, increased T_4 synthesis and secretion, decreased TSH level (by negative feedback), and classic symptoms of thyrotoxicosis.

6. There are three general approaches to the treatment of Graves' disease: (i) removal or destruction of the thyroid gland, (ii) inhibition of thyroid hormone synthesis with drugs, and (iii) blockade of the β_1-adrenergic effects of thyroid hormones that may cause a dangerous increase in arterial pressure.

   Thyroidectomy is a self-evident solution. Alternatively, the thyroid gland can be destroyed with radioactive I^- (much larger amounts than are used for the I^- uptake scan). **Propylthiouracil (PTU)** is an inhibitor of the **peroxidase enzyme** (see Fig. 6–4) that catalyzes all of the steps in thyroid hormone synthesis; **thiocyanate** is a competitive inhibitor of the Na^+-I^- pump in the thyroid gland. Thus, both PTU and thiocyanate decrease the synthesis of thyroid hormones. **Propranolol** is a β-adrenergic antagonist that blocks the positive **inotropic effect** and positive chronotropic effect of thyroid hormones that result from up-regulation of myocardial β_1 receptors. Thus, propranolol would be expected to offset the increases in cardiac output and arterial pressure that are caused by excess thyroid hormones.

7. Natasha developed **hypocalcemia** because the surgeon must have inadvertently destroyed or removed her parathyroid glands along with her thyroid gland. **Parathyroid hormone (PTH)** increases blood Ca^{2+} concentration by coordinated actions on kidney, bone, and intestine. In the absence of PTH, the blood Ca^{2+} concentration falls. Low blood Ca^{2+} concentration causes muscle cramps, a positive **Chvostek sign** (twitching of facial muscles elicited by tapping on the facial nerve), the **Trousseau sign** (carpopedal spasm after inflation of a blood pressure cuff), and tingling and numbness (by direct effects of low extracellular Ca^{2+} concentration on sensory nerves).

8. **Hypoparathyroidism** is treated with a combination of vitamin D and a high-Ca^{2+} diet. (Although it would seem logical to administer synthetic PTH, such preparations are not available.) Several forms of vitamin D are available, and knowledge of the hormonal regulation of Ca^{2+} homeostasis helps in choosing the appropriate form (Fig. 6–5). PTH stimulates the renal production of **1,25-dihydroxycholecalciferol** (the active form of vitamin D) in the kidney; in hypoparathyroidism, this activation step is diminished. Therefore, Natasha should receive the *active* form of vitamin D (1,25-dihydroxycholecalciferol), along with dietary Ca^{2+} supplementation. Neither cholecalciferol (vitamin D_3) nor 25-hydroxycholecalciferol would correct her hypocalcemia because each substance must be activated in the kidney, which requires PTH.

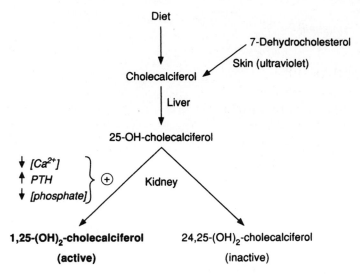

Figure 6–5 Steps and regulation of the synthesis of 1,25-dihydroxycholecalciferol. (PTH, parathyroid hormone.) (Reprinted, with permission, from Costanzo LS. *BRS Physiology* 4th ed. Baltimore: Lippincott Williams & Wilkins; 2007:263.)

Key topics

Arterial pressure (P_a)

Basal metabolic rate (BMR)

β_1 receptors, or β_1-adrenergic receptors

Cardiac output

Chronotropic effect

Chvostek sign

Contractility

1,25-dihydroxycholecalciferol

Factitious hyperthyroidism

Goiter

Graves' disease

Hypocalcemia

Hypoparathyroidism

I^- uptake by the thyroid gland

Inotropic effect

Na^+-I^- pump

Parathyroid hormone (PTH)

Peroxidase enzyme

Pituitary adenoma

Propylthiouracil (PTU)

Pulse pressure

Stroke volume

T_3 resin uptake

Thiocyanate

Key topics *(continued)*

Thyroid hormones

Thyroid-binding globulin (TBG)

Thyroid-stimulating hormone (TSH)

Thyroid-stimulating immunoglobulin (TSI)

Thyrotoxicosis

Thyrotropin-releasing hormone (TRH)

Thyroxine (T$_4$)

Triiodothyronine (T$_3$)

Trousseau sign

Case 51

Hypothyroidism: Autoimmune Thyroiditis

Shirley Tai is a 43-year-old elementary school teacher. At her annual checkup, Shirley complained that, despite eating less, she had gained 16 lb in the past year. Her physician might have attributed this weight gain to "getting older" except that Shirley also complained that she has very little energy, always feels cold (when everyone else is hot), is constipated, and has heavy menstrual flow every month. In addition, the physician noticed that Shirley's neck was very full. The physician suspected that Shirley had hypothyroidism and ordered laboratory tests (Table 6–4).

TABLE 6–4	Shirley's Laboratory Values and Test Results
T_4	3.1 µg/dL (normal, 5–12 µg/dL)
TSH	85 mU/L (normal, 0.3–5 mU/L)
T_3 resin uptake	Decreased
Thyroid antimicrosomal antibodies	Increased

T_4, thyroxine; T_3, triiodothyronine; TSH, thyroid-stimulating hormone.

Based on the physical findings and laboratory results, Shirley's physician concluded that Shirley had autoimmune (Hashimoto) thyroiditis and prescribed oral administration of synthetic T_4 (L-thyroxine). The physician planned to determine the correct dosage of T_4 by monitoring the TSH level in Shirley's blood.

 QUESTIONS

1. How were Shirley's symptoms of weight gain and cold intolerance consistent with a diagnosis of hypothyroidism?

2. Review the regulation of thyroid hormone secretion by the hypothalamic–anterior pituitary–thyroid axis. List the potential mechanisms that could result in decreased secretion of thyroid hormones. How might you distinguish between these mechanisms as potential causes for her hypothyroidism?

3. Based on the laboratory results, what is the etiology of Shirley's hypothyroidism? Why was her T_4 level decreased?

4. Why was the triiodothyronine (T_3) resin uptake decreased?

5. Why was her thyroid-stimulating hormone (TSH) level increased?

6. Shirley's neck appeared full because she had an enlarged thyroid gland (goiter). If Shirley had *hypo*thyroidism, why was her thyroid gland enlarged?

7. Shirley is receiving hormone replacement therapy in the form of synthetic T_4. How does her body process this T_4? How is synthetic T_4 expected to ameliorate her symptoms?

8. How was Shirley's serum TSH level used to adjust the dosage of synthetic T_4?

9. What symptoms might Shirley experience if the dosage of T_4 is too high?

ANSWERS AND EXPLANATIONS

1. To understand the symptoms of hypothyroidism, we need to review the actions of thyroid hormone and then predict the consequences of hormone deficiency. Like steroid hormones, thyroid hormone acts by inducing the synthesis of new proteins. These proteins are responsible for the various hormone actions, many of which are metabolic. Thyroid hormone increases both the **basal metabolic rate (BMR)** and O_2 consumption (in part because it increases the synthesis of Na^+-K^+ ATPase). Increases in BMR and O_2 consumption lead to increased **heat production.** To provide additional substrates for oxidative metabolism, thyroid hormone increases the absorption of glucose from the gastrointestinal tract and induces the synthesis of key metabolic enzymes, including cytochrome oxidase, NADPH cytochrome C reductase, α-glycerophosphate dehydrogenase, and malic enzyme. To supply more O_2 for aerobic metabolism, thyroid hormone also increases cardiac output and ventilation rate. In adults, thyroid hormone is required for **normal reflexes** and **mentation.** In the perinatal period, thyroid hormone is absolutely required for normal development of the central nervous system.

Shirley had classic symptoms of **hypothyroidism** (deficiency of thyroid hormones): her BMR was decreased, she had gained weight despite stable caloric intake, she was always cold (when others were hot), and she lacked energy.

2. Refer back to Figure 6–3, which shows how the hypothalamic–anterior pituitary axis regulates thyroid hormone secretion. The hypothalamus secretes a tripeptide **(thyrotropin-releasing hormone, or TRH)** that stimulates the thyrotrophs of the anterior pituitary to secrete **thyroid-stimulating hormone (TSH).** TSH (a glycoprotein) circulates to the thyroid gland, where it has two actions. (i) It increases the synthesis and secretion of thyroid hormones (T_4 and T_3) by stimulating each step in the biosynthetic process. (ii) It causes hypertrophy and hyperplasia of the thyroid gland.

The system is regulated primarily through negative feedback effects of thyroid hormone on TSH secretion. Specifically, T_3 down-regulates TRH receptors on the thyrotrophs of the anterior pituitary, decreasing their responsiveness to TRH. Thus, when thyroid hormone levels are increased, TSH secretion is inhibited. Conversely, when thyroid hormone levels are decreased, TSH secretion is stimulated.

We can use Figure 6–3 to postulate three potential mechanisms for decreased thyroid hormone secretion: (i) primary failure of the hypothalamus to secrete TRH, which would decrease TSH secretion by the anterior pituitary; (ii) primary failure of the anterior pituitary to secrete TSH; and (iii) a primary defect in the thyroid gland itself (e.g., autoimmune destruction or removal of the thyroid).

The three mechanisms that cause hypothyroidism are *not* distinguishable by their effects on circulating thyroid hormone levels or by their symptoms. In each case, circulating levels of T_3 and T_4 are decreased, and symptoms of hypothyroidism occur. However, the mechanisms *are* distinguishable by the circulating levels of TRH and TSH. In **hypothalamic failure** (very rare), secretion of both TRH and TSH is decreased, leading to decreased secretion of thyroid hormones. In **anterior pituitary failure**, secretion of TSH is decreased, leading to decreased secretion of thyroid hormones. In **primary failure of the thyroid gland** (most common), secretion of thyroid hormones is decreased, but secretion of TSH by the anterior pituitary is *increased*. In this scenario, the anterior pituitary gland is normal; TSH secretion is increased because of diminished feedback inhibition by thyroid hormones.

Thus, the most common cause of hypothyroidism (a primary defect in the thyroid gland) is clearly distinguishable from the second most common cause (a defect in the anterior pituitary) by their respective TSH levels. If the defect is in the anterior pituitary, TSH levels are decreased; if the defect is in the thyroid, TSH levels are increased.

3. Shirley's laboratory results supported the conclusion that her hypothyroidism was caused by a primary defect in her thyroid gland (decreased T_3 level and increased TSH level). Significantly, she had increased levels of **thyroid antimicrosomal antibodies**, which are antibodies to the **peroxidase enzyme** in the thyroid gland (see Fig. 6–4). The peroxidase enzyme catalyzes the major reactions in the synthesis of thyroid hormones (i.e., reactions involving oxidation of I⁻ to I_2, organification of I_2 into **monoiodotyrosine [MIT]** and **diiodotyrosine [DIT]**, and coupling of MIT and DIT to form T_3 and T_4). Because the circulating antibodies inhibited her peroxidase enzyme, Shirley's thyroid gland did not produce sufficient amounts of thyroid hormones. This form of primary hypothyroidism is called **autoimmune thyroiditis (Hashimoto's thyroiditis)**.

4. **Triiodothyronine (T_3) resin uptake** was decreased because Shirley's circulating T_3 levels were decreased. T_3 resin uptake is determined by mixing radioactive T_3 with a synthetic binding resin and a sample of the patient's blood. The radioactive T_3 first binds to thyroid-binding globulin (TBG) in the patient's blood; any remaining radioactive T_3 binds to the synthetic resin (i.e., resin uptake). The more radioactive T_3 that is left over, the greater the resin uptake. Thus, T_3 resin uptake is decreased when circulating levels of TBG are increased (more of the patient's TBG binding sites are available, with less spillover to the resin) or when the patient's T_3 levels are decreased (less of the patient's own T_3 occupies binding sites on TBG; more radioactive T_3 binds to TBG and radioactive T_3 resin uptake is decreased).

5. Earlier, we discussed why Shirley's **TSH** level was increased. Briefly, a primary defect in her thyroid gland led to decreased blood levels of T_4 and T_3. As a result, there was less negative feedback inhibition by thyroid hormones on her anterior pituitary, resulting in increased TSH secretion.

6. Because Shirley had *hypo*thyroidism, perhaps you are surprised that she had a **goiter** (enlarged thyroid gland). In fact, goiter can occur in both hyperthyroidism (hyperactive gland) and hypothyroidism (hypoactive gland). In Shirley's case, decreased secretion of thyroid hormones led to increased secretion of TSH. Through its trophic effects on the thyroid gland, TSH caused hypertrophy, hyperplasia, and enlargement of the gland (even though synthesis and secretion of thyroid hormones was diminished).

7. **Synthetic T_4** (or L-thyroxine) is processed in the body just like endogenous T_4. In the target tissues, T_4, whether endogenous or synthetic, is converted either to T_3 or to reverse T_3 (rT_3). T_3 is the most active form of thyroid hormone, and rT_3 is inactive. Therefore, this conversion step in the target tissues modulates how much active hormone is produced.

   In Shirley's target tissues, synthetic T_4 was converted to T_3, which then executed all of the physiologic effects of thyroid hormones, including increases in BMR, O_2 consumption, and heat production, and restoration of normal reflexes and central nervous system function.

   If T_3 is the active form of thyroid hormone, you may wonder why it isn't administered directly. Patients with hypothyroidism are more often treated with T_4 because it has a much longer half-life than T_3 and, therefore, it can be taken less frequently.

8. The serum TSH level is used to adjust the dosage of synthetic T_4 because TSH secretion is sensitive to feedback inhibition by thyroid hormones. If the replacement dose of T_4 is correct, TSH levels will decrease to normal. If too little T_4 is given, TSH levels will remain elevated. If too much T_4 is given, TSH levels will decrease to below normal.

9. Excessive replacement of T_4 causes the classic symptoms of *hyper*thyroidism: weight loss despite adequate food intake, heat intolerance, nervousness, diarrhea, and amenorrhea.

Key topics

Autoimmune thyroiditis

Basal metabolic rate (BMR)

Diiodotyrosine (DIT)

Goiter

Hashimoto's thyroiditis

Hypothyroidism

Monoiodotyrosine (MIT)

Peroxidase enzyme

T_3 resin uptake

Thyroid antimicrosomal antibodies

Thyroid-stimulating hormone (TSH)

Thyrotropin-releasing hormone (TRH)

Thyroxine (T_4)

Triiodothyronine (T_3)

Case 52

Adrenocortical Excess: Cushing's Syndrome

Harold Potts is a 48-year-old employee of a local moving company. Over the past 2 years, he had gained 30 pounds, mostly around his "middle," face, and shoulders, although his arms and legs had become very thin. In addition, he had purple stretch marks on his abdomen. His appetite had always been good, but in the past 2 years, it had become enormous! He made an appointment to see his physician because he was having trouble doing the heavy lifting that is required in his job.

In the physician's office, Harold's blood pressure was significantly elevated at 165/105. He had centripetal (truncal) obesity with thin extremities, a buffalo hump (interscapular fat accumulation), a "moon" face, and purple stretch marks (striae) on his abdomen. Table 6–5 shows the laboratory results obtained in the fasting state.

TABLE 6–5	Harold's Laboratory Values	
Serum Na$^+$		140 mEq/L (normal, 140 mEq/L)
Serum K$^+$		3.0 mEq/L (normal, 4.5 mEq/L)
Fasting glucose		155 mg/dL (normal, 70–110 mg/dL)
Serum cortisol		Increased
Serum ACTH		Undetectable

ACTH, adrenocorticotropic hormone.

When a low-dose of dexamethasone (a synthetic glucocorticoid) was administered, Harold's serum cortisol level remained elevated. Harold's physician ordered a computed tomography scan, which showed a 7-cm mass (adenoma) on the right adrenal gland. The adenoma was surgically removed 1 week later.

 QUESTIONS

1. Harold had Cushing's syndrome. He had an adrenal adenoma that secreted large amounts of adrenocortical hormones, primarily cortisol and aldosterone. The increased levels of cortisol were responsible for Harold's centripetal obesity, buffalo hump, muscle wasting, striae, and hyperglycemia (increased blood glucose concentration). How is each of these abnormalities caused by increased circulating levels of cortisol?

2. Why was Harold's serum adrenocorticotropic hormone (ACTH) level so low? Which etiologies of hypercortisolism were ruled out by his decreased serum ACTH level?

3. How would a healthy person respond to a low-dose dexamethasone test? Was Harold's response normal? If not, why not?

4. Why was Harold's arterial pressure increased?

5. Why was Harold's serum K$^+$ concentration decreased?

6. In women, Cushing's syndrome causes masculinization, with increased body hair, acne, and irregular menses. Why does Cushing's syndrome have these effects in women?

7. If Harold's surgery had been delayed, his physician could have prescribed a drug that inhibits the synthesis of adrenocortical steroids. What drug might he have prescribed, and what is its mechanism of action?

ANSWERS AND EXPLANATIONS

1. **Cortisol** has diverse actions, several of which are metabolic. One essential role of cortisol is to promote **gluconeogenesis** by altering protein and fat metabolism and directing substrates toward glucose synthesis. Thus, cortisol decreases lipogenesis and stimulates lipolysis, providing gluconeogenic substrates to the liver. Cortisol also increases protein catabolism and decreases new protein synthesis, providing more amino acids to the liver for gluconeogenesis.

   Because Harold had **Cushing's syndrome**, his serum cortisol level was increased. In him, each of the normal physiologic actions of cortisol was exaggerated. He was **hyperglycemic** (had a higher than normal fasting blood glucose) because his liver synthesized too much glucose. He had **muscle wasting** (thin arms and legs) because of the protein catabolic effect of excess cortisol. The **striae** were caused by decreased synthesis of collagen proteins (resulting in fragility of subcutaneous tissues).

   The tendency to accumulate fat around the trunk **(centripetal fat)**, face, neck, and back **(buffalo hump)** is characteristic of hypercortisolism. This characteristic is puzzling because cortisol stimulates lipolysis (increased fat breakdown). However, cortisol also stimulates the appetite; for reasons that are not entirely understood, the increased caloric intake causes fat to be deposited in these specific regions of the body. The centripetal fat distribution is also visually exaggerated because of muscle wasting in the arms and legs.

2. Harold had a very low (undetectable) circulating level of **adrenocorticotropic hormone (ACTH)** secondary to the high levels of cortisol secreted by the adrenal adenoma. High levels of cortisol inhibit ACTH secretion from the anterior pituitary gland by negative feedback (Fig. 6–6).

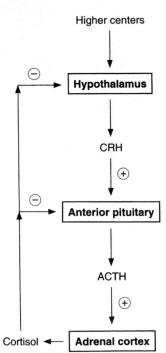

Figure 6–6 Control of glucocorticoid secretion. (ACTH, adrenocorticotropic hormone; CRH, corticotropin-releasing hormone.) (Reprinted, with permission, from Costanzo LS. *BRS Physiology* 4th ed. Baltimore: Lippincott Williams & Wilkins; 2007:251.)

Harold's decreased ACTH level ruled out three potential causes of hypercortisolism: a hypothalamic tumor that secretes **corticotropin-releasing hormone (CRH)**, an anterior pituitary tumor that secretes ACTH, and an ectopic tumor that secretes ACTH. In each of these potential causes of hypercortisolism, circulating levels of ACTH are *increased*. For example, the hypothalamic tumor oversecretes CRH, which drives the anterior pituitary to oversecrete ACTH, which drives the adrenal cortex to oversecrete cortisol. In the case of the anterior pituitary tumor or the ectopic ACTH-secreting tumor, the high levels of ACTH drive the adrenal cortex to oversecrete cortisol. The bottom line is that none of these potential causes was possible in Harold because his ACTH level was decreased, not increased.

3. **Dexamethasone** is a synthetic glucocorticoid that has all of the effects of cortisol, including inhibition of ACTH secretion from the anterior pituitary. In healthy persons, a low dose of dexamethasone inhibits ACTH secretion, which inhibits endogenous cortisol secretion. Accordingly, in healthy persons, dexamethasone causes both ACTH and cortisol levels in the blood to decrease.

   Harold's response to the low-dose dexamethasone test was *abnormal* (his serum cortisol level remained elevated) because his adrenal adenoma autonomously secreted large amounts of cortisol. These high levels of cortisol completely suppressed ACTH secretion. When more glucocorticoid was added to the blood in the form of synthetic dexamethasone, further inhibition of ACTH secretion did not occur because it was already completely inhibited.

4. Harold's **arterial pressure** was increased (160/105) for two reasons: (i) increased circulating levels of cortisol and (ii) increased circulating levels of aldosterone. **Cortisol** increases arterial pressure by up-regulating α_1-adrenergic receptors on vascular smooth muscle. In this way, cortisol increases the sensitivity of blood vessels, particularly arterioles, to the vasoconstrictor actions of catecholamines (e.g., norepinephrine). **Aldosterone** increases arterial pressure through its effect on renal Na^+ reabsorption. Aldosterone increases Na^+ reabsorption, which leads to increased extracellular fluid volume and blood volume. Increased blood volume leads to increased preload, increased cardiac output, and increased arterial pressure.

5. Harold's serum K^+ concentration was decreased (3.0 mEq/L) because the adrenal adenoma secreted large amounts of **aldosterone.** One major action of aldosterone is to increase K^+ secretion by the renal principal cells, and this increased secretion results in negative K^+ balance and **hypokalemia.**

6. In addition to cortisol and aldosterone, the adrenal cortex secretes the androgens **dehydroepiandrosterone (DHEA)** and **androstenedione** (Fig. 6–7). In women, the adrenal cortex is the major source of androgens. In women who have Cushing's syndrome, the hyperactive adrenal cortex secretes increased amounts of adrenal androgens, which have masculinizing effects (e.g., increased body hair). In men with Cushing's syndrome, secretion of adrenal androgens is increased, but this increase is only a "drop in the (androgen) bucket" because the testes secrete large amounts of their own androgen (testosterone).

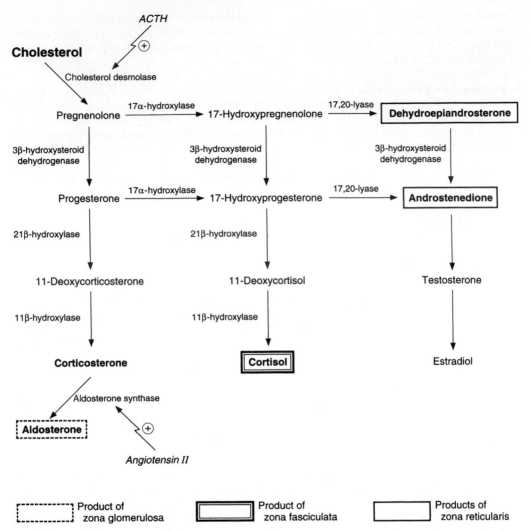

Figure 6–7 Synthetic pathways for glucocorticoids, androgens, and mineralocorticoids in the adrenal cortex. (ACTH, adrenocorticotropic hormone.) (Reprinted, with permission, from Costanzo LS. *BRS Physiology* 4th ed. Baltimore: Lippincott Williams & Wilkins; 2007:250.)

7. If surgery had been delayed, Harold could have been treated with **ketoconazole**, an inhibitor of **cholesterol desmolase** (the enzyme that catalyzes the first step in the biosynthesis of adrenocortical steroids). Ketoconazole treatment would have decreased the production of cortisol and aldosterone by the adrenal adenoma and decreased the symptoms caused by hypercortisolism and hyperaldosteronism.

Key topics

Adrenocorticotropic hormone (ACTH)

Aldosterone

Androstenedione

Arterial pressure

Buffalo hump

Centripetal obesity

Cholesterol desmolase

Corticotropin-releasing hormone (CRH)

Cortisol

Cushing's syndrome

Dehydroepiandrosterone (DHEA)

Dexamethasone

Hyperglycemia

Hypokalemia

Ketoconazole

Striae

Case 53

Adrenocortical Insufficiency: Addison's Disease

Susan Oglesby is a 41-year-old divorced mother of two teenagers. She has always been in excellent health. She recently saw her physician because of several unexplained symptoms, including weight loss of 15 lb, extreme fatigue, and decreased body hair in the axillary and pubic regions. In addition, her skin was very tanned, even though she had not been in the sun. Susan hadn't had a menstrual period in 3 months; she knew she wasn't pregnant and wondered whether she was experiencing early menopause.

In her physician's office, Susan appeared very thin, with sunken eyes and decreased skin turgor. When she was supine (lying), her blood pressure was 90/60 and her pulse rate was 95 beats/min. When she was standing, her blood pressure was 70/35 and her pulse rate was 120 beats/min. Her skin was deeply pigmented, especially her nipples and the creases in the palms of her hands. Susan's physician ordered laboratory tests (Table 6–6).

TABLE 6–6	Susan's Laboratory Values

Venous Blood

Na^+	126 mEq/L (normal, 140 mEq/L)
K^+	5.7 mEq/L (normal, 4.5 mEq/L)
Osmolarity	265 mOsm/L (normal, 290 mOsm/L)
Glucose (fasting)	50 mg/dL (normal, 70–100 mg/dL)
Cortisol	Decreased
Aldosterone	Decreased
ACTH	Increased

Arterial Blood

pH	7.32 (normal, 7.4)
HCO_3^-	18 mEq/L (normal, 24 mEq/L).

ACTH, adrenocorticotropic hormone.

Results of an adrenocorticotropic hormone (ACTH) stimulation test were negative (i.e., there was no increase in the serum level of cortisol or aldosterone). Based on the symptoms, physical examination, laboratory values, and results of the ACTH stimulation test, Susan was diagnosed with primary adrenal insufficiency (Addison's disease). Susan's physician prescribed daily treatment with hydrocortisone (a synthetic glucocorticoid) and fludrocortisone (a synthetic mineralocorticoid). Susan was instructed to take hydrocortisone in two divided doses, with a larger dose at 8 AM and a smaller dose at 1 PM.

At a follow-up visit 2 weeks later, Susan's circulating ACTH level was normal. She had gained 5 lb, her blood pressure was normal (both supine and standing), her tan had started to fade, and she had much more energy.

 QUESTIONS

1. Why were Susan's serum cortisol, aldosterone, and ACTH levels consistent with primary adrenocortical insufficiency? How did her negative response to the ACTH stimulation test confirm this diagnosis?

2. How did adrenocortical insufficiency cause Susan's decreased arterial pressure? Why did her blood pressure decrease further when she moved from a supine position to a standing position?

3. Why was her pulse rate increased? Why was her pulse rate higher when she was standing than when she was supine?

4. Why was Susan's fasting blood glucose level lower than normal?

5. Why was her serum K^+ concentration elevated (hyperkalemia)?

6. Why was her serum Na^+ concentration decreased (hyponatremia)?

7. What acid–base abnormality did Susan have, and what was its cause? If her P_{CO_2} had been measured, would you expect it to be normal, increased, or decreased? Why?

8. Why did Susan's skin appear tanned (hyperpigmentation)?

9. Why did she have decreased pubic and axillary hair?

10. Why did Susan's ACTH level return to normal within 2 weeks of starting treatment?

11. Why was Susan instructed to take the hydrocortisone in two divided doses, with a larger dose at 8 AM?

ANSWERS AND EXPLANATIONS

1. Susan's decreased serum levels of **cortisol** and **aldosterone** and increased serum level of **adrenocorticotropic hormone (ACTH)** were consistent with primary adrenocortical insufficiency **(Addison's disease)**. In this disease, the adrenal cortex is destroyed (usually secondary to an autoimmune process). As a result, the adrenal cortex can no longer secrete its steroid hormones cortisol, aldosterone, and the adrenal androgens dehydroepiandrosterone (DHEA) and androstenedione.

   The circulating **ACTH** level can be used to distinguish primary adrenocortical insufficiency from secondary adrenocortical insufficiency (refer back to Fig. 6–6 in Case 52). In the *primary* form, the defect is in the adrenal cortex itself; the serum ACTH level is *increased* because the low level of cortisol reduces negative feedback inhibition of ACTH secretion by the anterior pituitary, thereby increasing ACTH levels. In the *secondary* form (hypothalamic or anterior pituitary failure), serum ACTH levels are *decreased* (which leads to decreased cortisol secretion).

   The **ACTH stimulation test** evaluates the responsiveness of cortisol secretion to an injection of exogenous ACTH. The test confirmed that Susan's disease was caused by primary adrenal failure. Even the large amount of ACTH in the injection couldn't stimulate her adrenal cortex to secrete cortisol!

2. Decreased circulating levels of cortisol and aldosterone were responsible for Susan's **decreased arterial pressure** (90/60 supine), as follows. (i) One action of cortisol is up-regulation of α_1-adrenergic receptors on vascular smooth muscle, resulting in increased responsiveness of blood vessels to catecholamines. In the absence of cortisol, the responsiveness of blood vessels to catecholamines is decreased. As a result, there is a decrease in **total peripheral resistance** and arterial pressure. (ii) A major action of aldosterone is increased Na^+ reabsorption by the renal principal cells, leading to increases in extracellular fluid volume and blood volume, venous return, cardiac output, and arterial pressure. In the absence of aldosterone, there is decreased Na^+ reabsorption, decreased extracellular fluid volume and blood volume, and decreased arterial pressure.

   The further decrease in Susan's arterial pressure when she was upright **(orthostatic hypotension)** is characteristic of hypovolemia (decreased blood volume). When Susan stood up, blood pooled in the veins of the legs, further compromising venous return, cardiac output, and arterial pressure.

3. Susan's pulse rate was elevated (95 beats/min) because decreases in arterial pressure activate the **baroreceptor reflex.** This reflex directs an increase in sympathetic outflow to the heart and blood vessels. One of these sympathetic responses is an increase in heart rate mediated by β_1-adrenergic receptors in the sinoatrial node.

   When Susan stood up, her pulse rate increased because her blood pressure had decreased further. The even lower arterial pressure triggered an even stronger response of the baroreceptor reflex.

4. Susan was **hypoglycemic** (fasting blood glucose level, 50 mg/dL) as a result of her decreased cortisol level. One action of cortisol is to increase the blood glucose concentration by promoting gluconeogenesis and decreasing glucose uptake by the tissues. Thus, in cortisol deficiency, gluconeogenesis decreases, glucose uptake by the tissues increases, and as a result, the blood glucose concentration decreases.

5. Susan's serum K^+ concentration was elevated **(hyperkalemia)** secondary to her decreased aldosterone level. In addition to stimulating Na^+ reabsorption, aldosterone stimulates K^+

secretion by the renal principal cells. Thus, in aldosterone deficiency, K^+ secretion is decreased, which leads to positive K^+ balance and hyperkalemia.

6. You may have proposed that Susan was **hyponatremic** because aldosterone deficiency caused her to excrete too much Na^+ in urine. While this explanation seems logical, it is not complete. Susan was hyponatremic because she had *excess water* in her body relative to Na^+; the excess water diluted her serum Na^+ concentration.

   Now we are faced with a more difficult question: Why did Susan retain excess water? There are two major reasons why an increase in body water occurs: (i) the person drinks more water than the kidneys can excrete or (ii) there is increased water reabsorption by the kidneys. The first mechanism (primary polydipsia) is a rare cause of hyponatremia. It is much more likely that Susan's kidneys reabsorbed too much water because of a high circulating level of **antidiuretic hormone (ADH)**. Recall that ADH secretion is stimulated by both hyperosmolarity and hypovolemia, and that the hypovolemic stimulus will "override" the osmotic stimulus. Thus, Susan's hyponatremia was caused by the following sequence of events: decreased Na^+ reabsorption (as a result of aldosterone deficiency), decreased extracellular fluid volume, decreased blood volume, increased ADH secretion (secondary to hypovolemia), and increased reabsorption of water by the renal collecting ducts.

   You may ask whether this high ADH secretion was appropriate given Susan's low serum osmolarity. Shouldn't her low serum osmolarity have turned off ADH secretion? Yes, it should have! Again, the hypovolemic stimulus for ADH secretion overrides the osmotic stimulus.

7. With an arterial pH of 7.32 and an HCO_3^- concentration of 18 mEq/L, Susan had **metabolic acidosis.** (Recall from acid–base physiology that metabolic acidosis begins with a decrease in HCO_3^- concentration, which decreases pH.) If her arterial P_{CO_2} had been measured, it would have been decreased secondary to respiratory compensation for metabolic acidosis (i.e., **hyperventilation**).

   The likely cause of Susan's metabolic acidosis is **aldosterone deficiency.** In addition to increasing Na^+ reabsorption and K^+ secretion in the renal principal cells, aldosterone increases H^+ secretion and "new" HCO_3^- reabsorption in the renal intercalated cells. Thus, aldosterone deficiency leads to decreased Na^+ reabsorption (leading to decreased extracellular fluid volume), decreased K^+ secretion (leading to hyperkalemia), and decreased H^+ secretion and new HCO_3^- reabsorption (leading to metabolic acidosis). This form of metabolic acidosis (secondary to aldosterone deficiency) is called **type 4 renal tubular acidosis.** Specifically, aldosterone deficiency causes hyperkalemia, which **inhibits renal NH_3 synthesis**, the decreased supply of NH_3, combined with decreased H^+ secretion, leads to a decrease in NH_4^+ excretion and metabolic acidosis.

8. Susan's **hyperpigmentation** was a consequence of the negative feedback regulation of ACTH secretion. Susan had primary adrenocortical failure, which led to decreased serum levels of cortisol. Decreased levels of cortisol led to decreased negative feedback inhibition of **pro-opiomelanocortin (POMC)** synthesis by the anterior pituitary. POMC, the precursor for ACTH, is a complex molecule that contains **melanocyte-stimulating hormone (MSH)** fragments. Thus, when POMC levels are increased, so are the levels of MSH, which pigments the skin.

9. Susan had decreased pubic and axillary hair because, in addition to deficiencies of cortisol and aldosterone, she had a **deficiency of adrenal androgens.** In women, the adrenal cortex is the major source of androgens (DHEA and androstenedione), which are responsible for body hair and libido.

10. Susan's ACTH level returned to normal within 2 weeks of the initiation of hormone replacement treatment with hydrocortisone (a glucocorticoid) and fludrocortisone (a mineralocorticoid). Like endogenous cortisol, exogenous glucocorticoid has a negative feedback effect on the secretion of ACTH from the anterior pituitary.

11. Susan was instructed to take hydrocortisone (glucocorticoid) in two divided doses, with a larger dose at 8 AM and a smaller dose at 1 PM to replicate the body's **diurnal pattern** of cortisol secretion. Endogenous cortisol secretion is **pulsatile** (occurs in bursts), with the largest burst occurring just before awakening (e.g., at 8 AM). Several smaller bursts occur in the afternoon, and the lowest rates of cortisol secretion occur in the evening and just after falling asleep.

Key topics

Addison's disease

Adrenocortical insufficiency

Adrenocorticotropic hormone (ACTH)

Aldosterone

Antidiuretic hormone (ADH)

Arterial pressure

Baroreceptor reflex

Cortisol

Diurnal pattern (of cortisol secretion)

Hyperkalemia

Hyperpigmentation

Hypoglycemia

Hyponatremia

Melanocyte-stimulating hormone (MSH)

Metabolic acidosis

Orthostatic hypotension

Pro-opiomelanocortin (POMC)

Type 4 renal tubular acidosis

Case 54

Congenital Adrenal Hyperplasia: 21β-Hydroxylase Deficiency

Lauren and Tim Anderson recently had their second child, a girl whom they named Anne Carter. A day after the delivery, the pediatrician told the Andersons that Anne Carter's clitoris was enlarged. The pediatrician ordered a chromosomal evaluation, which confirmed an XX (female) genotype. Other tests showed that she has ovaries, a uterus, and no testes. Table 6–7 gives the results of laboratory tests.

TABLE 6–7	*Anne Carter's Laboratory Values*
Blood glucose	70 mg/dL (normal fasting, 70–100 mg/dL)
Serum cortisol	Low-normal
Serum ACTH	Increased
17-ketosteroid excretion	Increased

ACTH, adrenocorticotropic hormone.

The consulting pediatric endocrinologist made a diagnosis of congenital adrenal hyperplasia secondary to 21β-hydroxylase deficiency. It was recommended that Anne Carter receive hormone replacement therapy and that she undergo surgery to reduce the size of her clitoris.

 QUESTIONS

1. Using your knowledge of the biosynthetic pathways of the adrenal cortex, predict the consequences of 21β-hydroxylase deficiency. Which adrenocortical hormones will be deficient? Which hormones will be produced in excess?

2. What are the expected physiologic consequences of the hormonal deficiencies you predicted in Question 1?

3. Why was Anne Carter's serum adrenocorticotropic hormone (ACTH) level increased?

4. Anne Carter's blood glucose and serum cortisol levels were both low-normal. Why weren't these values more obviously abnormal?

5. What was the significance of her increased urinary excretion of 17-ketosteroids?

6. Why was Anne Carter's clitoris enlarged at birth?

7. Did she have partial or complete deficiency of 21β-hydroxylase?

8. What hormone replacement therapy did she receive?

9. In terms of later development, what might have happened if Anne Carter's condition had not been diagnosed (and she did not receive hormone replacement therapy)?

ANSWERS AND EXPLANATIONS

1. Refer back to Figure 6–7, which shows the biosynthetic pathways of the adrenal cortex. Briefly, the first step in the pathway is conversion of cholesterol to pregnenolone, which is catalyzed by the enzyme **cholesterol desmolase**. After pregnenolone is generated, it either proceeds through a series of steps to **aldosterone**, or it is hydroxylated at C-17. 17-Hydroxylated compounds are precursors of cortisol and adrenal androgens as follows. If the two-carbon side chain is cleaved at C-17 (by 17,20 lyase), **adrenal androgens dehydroepiandrosterone (DHEA)** and **androstenedione** are generated; if the side chain is not cleaved, **cortisol** is generated.

   Figure 6–7 shows that **21β-hydroxylase** is *required for synthesis of aldosterone and cortisol*. In the aldosterone pathway, it catalyzes the conversion of progesterone to 11-deoxycorticosterone. In the cortisol pathway, it catalyzes the conversion of 17-hydroxyprogesterone to 11-deoxycortisol. If 21β-hydroxylase is absent, both pathways are blocked, and neither aldosterone nor cortisol is synthesized. In addition, steroid intermediates (progesterone, pregnenolone, 17-hydroxypregnenolone, and 17-hydroxyprogesterone) "build up" proximal to the blockage. These intermediates are precursors for, and are shunted toward, the synthesis of adrenal androgens, which are then produced in excess. Therefore, the short answer to the question is that, in addition to a *deficiency* of aldosterone and cortisol, there will be an *excess* of adrenal androgens.

2. The physiologic consequences of aldosterone and cortisol deficiency can be inferred from the established actions of the hormones. The major actions of cortisol are gluconeogenesis, anti-inflammatory effects, immune suppression, and vascular responsiveness to catecholamines (which increases arterial pressure). The major actions of aldosterone are increased Na^+ reabsorption (which leads to increased extracellular fluid volume and increased arterial pressure), increased K^+ secretion, and increased H^+ secretion and "new" HCO_3^- reabsorption. Thus, cortisol deficiency leads to **hypoglycemia** and **hypotension**. Aldosterone deficiency leads to hypotension, **hyperkalemia**, and **metabolic acidosis**.

3. Anne Carter's serum **adrenocorticotropic hormone (ACTH)** level was elevated as a result of her low-normal level of cortisol. Based on the diagnosis of 21β-hydroxylase deficiency, we can presume that, initially, her adrenal cortex produced insufficient amounts of cortisol. Decreased levels of cortisol caused increased secretion of ACTH by reducing negative feedback inhibition on the anterior pituitary (see Fig. 6–6).

4. Initially, it may be puzzling why Anne Carter's blood glucose and cortisol levels were not decreased more significantly. Both values were at the low end of the normal range. However, if she is deficient in 21β-hydroxylase, why weren't these levels even lower? The answer lies in the high levels of ACTH that resulted from her decreased serum cortisol. This increased level of ACTH caused hyperplasia of the adrenal cortex. The hyperplastic adrenal cortex was stimulated to synthesize more cortisol, partially offsetting the original deficiency. (In recognition of this phenomenon, the syndrome is also called **congenital adrenal hyperplasia**.)

5. Adrenal androgens have a ketone group at C-17 that distinguishes them from cortisol, aldosterone, and testosterone. (Cortisol and aldosterone have side chains at C-17. Testosterone, an androgen produced in the testes, has a hydroxyl group at C-17.) Thus, adrenal androgens are called 17-ketosteroids. In Anne Carter's case, increased excretion of **17-ketosteroids** reflected increased synthesis of *adrenal* androgens. This increased synthesis was caused by shunting of steroid intermediates toward androgens and hyperplasia of the adrenal cortex secondary to high levels of ACTH.

6. Anne Carter's clitoris was enlarged because excess adrenal androgens masculinized her external genitalia. In recognition of this masculinizing effect in girls, the disorder is also called **adrenogenital syndrome**. In boys who have 21β-hydroxylase deficiency, the effects of excess

adrenal androgens are not obvious at birth; however, these boys may have early masculinization and precocious puberty.

7. Presumably, Anne Carter had a *partial* deficiency of 21β-hydroxylase. This conclusion is supported by the finding that her adrenal cortex maintained low-normal levels of cortisol secretion. *Some* enzyme activity must have been present because her adrenal cortex secreted *some* cortisol. If she had *complete* enzyme deficiency, she would have secreted *no* cortisol and *no* aldosterone. (A complete deficiency of 21β-hydroxylase would have caused a life-threatening crisis with severe hypotension and hypoglycemia at delivery.)

8. Anne Carter was treated with **glucocorticoid replacement** therapy (e.g., hydrocortisone). You may wonder whether this treatment was necessary since her hyperplastic adrenal cortex, driven by the high ACTH levels, was already capable of maintaining cortisol synthesis. Indeed, this treatment *was* necessary because adrenocortical hyperplasia also caused excessive production of androgens (which is undesirable in females). Therefore, the rationale for giving Anne Carter exogenous glucocorticoid treatment was to inhibit ACTH secretion, prevent adrenal hyperplasia, and reduce adrenocortical production of androgens.

   Anne Carter may also need **mineralocorticoid replacement** therapy (e.g., fludrocortisone). As with cortisol, she maintained sufficient levels of aldosterone because her adrenal cortex was hyperplastic. However, treatment with exogenous glucocorticoid would be expected to reduce both ACTH secretion and the size of the adrenal cortex. Once the adrenal cortex was reduced in size, it would no longer secrete sufficient quantities of aldosterone (because of the 21β-hydroxylase deficiency) and mineralocorticoid replacement would be required.

9. If not for the clue of clitoromegaly, Anne Carter's condition might not have been diagnosed. If she had not been diagnosed, she would have become further masculinized by the high levels of adrenal androgens. In the prepubertal years, she would have had accelerated linear growth, increased muscle mass, and increased body hair. At puberty, she would have experienced irregular menses or even amenorrhea. Finally, because androgens cause closure of the epiphyseal growth plates, her final adult height would have been shorter than average.

Key topics

Adrenocorticotropic hormone (ACTH)

Adrenogenital syndrome

Aldosterone

Androstenedione

Cholesterol desmolase

Congenital adrenal hyperplasia

Cortisol

Dehydroepiandrosterone (DHEA)

21β-hydroxylase

Hyperkalemia

Hypoglycemia

Hypotension

17-ketosteroids

Metabolic acidosis

Case 55

Primary Hyperparathyroidism

Carl Felicetti is a 53-year-old violinist with a local symphony orchestra. He had always been in excellent health. However, after two sets of tennis on a hot day in July, he suddenly experienced the worst pain of his life. The pain came in waves that started in his right flank and radiated into his groin. When he went to the bathroom, he voided bright red urine. His tennis partner drove him to the emergency room, where an intravenous pyelogram showed several ureteral stones. He was sent home with a prescription for narcotics and instructions to drink lots of water and "wait it out." Fortunately, Carl didn't need to wait long; that evening, he voided more bright red urine and two hard, brown stones. He saved the stones, as instructed, for chemical analysis.

Carl saw his physician the next day. There was nothing unusual in his history, except for constipation and his wife's new "health kick." (She was taking multivitamins and Ca^{2+} supplementation and had convinced Carl that he should take the supplements, too.) Table 6–8 shows the results of laboratory tests.

TABLE 6–8	*Carl's Laboratory Values*	
Serum Ca^{2+}		11.5 mg/dL (normal, 10 mg/dL)
Serum phosphate		2 mg/dL (normal, 3.5 mg/dL)
Serum parathyroid hormone		125 pg/mL (normal, 10–65 pg/mL)
Serum albumin		Normal
Alkaline phosphatase		Elevated
Urinary Ca^{2+} excretion		Elevated
Urinary stone composition		Calcium oxalate

Based on the laboratory findings, Carl was diagnosed with primary hyperparathyroidism and scheduled for exploratory neck surgery. While awaiting surgery, he was instructed to discontinue all Ca^{2+} and vitamin supplementation and to drink at least 3 L water each day. At surgery, a single parathyroid adenoma was identified and removed. Carl recovered well; his serum Ca^{2+}, phosphate, and parathyroid hormone (PTH) levels returned to normal, and he had no recurrences of urinary stones.

 QUESTIONS

1. What are the forms of Ca^{2+} in serum? Which forms are biologically active?

2. What are the physiologic actions of PTH on bone, kidney, and intestine?

3. Carl's physician made a diagnosis of primary hyperparathyroidism on the basis of Carl's serum Ca^{2+}, phosphate, and PTH levels. How were these values consistent with primary hyperparathyroidism?

4. What was the significance of Carl's elevated alkaline phosphatase level?

5. In making the correct diagnosis, it was important to know that Carl's serum albumin level was normal. Why?

6. Why was Carl's urinary Ca^{2+} excretion elevated (hypercalciuria)?

7. What was the relationship between Carl's recent history of dietary Ca^{2+} supplementation and his hypercalciuria?

ANSWERS ON NEXT PAGE

ANSWERS AND EXPLANATIONS

1. The normal value for total serum Ca^{2+} concentration is 10 mg/dL. This total Ca^{2+} has three components: (i) Ca^{2+} that is bound to albumin (40%), (ii) Ca^{2+} that is complexed to anions (e.g., phosphate, citrate) (10%), and (iii) free, ionized Ca^{2+} (50%). Free, **ionized Ca^{2+}** is the only form that is biologically active.

2. The actions of **parathyroid hormone (PTH)** on bone, kidney, and intestine are coordinated to increase the serum ionized Ca^{2+} concentration and decrease the serum phosphate concentration.

   In **bone**, PTH works synergistically with 1,25-dihydroxycholecalciferol to stimulate **osteoclasts** and increase **bone resorption.** As a result, both Ca^{2+} and phosphate are released from mineralized bone into the extracellular fluid. By itself, this effect on bone would not increase the serum ionized Ca^{2+} concentration because the phosphate that is released from bone complexes with Ca^{2+}.

   In the **kidney**, PTH has two actions, both of which are mediated by the activation of **adenylyl cyclase** and production of cyclic AMP. (i) In the early proximal tubule, PTH inhibits the **Na^+-phosphate cotransporter** that is responsible for phosphate reabsorption, thus causing an increase in urinary phosphate excretion. This **phosphaturic** effect of PTH is particularly important because the phosphate that was resorbed from bone is then excreted in the urine, thus allowing the serum ionized Ca^{2+} to increase. (ii) PTH stimulates Ca^{2+} reabsorption in the distal tubule.

   In the **intestine**, PTH acts indirectly to increase Ca^{2+} absorption by stimulating renal synthesis of **1,25-dihydroxycholecalciferol**, the active form of vitamin D.

3. The diagnosis of **primary hyperparathyroidism** was consistent with Carl's serum Ca^{2+}, phosphate, and PTH levels. He was hypercalcemic (his serum Ca^{2+} was elevated at 11.5 mg/dL) and hypophosphatemic (his serum phosphate was decreased at 2 mg/dL). In addition, he had an elevated circulating level of PTH. The parathyroid adenoma secreted excessive amounts of PTH that had all of the expected actions: increased bone resorption, decreased renal phosphate reabsorption, increased renal Ca^{2+} reabsorption, and increased intestinal Ca^{2+} absorption (through 1,25-dihydroxycholecalciferol). Thus, Carl's **hypercalcemia** resulted from increased bone resorption, increased renal Ca^{2+} reabsorption, and increased intestinal Ca^{2+} absorption. His resulted from decreased renal phosphate reabsorption (phosphaturia).

   Primary hyperparathyroidism is sometimes characterized as "**stones, bones, and groans**": "stones" from hypercalciuria (discussed later), "bones" from the increased bone resorption, and "groans" from the constipation caused by hypercalcemia.

   You may wonder why Carl's hypercalcemia didn't inhibit PTH secretion. PTH secretion by normal parathyroid tissue *is* inhibited by hypercalcemia. However, PTH secretion by the adenoma is autonomous and, therefore, is not under negative feedback regulation. Thus, the adenoma continued to secrete PTH unabated, even in the face of hypercalcemia.

4. The major sources of alkaline phosphatase are liver and bone. Increased levels of **alkaline phosphatase** in bone are associated with increased **osteoblastic** activity and high bone turnover (e.g., primary hyperparathyroidism).

5. In considering the etiology of Carl's elevated serum Ca^{2+} concentration, it was important to know that his serum albumin level was normal. From our previous discussion, recall that the total Ca^{2+} concentration is the sum of protein-bound Ca^{2+} (40%), complexed Ca^{2+} (10%), and ionized Ca^{2+} (50%). Although *ionized* Ca^{2+} is the only form that is biologically active, *total*

serum Ca^{2+} is more commonly measured. Carl's *total* Ca^{2+} was elevated (11.5 mg/dL). We need to know whether this increase in total Ca^{2+} was simply the result of an increase in serum albumin concentration or whether it was the result of an abnormality in Ca^{2+} homeostasis. Carl's serum albumin level was normal, suggesting that the increase in total Ca^{2+} concentration was caused by an increase in ionized, biologically active Ca^{2+}.

6. Carl's increased urinary Ca^{2+} excretion **(hypercalciuria)** led to the formation of painful urinary calcium oxalate stones. Inevitably, students ask why, if PTH increases renal Ca^{2+} reabsorption, does primary hyperparathyroidism cause increased urinary Ca^{2+} excretion? Shouldn't Ca^{2+} excretion be decreased? It is true that a major action of PTH is to increase Ca^{2+} reabsorption in the distal tubule, which contributes to the development of hypercalcemia. However, as the serum Ca^{2+} concentration increases, the filtered load of Ca^{2+} also increases. Thus, despite increased Ca^{2+} reabsorption, the filtered load of Ca^{2+} eventually overwhelms the reabsorptive capacity of the kidneys. Thus, in primary hyperparathyroidism, both the reabsorption *and* excretion of Ca^{2+} are increased.

7. Carl's primary hyperparathyroidism may have been present (although silent) for several years. Carl could be asymptomatic because, as his serum Ca^{2+} level gradually increased, his filtered load of Ca^{2+} also increased and the excess Ca^{2+} was excreted in the urine. By dumping Ca^{2+} in the urine, his serum was "protected" from dangerous increases in Ca^{2+} concentration. However, when Carl took Ca^{2+} and vitamin D supplements, the Ca^{2+} load to his kidneys sharply increased. The final "precipitating" event was dehydration on the tennis courts. Dehydration stimulated ADH secretion, and Carl's urine became concentrated. Carl's symptoms were caused by an increase in the urinary Ca^{2+} concentration and the precipitation of calcium oxalate stones.

Key topics

Adenylyl cyclase

Alkaline phosphatase

Bone resorption

Cyclic adenosine monophosphate (cyclic AMP)

1,25-dihydroxycholecalciferol

Hypercalcemia

Hypercalciuria

Hypophosphatemia

Na^+-phosphate cotransporter

Osteoblasts

Osteoclasts

Parathyroid hormone (PTH)

Phosphaturia

Primary hyperparathyroidism

Case 56

Humoral Hypercalcemia of Malignancy

Sam Kessler is a 69-year-old retired businessman. He and his wife had been looking forward to spending more time with their children and grandchildren. Unfortunately, 3 years ago, Mr. Kessler was diagnosed with lung cancer. Despite surgery, radiation therapy, and chemotherapy, his cancer returned. Mr. Kessler told his physicians that he did not want further treatment and preferred to spend his remaining time at home with his family, as pain-free as possible. In the past week, Mr. Kessler became very lethargic and had both polyuria (increased urine production) and polydipsia (increased water drinking). He was admitted to the hospital, where laboratory tests were performed (Table 6–9).

TABLE 6-9	Mr. Kessler's Laboratory Values
Serum Ca^{2+}	15.5 mg/dL (normal, 10 mg/dL)
Serum phosphate	1.8 mg/dL (normal, 3.5 mg/dL)
Serum albumin	4.1 g/dL (normal, 3.5–5.5 g/dL)
Serum PTH	4 pg/mL (normal, 10–65 pg/mL)
Serum alkaline phosphatase	Very elevated

PTH, parathyroid hormone.

During a test involving 4 hours of water deprivation, Mr. Kessler's serum osmolarity was 305 mOsm/L (normal, 290 mOsm/L) and his urine osmolarity was 90 mOsm/L.

The physicians concluded that Mr. Kessler had humoral hypercalcemia of malignancy because his lung cancer cells were secreting parathyroid hormone (PTH)-related peptide (PTH-rp). He was treated with a saline infusion and furosemide (a loop diuretic), which caused his serum Ca^{2+} to decrease to 10.8 mg/dL. He returned home with a prescription for pamidronate, an inhibitor of bone resorption that was expected to keep his serum Ca^{2+} in the normal range.

 QUESTIONS

1. PTH-rp, secreted by certain malignant tumors, is chemically homologous with PTH that is secreted by the parathyroid glands. PTH-rp has all of the biologic actions of PTH on bone and kidney. Given this information, why was Mr. Kessler hypercalcemic (increased serum Ca^{2+}) and hypophosphatemic (decreased serum phosphate)? Why was his alkaline phosphatase level elevated?

2. What was the significance of Mr. Kessler's normal serum albumin level?

3. Why was Mr. Kessler's serum PTH level decreased?

4. After the 4-hour water deprivation test, Mr. Kessler's serum osmolarity was 305 mOsm/L (normal, 290 mOsm/L) and his urine osmolarity was 90 mOsm/L. Administration of an ADH analogue (dDAVP) by nasal spray did not alter his serum or urine osmolarity. The physician concluded that Mr. Kessler had nephrogenic diabetes insipidus. Why? What might be the cause of this condition?

5. Why did Mr. Kessler have polyuria and polydipsia?

6. How did treatment with saline and furosemide decrease his serum Ca^{2+} concentration?

7. How was pamidronate expected to keep Mr. Kessler's serum Ca^{2+} in the normal range?

ANSWERS ON NEXT PAGE

ANSWERS AND EXPLANATIONS

1. **Parathyroid hormone-related peptide (PTH-rp)** is a peptide that is secreted by certain malignant tumor cells (e.g., lung, breast). It is homologous with, and has all of the biologic actions of, **PTH** that is secreted by the parathyroid glands. Therefore, if we know the biologic actions of PTH on bone and kidney, we also know the biologic actions of PTH-rp that caused Mr. Kessler's **hypercalcemia** and **hypophosphatemia.** These actions are as follows. (i) PTH and PTH-rp stimulate **osteoclasts** and increase **bone resorption,** bringing Ca^{2+} and phosphate from bone into the extracellular fluid. (ii) PTH and PTH-rp inhibit Na^+- phosphate cotransport and renal phosphate reabsorption and cause **phosphaturia.** (iii) PTH and PTH-rp stimulate renal Ca^{2+} reabsorption. Together, the effects of PTH-rp on bone and kidney increase the serum Ca^{2+} concentration **(humoral hypercalcemia of malignancy)** and decrease the serum phosphate concentration (hypophosphatemia). Increased **alkaline phosphatase** activity is associated with increased osteoblastic activity in states of high bone turnover.

2. Although Mr. Kessler's serum albumin was normal, his total serum Ca^{2+} was elevated. Therefore, the increase in his total serum Ca^{2+} was not caused by an increase in protein-bound Ca^{2+}, but rather by an increase in serum ionized Ca^{2+}.

3. Mr. Kessler's circulating level of PTH was decreased secondary to his hypercalcemia. PTH secretion by the parathyroid glands is feedback-regulated by the serum Ca^{2+} concentration. When serum Ca^{2+} is decreased, PTH secretion is stimulated; when serum Ca^{2+} is increased (in this case, by PTH-rp), PTH secretion is inhibited.

   This question points out a critical difference between hypercalcemia caused by primary hyperparathyroidism (see Case 55) and hypercalcemia of malignancy. In primary hyperparathyroidism, by definition, PTH levels are increased. In humoral hypercalcemia of malignancy, PTH levels are decreased by feedback inhibition on the parathyroid gland.

4. After a **water deprivation test,** Mr. Kessler's **serum osmolarity** was elevated at 305 mOsm/L (normal, 290 mOsm/L). In the face of this elevated serum osmolarity, his **urine osmolarity** was very dilute (hyposmotic) at 90 mOsm/L. Something is wrong with this picture! Shouldn't Mr. Kessler be making concentrated (hyperosmotic) urine when his serum osmolarity is elevated? This abnormal pattern suggests that Mr. Kessler had **diabetes insipidus** caused by ADH deficiency (central diabetes insipidus) or by ADH resistance of the collecting ducts (nephrogenic diabetes insipidus).

   Results of the test with **dDAVP** nasal spray (an ADH analogue) confirmed that Mr. Kessler had **nephrogenic diabetes insipidus**—even exogenous ADH couldn't cause his urine to become concentrated. His nephrogenic diabetes insipidus (or ADH resistance) was caused by hypercalcemia. In this condition, Ca^{2+} deposition in the inner medulla of the kidney inhibits ADH-dependent adenylyl cyclase and prevents the ADH action to increase water permeability of the collecting ducts. Thus, even in the presence of exogenous ADH, the urine cannot be concentrated.

5. Mr. Kessler had polyuria (increased urine production) and polydipsia (increased water drinking) secondary to nephrogenic diabetes insipidus. **Polyuria** occurred because his collecting ducts were resistant to the action of ADH and therefore were impermeable to water. Water that was not reabsorbed by the collecting ducts was excreted in the urine. **Polydipsia** occurred because increased urinary water excretion made his body fluids (including the serum) more concentrated. Increased serum osmolarity is a potent stimulus for thirst and drinking behavior through osmoreceptors in the hypothalamus.

6. In the hospital, Mr. Kessler was given saline and furosemide to decrease his serum Ca^{2+} concentration. **Furosemide** inhibits the **Na^+-K^+-$2Cl^-$ cotransporter** in the thick ascending limb

and therefore inhibits renal Na^+ reabsorption. Furosemide also inhibits Ca^{2+} reabsorption in the thick ascending limb, which is explained as follows. The Na^+-K^+-$2Cl^-$ cotransporter normally generates a **lumen-positive potential difference** in the thick ascending limb that drives Ca^{2+} reabsorption from the lumen to the blood through a paracellular route. (The positive charge in the lumen repels the positive charges on Ca^{2+}.) By inhibiting the Na^+-K^+-$2Cl^-$ cotransporter, furosemide eliminates the lumen-positive potential, thereby inhibiting paracellular Ca^{2+} reabsorption. Thus, a portion of the filtered Ca^{2+} that would otherwise have been reabsorbed was excreted in the urine, decreasing Mr. Kessler's serum Ca^{2+} concentration. Saline was administered with the furosemide to prevent extracellular volume contraction.

7. **Pamidronate** is a **bisphosphonate** compound that inhibits osteoclastic bone resorption. This inhibitor of bone resorption was given to offset the osteoclast-stimulating action of PTH-rp.

Key topics

Alkaline phosphatase

Bisphosphonates

Bone resorption

Central diabetes insipidus

dDAVP

Furosemide

Humoral hypercalcemia of malignancy

Hypercalcemia

Hypophosphatemia

Na^+-K^+-$2Cl-$ cotransporter

Na^+-phosphate cotransport

Nephrogenic diabetes insipidus

Osteoclasts

Pamidronate

Parathyroid hormone-related peptide (PTH-rp)

Parathyroid hormone (PTH)

Phosphaturia

Polydipsia

Polyuria

Serum osmolarity

Urine osmolarity

Water deprivation test

Case 57

Hyperglycemia: Type I Diabetes Mellitus

David Mandel was diagnosed with type I (insulin-dependent) diabetes mellitus when he was 12 years old (see Cases 31 and 36). At the time of his diagnosis, David was in middle school. He was an excellent student and had many friends. At a sleepover party, the unimaginable happened: David wet his sleeping bag! He might not have told his parents except that he was worried about other symptoms he was having. He was constantly thirsty and was urinating every 30 to 40 minutes. Furthermore, despite a voracious appetite, he seemed to be losing weight; all of his pants had become loose in the waist. David's parents panicked because they knew that these were classic symptoms of diabetes mellitus. They took David to see his pediatrician immediately. The pediatrician performed a physical examination and ordered laboratory tests (Table 6–10).

TABLE 6–10	David's Physical Examination and Laboratory Results
Height	5 ft, 3 in
Weight	100 lb (decreased 5 lb from his annual checkup 2 months earlier)
Blood pressure	90/55 (lying down), 75/45 (standing up)
Fasting plasma glucose	320 mg/dL (normal, 70–110 mg/dL)
Plasma ketones	1+ (normal, none)
Urinary glucose	4+ (normal, none)
Urinary ketones	2+ (normal, none)

All of the findings were consistent with a diagnosis of type I (insulin-dependent) diabetes mellitus. David immediately started taking injectable insulin and learned how to monitor his blood glucose level with a fingerstick. He excelled in high school and won a scholarship to the state university, where he is currently a premedical student and is planning a career in pediatric endocrinology. He has periodic checkups with his endocrinologist, who closely monitors his renal function.

 QUESTIONS

1. How did insulin deficiency lead to an increase in David's blood glucose concentration?

2. How did insulin deficiency lead to the finding of ketones in David's blood and urine?

3. Why did David have glucose in his urine (glucosuria)?

4. Why did David have increased urine production (polyuria)? Why was he drinking so much (polydipsia)?

5. Why was David's blood pressure lower than normal? Why did it decrease further when he stood up?

6. David takes his insulin parenterally (by subcutaneous injection). Why can't he take insulin orally?

7. The endocrinologist closely monitors David's renal function. What is the major nephrologic complication of type I diabetes mellitus?

ANSWERS ON NEXT PAGE

ANSWERS AND EXPLANATIONS

1. David has **type I diabetes mellitus**—his pancreatic β cells do not make sufficient insulin. Two consequences of **insulin deficiency** made David **hyperglycemic**: decreased uptake of glucose by cells and increased gluconeogenesis. These consequences are best understood by reviewing the normal actions of insulin and then considering what happens with insulin deficiency.

- One important action of insulin is to direct insertion of a facilitated transporter for glucose (GLUT4) into cell membranes of muscle and adipose tissue. This transporter causes the uptake of glucose from blood into the cells. When insulin is deficient, GLUT4 transporters are not inserted into cell membranes, glucose is not transported into the cells, and the blood glucose concentration increases.

- Insulin increases the storage of nutrients, including carbohydrates, proteins, and fats. Thus, insulin promotes glycogen formation (and inhibits gluconeogenesis), protein synthesis, and fat deposition (and inhibits lipolysis). When insulin is deficient, both protein catabolism (which generates amino acids) and lipolysis (which generates glycerol and fatty acids) are increased. Thus, insulin deficiency provides more amino acid and glycerol substrates for glucose synthesis (i.e., **increased gluconeogenesis**; Fig. 6–8).

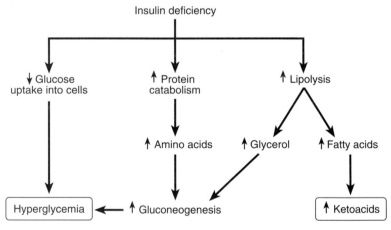

Figure 6–8   Metabolic effects of insulin deficiency.

2. David's blood and urine contained ketones because insulin deficiency increased the blood levels of fatty acids, which are the biosynthetic precursors of ketoacids. Insulin deficiency promotes catabolism of all nutrients, including fats (Fig. 6–8). Increased lipolysis leads to increased blood levels of fatty acids that are converted in the liver to **ketoacids**, β-hydroxybutyric acid and acetoacetic acid. As the concentration of ketoacids increases in the blood, they are filtered across the glomerular capillaries and appear in the urine.

3. David had **glucosuria** (glucose in his urine) because he was hyperglycemic. His blood glucose concentration became so high that the amount of glucose filtered across the glomerular capillaries exceeded the reabsorptive capacity of the renal proximal tubule. Any glucose that was not reabsorbed was excreted in the urine. (For a more complete discussion of renal glucose reabsorption, see Case 31.)

4. David had **polyuria** (increased urine production) because his urine contained glucose. As discussed in the previous question, the filtered load of glucose was greater than the reabsorptive

capacity of the proximal tubule and, as a result, glucose was excreted in the urine. The unreabsorbed glucose acted as an **osmotic diuretic,** causing a "back-flux" of Na^+ and water into the proximal tubule. Thus, along with glucose, increased quantities of Na^+ and water were excreted.

David had **polydipsia** because the hyperglycemia caused an increase in his serum osmolarity, which stimulated osmoreceptors in the anterior hypothalamus that increase thirst and promote drinking behavior.

5. David's **arterial pressure** was decreased secondary to the osmotic diuresis that was caused by glucose in his urine. Increased excretion of Na^+ and water decreased his extracellular fluid volume and his blood volume. Decreased blood volume led to a decrease in venous return to the heart, decreased cardiac output (by the Frank-Starling mechanism), and decreased arterial pressure. David's arterial pressure decreased further when he stood up **(orthostatic hypotension)** because, as blood pooled in the veins of the legs, venous return and cardiac output were compromised further.

6. Insulin is a protein; therefore, it must be administered parenterally (i.e., by routes other than the gastrointestinal tract). If given orally, it would be digested by intestinal peptidases to amino acids and di- and tripeptides. Once digested, it would no longer be insulin! Subcutaneous injection of insulin bypasses these degradative steps in the gastrointestinal tract.

7. A serious complication of type I diabetes mellitus is **diabetic nephropathy.** This condition can progress to end-stage renal failure that requires dialysis or renal transplantation. Therefore, David's renal function must be monitored for the rest of his life.

The earliest phase of diabetic nephropathy is characterized by an *increase* in the glomerular filtration rate (GFR) that roughly correlates with the adequacy of glycemic control. In this **hyperfiltration** phase, the better the control of blood glucose concentration with insulin injections, the smaller the increase in GFR. In the next phase of diabetic nephropathy (and a consequence of hyperfiltration), histologic changes occur in the glomerular capillary barrier. The mesangial cells expand, and the basement membrane thickens. Eventually, these changes lead to diffuse glomerular scarring. During this phase, which occurs 5 to 15 years from the onset of type I diabetes mellitus, progressive glomerular changes occur; although the GFR remains elevated and no frank protein is found in the urine, **microalbuminuria** can be detected. Finally, in the later phases of diabetic nephropathy, there is gross proteinuria, decreased GFR, hypertension, and renal failure.

David will be monitored closely for the presence of the microalbuminuria that signals the beginning of glomerular damage. If microalbuminuria is detected, David will be treated with an **angiotensin-converting enzyme (ACE) inhibitor,** which selectively dilates renal efferent arterioles and reduces glomerular filtration (offsetting the damaging hyperfiltration).

Key topics

Angiotensin-converting enzyme (ACE) inhibitor

Diabetes mellitus type I

Diabetic nephropathy

Gluconeogenesis

Glucosuria

GLUT4 transporter

Hyperfiltration

Insulin deficiency

Ketoacids

Microalbuminuria

Orthostatic hypotension

Osmotic diuresis

Polydipsia

Polyuria

Case 58

Primary Amenorrhea: Androgen Insensitivity Syndrome

Marcy Maloney is a 17-year-old junior in high school. She seemed to go through puberty at the same time as her peers; she had a growth spurt and her breasts developed. However, she has never had a menstrual period. Her mother's menstrual cycles started at age 13, and Marcy's 12-year-old sister recently began to menstruate. Marcy's mother made an appointment for a thorough gynecologic examination.

Marcy's history was unremarkable except for the absence of menstrual cycles (primary amenorrhea). On physical examination, Marcy appeared to be a healthy young woman. Her breasts and external genitalia appeared normal. However, she had a short, blind-ending vagina and no visible cervix. On bimanual examination, she had no palpable uterus or ovaries. She had no axillary or pubic hair, and very little hair on her arms and legs.

Marcy had a normal serum cortisol level, normal results on thyroid function tests, and a normal serum prolactin level. A pregnancy test was negative. However, her serum testosterone level was very elevated (even higher than the levels found in normal men).

Because of the findings on physical examination and the elevated serum testosterone level, Marcy's physician ordered a genotype, which was 46, XY. During exploratory surgery, the surgeons found intraabdominal testes, which were removed. Marcy was given estrogen replacement therapy.

The physicians explained to Marcy and her parents that she has androgen insensitivity syndrome (formerly called testicular feminizing syndrome). She has a male genotype (XY) and male gonads (testes), but a female phenotype. Marcy was counseled that, because she has no ovaries or uterus, she would never be able to bear children. However, she would continue to look like a woman. The physicians also explained that she could elect to undergo reconstructive surgery on her vagina to permit normal sexual intercourse.

 QUESTIONS

1. How does a fetus with an XY (male) genotype normally develop into the male phenotype? How does a fetus with an XX (female) genotype normally develop into the female phenotype?

2. Marcy looked like a female, but she was genetically and gonadally a male. Her disorder (testicular feminizing syndrome) is caused by a deficiency or lack of androgen receptors on target tissues. Which of the following characteristics are explained by the lack of androgen receptors: presence of female external genitalia, absence of a cervix and uterus, absence of body hair, and presence of testes?

3. Why was Marcy's serum testosterone level even higher than that found in normal men?

4. Why did Marcy develop breasts?

5. Marcy's testes were removed because a malignancy can develop in them. Why did she require estrogen replacement therapy after the surgery?

ANSWERS AND EXPLANATIONS

1. In the first 5 weeks of gestational life, the gonads are **bipotential** (can develop into either ovaries or testes). In the sixth gestational week, if the fetus is male, the testes begin to develop. In the ninth week, if the fetus is female, the ovaries begin to develop. Thus, genetic sex (either XY or XX) determines gonadal sex, which ultimately determines phenotypic sex (Fig. 6–9).

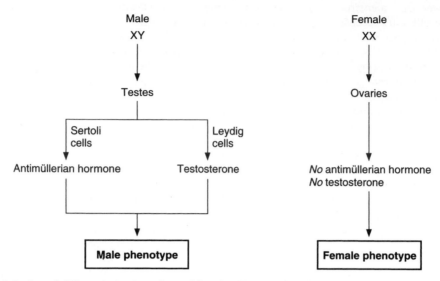

Figure 6–9 Sexual differentiation in males and females. (Reprinted, with permission, from Costanzo LS. *BRS Physiology* 4th ed. Baltimore: Lippincott Williams & Wilkins; 2007:264.)

A male fetus with an **XY genotype** develops into a gonadal and phenotypic male as follows. During gestational week 6, the SRY gene on the Y chromosome causes differentiation of the bipotential gonads into testes. These fetal testes produce testosterone and antimüllerian hormone, both of which are required for normal development of the male phenotype. **Testosterone**, which is produced by the fetal Leydig cells, stimulates differentiation and growth of the wolffian ducts. These ducts give rise to the internal male reproductive tract (epididymis, vas deferens, seminal vesicles, and ejaculatory ducts). At the same time, **antimüllerian hormone**, which is produced by the fetal Sertoli cells, causes atrophy of the müllerian ducts that otherwise would develop into the internal female genital tract. Finally, in gestational week 9, there is differentiation and growth of the male external genitalia (penis, scrotum); this process depends on the conversion of testosterone to **dihydrotestosterone** in these target tissues.

A female fetus with an **XX genotype** develops into a gonadal and phenotypic female as follows. At gestational week 9, the bipotential gonads develop into ovaries (because they did not develop into testes earlier). Because there are no testes, there is no secretion of testosterone or antimüllerian hormone. Thus, in females, there is *no* testosterone to promote differentiation and growth of the wolffian ducts into a male internal genital tract, and there is *no* antimüllerian hormone to suppress differentiation of the müllerian ducts into the female internal genital tract. Consequently, the **müllerian ducts** develop into the internal female genital tract (fallopian tubes, uterus, cervix, and upper one-third of the vagina). In addition, there is differentiation and growth of the external female genitalia (clitoris, labia majora, labia minora, and lower two-thirds of the vagina).

2. **Androgen insensitivity syndrome** is caused by **lack of androgen receptors** and a resultant androgen resistance of target tissues. In utero, Marcy's testes, which were normal, secreted both testosterone and antimüllerian hormone. Antimüllerian hormone suppressed differentiation of

the müllerian ducts into the internal female genital tract. As a result, Marcy has no fallopian tubes, uterus, or upper vagina. Testosterone (which should have caused differentiation of the wolffian ducts into the male internal genital tract) did not because the target tissues had no androgen receptors. In addition, dihydrotestosterone did not cause differentiation of the external male genitalia because those tissues also lacked androgen receptors. Therefore, by default, Marcy developed female external genitalia.

Only two of the characteristics listed are explained by lack of androgen receptors: the presence of female external genitalia (which differentiated because the male genitalia did not) and the absence of body hair (one of the biologic actions of androgens in adults). The absence of a cervix and a uterus was caused by antimüllerian hormone secreted from Marcy's fetal testes (which suppressed differentiation of the müllerian ducts). The presence of testes was determined by her genetic sex (XY).

3. Marcy's serum testosterone level was even higher than that found in men because feedback regulation of testosterone secretion involves testosterone receptors in the hypothalamus and anterior pituitary (Fig. 6–10). Although her testes secreted large amounts of testosterone, the testosterone could not feedback-regulate its own secretion because her hypothalamus and anterior pituitary had no testosterone receptors.

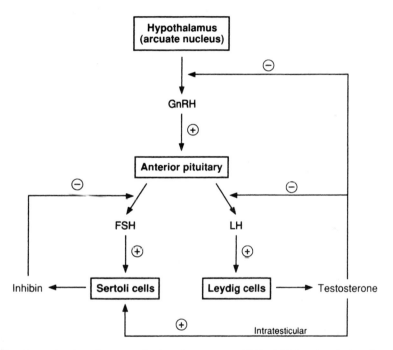

Figure 6–10 Control of male reproductive hormones. (FSH, follicle-stimulating hormone; GnRH, gonadotropin-releasing hormone; LH, luteinizing hormone.) (Reprinted, with permission, from Costanzo LS. *BRS Physiology* 4th ed. Baltimore: Lippincott Williams & Wilkins; 2007:266.)

4. Marcy developed **breasts** because the testes and adipose tissue contain the **aromatase** enzyme that converts testosterone to **estradiol.** Because Marcy's testosterone levels were so high, sufficient estradiol could be synthesized to cause breast development and female fat distribution. (Remember, the high levels of testosterone *do not* produce masculine characteristics because Marcy lacks androgen receptors.)

5. After the testes were removed, Marcy required **estrogen replacement therapy** to maintain her breasts and female fat distribution. The testes had served as the source of testosterone, which was the precursor for estradiol synthesis.

Key topics

Androgen insensitivity syndrome

Androgen receptors

Antimüllerian hormone

Aromatase

Dihydrotestosterone

Estradiol

Primary amenorrhea

Sexual differentiation

Testicular feminizing syndrome

Testosterone

Case 59

Male Hypogonadism: Kallmann's Syndrome

George Acevedo is the delivery man for a family-owned pharmacy and delicatessen. Although he is 22 years old, he looks more like a 12-year-old. He is still growing at the rate of approximately 0.5 inch per year, his arms appear very long for his body, and he has a prepubertal fat distribution. He has little body or facial hair, does not have erections, and is not sexually active. He has always had a very poor sense of smell. George's parents were concerned and scheduled a checkup with his family physician.

On physical examination, George had a very long arm span, sparse body and facial hair, and a small penis and testes. The results of laboratory tests are shown in Table 6–11.

TABLE 6–11	*George's Laboratory Values*	
Serum testosterone	120 ng/dL	(normal adult males, 300–1,000 ng/dL)
Serum luteinizing hormone	1.5 mU/mL	(normal adults, 3–18 mU/mL)

A gonadotropin-releasing hormone (GnRH) stimulation test caused a significant increase in George's serum luteinizing hormone (LH) and testosterone levels.

George was diagnosed with hypogonadotropic hypogonadism. His physician prescribed pulsatile GnRH treatment, which was delivered through a wearable infusion pump. On a follow-up visit 6 months after the start of treatment, George's height had stabilized, his muscle mass had increased, facial hair had started to grow, and he looked older. His penis had enlarged, and he was having erections and nocturnal emissions.

 QUESTIONS

1. George had hypogonadotropic hypogonadism of hypothalamic origin (Kallmann's syndrome). His hypothalamus secreted inadequate amounts of GnRH. How did decreased GnRH secretion cause decreased levels of LH and testosterone?

2. Explain George's prepubertal appearance. Why were his arms so long? Why was he still growing?

3. Decreased testosterone levels can result from a defect in the testes, the anterior pituitary, or the hypothalamus. How did George's physician know that George's low serum testosterone levels were caused by a hypothalamic problem (rather than a primary problem in the testes or in the anterior pituitary)?

4. Why did George have a poor sense of smell?

5. George was treated with pulsatile (rather than continuous or long-acting) GnRH. Why was pulsatile delivery important?

ANSWERS AND EXPLANATIONS

1. **Kallmann's syndrome (hypogonadotropic hypogonadism)** is caused by inadequate secretion of GnRH. In Kallmann's syndrome, which can be hereditary, the hypothalamus does not secrete Gonadotropin-releasing hormone (GnRH), although other hypothalamic functions are normal. In one hereditary form of the disorder, there is a defect in the **KAL peptide** that plays a role in normal neuronal migration; the neurons that secrete GnRH apparently do not migrate to their proper site in the hypothalamus and, therefore, are nonfunctional.

   George had a deficiency of GnRH that caused decreased secretion of the gonadotropins LH and follicle-stimulating hormone (FSH) from the anterior pituitary. Luteinizing hormone (LH) is responsible for testosterone synthesis in the Leydig cells of the testes. FSH is responsible for spermatogenesis and Sertoli cell functions. Thus, in the absence of GnRH, there was decreased LH and FSH secretion, decreased testosterone secretion, and decreased sperm production.

2. George had a childish appearance (little muscle mass, prepubertal fat distribution, lack of facial and body hair, small penis). Normally, a large increase in testosterone secretion by the testes occurs at puberty and causes the pubertal growth spurt, deepening of the voice, growth of body hair, growth of the penis, and development of libido. Because of his testosterone deficiency, George did not have these **secondary male sex characteristics.** His arms were very long because testosterone is required for closure of the epiphyseal growth plates (which stops the growth of the long bones). His arms continued to grow because his epiphyseal growth plates had not closed. He continued to grow in height for the same reason (failure of the epiphyseal plates to close, causing sustained growth of the long bones).

3. Because of the results of the **GnRH stimulation test,** George's physician concluded that George's decreased testosterone levels were caused by a problem with *hypothalamic* secretion of GnRH. In the test, administration of GnRH caused an increase in LH and testosterone secretion. Thus, George's anterior pituitary responded normally to GnRH (it secreted LH), and his testes responded normally to LH (they secreted testosterone). These responses implied that the defect resided in the hypothalamus, not in the anterior pituitary or the testes (see Fig. 6–10).

4. Kallmann's syndrome is responsible for George's poor sense of smell. Normally, GnRH-secreting neurons migrate from primordial olfactory tissue into their correct location in the hypothalamus. In Kallmann's syndrome, this migration does not occur. The defect results in a decreased sense of smell (hyposmia) or the complete absence of the sense of smell **(anosmia).**

5. George was treated with **pulsatile GnRH** to initiate puberty. It was expected that continued treatment with pulsatile GnRH would maintain gonadotropin secretion that would in turn maintain testosterone secretion and sperm production. Continuous (or long-acting) GnRH would *not* have been an effective treatment. In normal males (and females), the onset of *pulsatile* GnRH secretion from the hypothalamus initiates puberty by up-regulating GnRH receptors in the anterior pituitary, thus "sensitizing" the reproductive axis. When GnRH is given as a continuous infusion, the GnRH receptors in the anterior pituitary are actually down-regulated, which desensitizes the reproductive axis.

Key topics

Anosmia

Follicle-stimulating hormone (FSH)

GnRH stimulation test

Gonadotropin-releasing hormone (GnRH)

Hypogonadism

KAL peptide

Kallmann's syndrome

Luteinizing hormone (LH)

Male secondary sex characteristics

Puberty

Pulsatile GnRH

Testosterone

Case 60

Male Pseudohermaphroditism: 5α-Reductase Deficiency

Fourteen years ago, Wally and Wanda Garvey, who live in rural North Carolina, had their first child. The baby was delivered by a general practitioner, who said the baby was a girl. They named her Scarlett, from Wanda's favorite movie. From the beginning, Wally and Wanda felt something was wrong with Scarlett. She did not look like a normal baby girl (she had what looked like a very small penis), but it never would have occurred to Wally and Wanda to question a doctor's judgment.

By the time Scarlett was 13 years old, all of her girlfriends had developed breasts and were having periods. Scarlett was experiencing none of these changes and, alarmingly, her voice was deepening and she was becoming very muscular, like the boys. Her small penis (which she had kept secret) was growing larger. She and her girlfriends gossiped about the boys having wet dreams, but to Scarlett's embarrassment, *she* was having something like that. She was starting to feel like a boy, rather than a girl. Wally and Wanda noticed some of these changes, and they were very concerned. The doctor finally admitted that this case was beyond his expertise, and he referred the family to a medical school in another part of the state.

At the medical school, Scarlett was diagnosed with a form of male pseudohermaphroditism caused by a deficiency of 5α-reductase. On physical examination, she had no ovaries, no uterus, a blind vaginal pouch, a small prostate, a penis, descended testes, and hypospadias (urethral opening low on the underside of the penis). She had a male musculature, but no body hair, facial hair, or acne. Her genotype was confirmed as 46,XY, and blood work showed a high-normal level of testosterone and a low level of dihydrotestosterone. Tests on fibroblasts from genital skin showed an absence of 5α-reductase. The physician discussed treatment options, which would be different depending on whether Scarlett wanted to live the rest of her life as a woman or a man.

 QUESTIONS

1. In males, some androgenic actions depend on testosterone and some depend on dihydrotestosterone. What is the physiologic basis for this difference?

2. Which male target tissues respond to testosterone, and which require dihydrotestosterone?

3. Scarlett had a form of pseudohermaphroditism caused by 5α-reductase deficiency. At birth, which of the following characteristics were (are) a result of the enzyme deficiency, and why? Of the characteristics that were not (are not) a result of the enzyme deficiency, what was (is) their cause?

   a. 46,XY genotype
   b. Presence of testes
   c. Absence of uterus
   d. Blind-ending vagina
   e. Small penis

4. At puberty, which of the following characteristics result from Scarlett's high-normal levels of testosterone? Which characteristics result from her inability to produce dihydrotestosterone? Which characteristics are due to neither?

  a. Growth of penis
  b. Ejaculation
  c. Deepening of voice
  d. Lack of body and facial hair
  e. Lack of breast development

5. If Scarlett wishes to continue life as a woman, what is the appropriate treatment?

6. If Scarlett wishes to live the rest of her life as a man, what is the appropriate treatment?

ANSWERS AND EXPLANATIONS

1. The testes synthesize and secrete testosterone, which is converted, in *some* androgenic target tissues, to dihydrotestosterone by the action of the enzyme 5α-reductase. In target tissues that contain **5α-reductase**, dihydrotestosterone is synthesized and is responsible for androgenic activity. In those tissues, testosterone has little or no activity. Other androgenic target tissues do not contain 5α-reductase and do not synthesize dihydrotestosterone. In those tissues, testosterone is the active form.

2. Androgenic actions that utilize **dihydrotestosterone**, and thus *require* **5α-reductase,** include differentiation of the external male genitalia, male-pattern baldness, and growth of the prostate (Fig. 6–11). Androgenic actions that respond directly to **testosterone** and do *not* require 5α-reductase are differentiation of internal male genital tract (epididymis, vas deferens, seminal vesicles), muscle mass, pubertal growth spurt, growth of the penis, deepening of the voice, spermatogenesis, and libido.

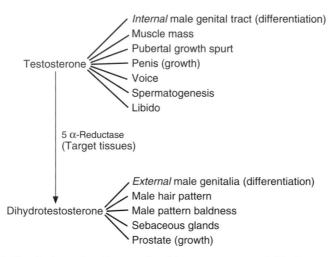

Figure 6–11   Androgenic actions mediated by testosterone and dihydrotestosterone.

3. It is helpful to organize your thoughts by considering the characteristics Scarlett did or did not have at birth. She is a genetic and gonadal male, who lacks the enzyme 5α-reductase (a form of **pseudohermaphroditism**). As a **genetic male** (46,XY), the presence of the Y chromosome determines that the bipotential gonads will develop into testes at gestational weeks 6 to 7. Scarlett's **testes are normal,** and thus prenatally, they synthesized both antimüllerian hormone and testosterone.

    Antimüllerian hormone suppresses development of the **müllerian ducts** into the internal female genital tract, so Scarlett has no fallopian tubes, uterus, or upper one-third of the vagina. **Testosterone** causes differentiation of the **wolffian ducts** into the internal male genital tract (epididymis, vas deferens, seminal vesicles), a process that does not require dihydrotestosterone and thus occurs in the absence of 5α-reductase. However, differentiation of the external male genitalia (e.g., penis and scrotum) requires dihydrotestosterone; thus, a **deficiency of 5α-reductase** meant that Scarlett's external genitalia were not normally developed.

    Based on this information, Scarlett's characteristics at birth are explained as follows.

    a. The 46,XY genotype is not a result of the enzyme deficiency.
    b. The presence of testes is determined by the Y chromosome, and is not a result of the enzyme deficiency.

c. Scarlett does not have a uterus because the normal testes produced antimüllerian hormone, which suppressed development of the müllerian ducts into an internal female genital tract. Thus, the absence of a uterus is not due to the enzyme deficiency.

d. Scarlett has a blind-ending vagina for the same reason she does not have a uterus—the testes produced antimüllerian hormone, which suppressed development of the internal female genital tract, including the upper one-third of the vagina.

e. The small penis is the result of the enzyme deficiency, because differentiation of the male external male genitalia is mediated by dihydrotestosterone.

4. Use the summary information from Answer 3 again to explain Scarlett's characteristics at puberty.

a. The penis grew at puberty because of the high-normal circulating level of testosterone, which apparently is sufficient to activate the androgen receptors that mediate growth of the external genitalia.

b. Both spermatogenesis and production of many components of the ejaculate are mediated by testosterone and do not require conversion to dihydrotestosterone.

c. Deepening of the voice is also mediated by testosterone and does not require conversion to dihydrotestosterone.

d. At puberty, despite acquiring many masculine characteristics, Scarlett did not develop body and facial hair. Specifically, the hair follicles require dihydrotestosterone.

e. At puberty, Scarlett did not develop breasts because she did not have ovaries. In females, the ovaries are the source of the estrogen that is needed for breast development.

5. If Scarlett chooses to continue life as a woman, it will be necessary to remove her testes, which are producing the testosterone that is causing her to be selectively masculinized (growth of penis, deepening of voice, etc.). In addition, because she lacks ovaries, Scarlett has no endogenous source of the estrogen that is needed for breast development and female fat distribution; thus, she will receive treatment with supplemental estrogen. She may elect to have surgical correction of the introitus; however, even with the surgery, she will not be able to bear children because she lacks ovaries and an internal female genital tract.

6. If Scarlett chooses to live the rest of her life as a man, she will be treated with androgenic compounds that do not require 5α-reduction for activity. The supplemental androgens will complete the masculinization process, including development of male body and facial hair, sebaceous gland activity, growth of the prostate, and in later life, male-pattern baldness.

Key topics

Antimüllerian hormone

Dihydrotestosterone

Müllerian ducts

Pseudohermaphroditism

5α-reductase

Testosterone

Wolffian ducts

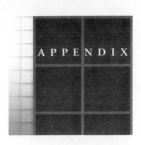

APPENDIX	Calculating Compensatory Responses to Simple Acid–Base Disorders		
Acid–Base Disturbance	**Primary Disturbance**	**Compensation**	**Predicted Compensatory Response**
Metabolic acidosis	$\downarrow [HCO_3^-]$	$\downarrow P_{CO_2}$	1 mEq/L decrease in HCO_3^- → 1.3 mm Hg decrease in P_{CO_2}
Metabolic alkalosis	$\uparrow [HCO_3^-]$	$\uparrow P_{CO_2}$	1 mEq/L increase in HCO_3^- → 0.7 mm Hg increase in P_{CO_2}
Respiratory acidosis			
Acute	$\uparrow P_{CO_2}$	$\uparrow [HCO_3^-]$	1 mm Hg increase in P_{CO_2} → 0.1 mEq/L increase in HCO_3^-
Chronic	$\uparrow P_{CO_2}$	$\uparrow [HCO_3^-]$	1 mm Hg increase in P_{CO_2} → 0.4 mEq/L increase in HCO_3^-
Respiratory alkalosis			
Acute	$\downarrow P_{CO_2}$	$\downarrow [HCO_3^-]$	1 mm Hg decrease in P_{CO_2} → 0.2 mEq/L decrease in HCO_3^-
Chronic	$\downarrow P_{CO_2}$	$\downarrow [HCO_3^-]$	1 mm Hg decrease in P_{CO_2} → 0.4 mEq/L decrease in HCO_3^-

Reprinted, with permission, from Costanzo LS. *BRS Physiology*. 4th ed. Baltimore: Lippincott Williams & Wilkins; 2006:185.

Index

Page numbers followed by t indicate table; those in *italics* indicate figure.